Psycho-Oncology

Edited by

Thomas N. Wise, M.D.

Massimo Biondi, M.D.

Anna Costantini, Ph.D.

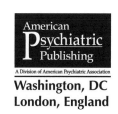

American **Psychiatric** Publishing

A Division of American Psychiatric Association

Washington, DC
London, England

Copyright © 2013 American Psychiatric Association
ALL RIGHTS RESERVED

Manufactured in the United States of America on acid-free paper
17   16   15   14   13   5   4   3   2   1
First Edition

Typeset in Warnock Pro and Optima.

American Psychiatric Publishing
A Division of American Psychiatric Association
1000 Wilson Boulevard
Arlington, VA 22209-3901
www.appi.org

Library of Congress Cataloging-in-Publication Data
Psycho-oncology / edited by Thomas N. Wise, Massimo Biondi, Anna Costantini. -- 1st ed.
      p. ; cm.
 Includes bibliographical references and index.
 ISBN 978-1-58562-423-2 (pbk. : alk. paper)
 I. Wise, Thomas N. II. Biondi, Massimo. III. Costantini, Anna, 1956- IV. American Psychiatric Association.
 [DNLM: 1. Neoplasms--psychology. 2. Neoplasms--therapy. QZ 200]
 RC270.8
 616.99'406--dc23
                              2013002652

British Library Cataloguing in Publication Data
A CIP record is available from the British Library.

Psycho-Oncology

Contents

Contributors

Lea Baider, Ph.D.
Professor of Medical Psychology, Faculty of Medicine, Hebrew University Medical School, Hadassah University Hospital; Director, Psycho-Oncology Unit, Sharett Institute of Oncology, Department of Radiation and Clinical Oncology, Hadassah University Hospital, Jerusalem, Israel

Walter F. Baile, M.D.
Professor of Behavioral Science and Psychiatry, Department of Faculty Development, The University of Texas MD Anderson Cancer Center, Houston, Texas

Francesco Saverio Bersani, M.D.
Resident Physician, Department of Neurology and Psychiatry, Sapienza University of Rome, Rome, Italy

Massimo Biondi, M.D.
Professor of Psychiatry, Department of Neurology and Psychiatry, Policlinico Umberto I—Sapienza University of Rome, Rome, Italy

Allison M. Burton-Chase, Ph.D.
Postdoctoral Research Fellow, Department of Behavioral Science, The University of Texas MD Anderson Cancer Center, Houston, Texas

Rosangela Caruso, M.D.
Fellow in Psychiatry and Psycho-Oncology, Doctoral School in Pharmacology and Molecular Oncology, and Section of Psychiatry, Department of Biomedical and Specialty Surgical Sciences, University of Ferrara, Ferrara, Italy

Anne Cawthorn, M.Sc., B.Sc., R.N.T., Dip. Hypno.
Macmillan Living Well Specialist Practitioner, The Living Well Centre, Blythe House Hospice, Derbyshire, United Kingdom

Anna Costantini, Ph.D.
Chief of Psycho-Oncology Unit and Professor of Psycho-Oncology, Department of Oncological Sciences, Sant'Andrea Hospital, Sapienza University of Rome, Rome, Italy; Board President, Italian Society of Psycho-Oncology; Certified Group Psychotherapist, American Group Psychotherapy Association

Matthew Doolittle, M.D.
Instructor in Psychiatry, Department of Psychiatry and Behavioral Sciences, Memorial Sloan-Kettering Cancer Center, New York, New York

Fabio Efficace, Ph.D.
Head, Health Outcomes Research Unit, Italian Group for Adult Hematologic Diseases (GIMEMA) Data Center, Rome, Italy

Johannes Giesinger, Ph.D.
Research Fellow, Department of Psychiatry and Psychotherapy, Innsbruck Medical University, Innsbruck, Austria

Luigi Grassi, M.D.
Professor and Chair of Psychiatry; Chair, Department of Biomedical and Specialty Surgical Sciences, University of Ferrara, Italy; Chair, IPOS Federation of Psycho-Oncology Societies

Ellen R. Gritz, Ph.D.
Professor and Chair, Olla S. Stribling Distinguished Chair for Cancer Research, Department of Behavioral Science, The University of Texas MD Anderson Cancer Center, Houston, Texas

Bernhard Holzner, Ph.D.
Associate Professor, Department of Psychiatry and Psychotherapy, Innsbruck Medical University, Innsbruck, Austria

David W. Kissane, M.D.
Professor of Psychiatry and Head of Discipline, School of Psychology and Psychiatry, Monash University, Victoria, Australia; Jimmie C. Holland Chair and Attending Psychiatrist, Memorial Sloan-Kettering Cancer Center; Adjunct Professor of Psychiatry, Weill Medical College of Cornell University, New York, New York

Sonia Krenz, Ph.D.
Psychiatric Liaison Service, University Hospital and University of Lausanne, Lausanne, Switzerland

Jon A. Levenson, M.D.
Associate Clinical Professor of Psychiatry, Division of Psychosomatic Medicine, Psychiatry Department, Columbia University Medical Center, New York, New York

Alex J. Mitchell, M.B.B.S., B.Med.Sci., M.Sc., M.R.C.Psych.
Consultant in Psycho-Oncology, Leicestershire Partnership Trust; Honorary Senior Lecturer in Psycho-Oncology, Department of Cancer and Molecular Medicine, Leicester Royal Infirmary, Leicester, United Kingdom

Maria Giulia Nanni, M.D.
Assistant Professor of Psychiatry, Section of Psychiatry, University of Ferrara, Department of Medical-Surgical Disciplines of Communication and Behavior, Ferrara, Italy

Massimo Pasquini, M.D.
Consultant Psychiatrist, Department of Neurology and Psychiatry, Policlinico Umberto I-Sapienza University of Rome, Rome, Italy

Susan K. Peterson, Ph.D., M.P.H.
Associate Professor, Department of Behavioral Science, The University of Texas MD Anderson Cancer Center, Houston, Texas

Carolyn Pitceathly, M.Sc.
Psycho-Oncology Service, Christie Hospital, Manchester, United Kingdom

Shannon R. Poppito, Ph.D.
Clinical Psychologist, Behavioral Health Optimization Program, LA Air Force Base 61 Medical Squadron, El Segundo, California

Friedrich Stiefel, M.D.
Psychiatric Liaison Service, University Hospital and University of Lausanne, Lausanne, Switzerland

Glendon R. Tait, M.D., M.Sc., F.R.C.P.C.
Assistant Professor of Psychiatry, Dalhousie University, Halifax, Nova Scotia, Canada; Adjunct Assistant Professor, University of Toronto, Toronto, Ontario, Canada

Maggie Watson, B.Sc., Ph.D., Dip.Clin.Psych.
Consultant Clinical Psychologist Royal Marsden Hospital; Head, Psychology Research Group Institute of Cancer Research; Honorary Professor, Research Department of Clinical, Health and Educational Psychology, University College, London, United Kingdom

Thomas N. Wise, M.D.
Professor of Psychiatry, George Washington University School of Medicine, Washington, D.C., and Johns Hopkins School of Medicine, Baltimore, Maryland; Medical Director of Behavioral Services, Inova Health Systems, Fairfax, Virginia

DISCLOSURE OF INTERESTS

All contributors affirm they have no financial interest in or other affiliation with a commercial supporter, manufacturer of a commercial product, provider of a commercial service, nongovernmental organization, and/or government agency that could represent or appear to represent a competing interest with their contributions to this book.

Introduction

RESEARCH HAS transformed many types of neoplastic disease into curable or chronic conditions rather than rapidly fatal diseases. With an increasing number of long-term treated "cancer survivors," there is greater recognition of the psychosocial and psychological reactions to and psycho-pathological consequences of confronting the threat of recurrence—the sequel of life-saving but traumatic and possibly disfiguring treatments. Despite such medical advances, surveys indicate that cancer is the most feared disease state (Rosentberg et al. 1987). Such interactions between a disease label and an emotional reaction, fear, underscore the profound psychosocial issues involved in oncology. Because more than 40% of individuals will experience a diagnosis of cancer during their lifetime, practitioners in all health care specialties and disciplines must have a knowledge base in oncology. Furthermore, any health professional involved in treating patients with oncological disease needs to understand the psychological aspects of cancer and either manage such problems or work within a team with the abilities and resources to allay this dimension of suffering.

The growing awareness of psychosocial issues within oncology was reviewed by Holland (1998), who cited Tolstoy's (1886/1960) *The Death of Ivan Ilych* as an early literary example of the isolation, fear, and lack of skill that individuals can face when coping with cancer. This short novel reminds the contemporary reader how cancer patients may experience isolation from family, friends, and caregivers, including the physician. Even in the 1960s, physicians rarely told cancer patients their diagnosis and rationalized that they themselves would not want to be told the diagnosis (Oken 1961). Fortunately, the situation has changed with the emergence of the field of psycho-oncology. Surbone's (2006) review noted that the withholding of accurate data has been less prevalent in more recent years but that cultural differences in some countries still limit such disclosure. The lack of comprehensive understanding and the limited availability of psychosocial treatments are highlighted in the Institute of Medicine's (2008) monograph *Cancer Care for the Whole Patient: Meeting Psychosocial Health Needs.* This important document calls for comprehensive cancer care. It is now considered imperative for any health care professional to consider all psychosocial domains in evaluation and treatment. To help meet this challenge, we have developed this volume, *Psycho-Oncology,* to provide a knowledge base and guide for the clinical imperative of attention and treatment of psychosocial elements within cancer care.

Psycho-oncology, which has developed as a field in and of itself, is a growing field that connects multiple disciplines, including oncology, psychiatry, psychology, surgery, radiotherapy, and palliative care, among others. This integrative discipline is a derivative of psychosomatic medicine, which is the current term for consultation-liaison psychiatry or health psychology. The International Psycho-Oncology Society embodies the complex aspects of this field in that the organization has contributions from many disciplines and a biopsychosocial approach (www.ipos-society.org). The involvement of various national organizations within this broad coalition reifies the international recognition of the importance of a biopsychosocial approach to the patient with cancer. Serial publications such as the journal *Psycho-Oncology* are dedicated to the field. Many educational programs now focus on physicians' communication skills, to help improve the patient-doctor relationship, the manner of giving of bad news, the transition of the patient to palliative care or hospice, and the relationship with the dying patient.

The contributors to our book *Psycho-Oncology* are international experts in the field. The volume offers an overview of the clinical elements in this field, with a core focus on the essential caregiver-patient dyad. The book is intended to provide not merely a systematic review of each topic but a discussion of the established evidence base of psycho-oncology together with emerging clinical developments, thereby offering a "bench-to-bedside" approach to benefit the everyday clinical practice for all health professionals who treat patients with neoplastic disease.

Each chapter in this volume can stand alone, but together they provide a coherent and sequential discussion about management of the patient with cancer as well as his or her significant others. This book utilizes the framework of psychosocial staging (Weisman 1979) to offer a pathway to better organize the unique challenges for each patient. The discovery of cancer—the initial diagnostic phase—signals a dramatic reminder of mortality to the patient. This phase, which demands careful evaluation and waiting for ascertainment of the staging of the neoplasm, is usually a time of great anxiety. The patient's family and extended support system may serve as a source of support or as an agent to promote blame and guilt. Therefore, the health care professional needs to understand the meaning of this diagnosis to each patient and family. Communication with both patient and family are essential skills for assessing both the patient and his or her significant others. In addition to these verbal skills by the physicians, nurses, and other health care professionals, psychometric screening methods may help in identifying patients who have psychiatric disorders. During this initial phase, the clinician must consider various questions: How was the neoplasm discovered? Did delay of symptoms play a factor in the course of the cancer? What does the cancer "mean" to the patient? What ideas does the patient possess to explain his or her illness? How does the patient react to the medical and surgical treatments, which often have significant side effects? The clinician needs to involve family members in discussions to allow them to verbalize their fears, as well as to gain important information about the patient. When patients and families ask "why" the cancer occurred, as well as when data indicate that the patient's neoplastic state may have genetic contributions, genetic counseling is particularly salient. During this early phase, delay or denial of necessary screening should be resolved with family members.

Treatment for a neoplasm, the second phase, is the next great challenge to the patient's homeostasis. Concurrent assessment for a psychiatric diagnosis is important and can be aided by psychometric assessment. A review of psychopharmacological interventions in the oncology patient will help clinicians of all disciplines. The concurrent effects of medications or surgeries can foster cognitive changes, mood disorders, or demoralization. The clinician, whether oncologist, psychiatrist, or bedside nurse, must be able to differentiate delirium from depression. Demoralization and depression are common reactions to the plight of the cancer patient and require attention (Clarke and Kissane 2002). Clinicians need to understand the nature of demoralization, in which the individual is coping with helplessness and subjective incompetence, and how it may differ from a major depressive episode. Simultaneously, clinicians need to focus on monitoring patients' quality of life. Treatments include milieu management for the delirious patient as well as medication. Families should understand that organic reactions of the family member who is delirious or has dementia with significant anxiety or cognitive changes are due to the disease or its treatments and are not a reflection of willful behavior. Rational psychopharmacology and psychotherapy are important in treating anxiety disorders, depression, and demoralization within such patient populations. If the initial treatment is successful, remission is a time of waiting and can lead to ongoing anxiety or denial of the implications of the disorder. Recurrence often renews fears that mandate psychosocial attention. The obvious psychological challenges of the terminal phase for such patients are often overlooked by clinicians who assume that depression or confusion is "understandable"—but these challenges mandate clinical attention (Chochinov et al. 2002; Hales 1980).

Thus, this clinically focused book covers broad issues, as well as specific categories of psychosocial distress and various psychiatric treatment methods.

Individual and family assessment and psychotherapy are important. The book concludes with developing trends in psycho-oncology. Clearly, international standards of care for the cancer patient mandate competent psychosocial assessment and treatment. We hope that this volume will aid clinicians in achieving that goal.

Massimo Biondi
Anna Costantini
Thomas Wise

References

Chochinov HM, Hack T, Hassard T, et al: Dignity in the terminally ill: a cross-sectional, cohort study. Lancet 360: 2026–2030, 2002

Clarke DM, Kissane DW: Demoralization: its phenomenology and importance. Aust N Z J Psychiatry 36:733–742, 2002

Hales RE: Dying patients: a challenge to their physicians and consultation psychiatry. Mil Med 145:674–680, 1980

Holland JC: Societal views of cancer and the emergence of psycho-oncology, in Psycho-oncology. Edited by Holland JC. New York, Oxford University Press, 1998, pp 3–15

Institute of Medicine: Cancer care for the whole patient: meeting psychosocial health needs. Edited by Adler NE, Page AEK. Washington, DC, National Academies Press, 2008

Oken D: What to tell cancer patients: a study of medical attitudes. JAMA 175:1120–1128, 1961

Rosentberg SJ, Hayes JR, Peterson RA: Revising the Seriousness of Illness Rating Scale: modernization and re-standardization. Int J Psychiatry Med 17:85–92, 1987

Surbone A: Telling the truth to patients with cancer: what is the truth? Lancet Oncol 7:944–950, 2006

Tolstoy L: The Death of Ivan Ilych (1886). New York, Signet Classics, 1960, pp 95–156

Weisman AD: A model for psychosocial phasing in cancer. Gen Hosp Psychiatry 1:187–195, 1979

CHAPTER 1

The Crisis of Discovery

Psychological and Psychopathological Reaction to the Disease

Anna Costantini, Ph.D.

Jon A. Levenson, M.D.

Francesco Saverio Bersani, M.D.

ONCOLOGICAL DISEASES are among the most prevalent ill-nesses globally and remain a leading cause of death and debility. Worldwide, there were close to 13 million new cancer cases in 2008, with an estimated projection of 21 million cases annually by 2030 (GLOBOCAN 2008). With new therapeutic technologies, many cancer patients are being cured, and many other patients are living longer with increasingly complicated, multi-modality treatment regimens.

Assessment of psychosocial and psychiatric needs related to cancer and its treatment, as well as the formulation of appropriate treatment plans, is increasingly recognized as an essential and critical cornerstone of compre-hensive cancer care (Adler and Page 2007). Although the first clinical descriptions from the psycho-oncology literature date back to 1952 (Suther-land et al. 1952), only in the past three decades has this attention to the psy-chosocial aspects of cancer care blossomed into its own distinct subspecialty, referred to as psycho-oncology (Holland 2002).

The focus of this chapter is on how the patient with a new diagnosis of cancer copes with the crisis of initial discovery of the illness, as well as the emotional challenges and demands associated with beginning oncological treatment. How well or how poorly a patient copes when he or she first learns of a new cancer diagnosis, or suspects a cancer from new suspicious signs or symptoms, is highly variable, with many factors at play. It is important for clinicians to appreciate these different factors, which collectively contribute to how an individual will cope and manage at the time of a cancer discovery and as treatment and evaluation proceed.

Universal major concerns that an individual faces at the time of initial diagnosis of cancer include fear of death, fear of permanent disability, worry about life trajectory disruptions from cancer, and especially fears about the effects from treatment that lead to dependence (Table 1–1). Finally, the fear of disfigurement is a common existential threat (Holland and Friedlander 2006). The challenge for patients is that they must proceed with prompt medical evaluation and make critically important treatment decisions about their care, all while comanaging their own distress level (Massie and Holland 1989).

The psycho-oncology literature is rich in data regarding the prevalence of anxiety and depression following the diagnosis of cancer (Mitchell et al. 2011). An analysis of the percentages of reactive depression or anxiety states is very important to explain the reaction to the disease, but such categorical labels are not enough to adequately understand how a person perceives the risk of suffering from pain and disfigurement as well as the spectre of death; these fears are what cancer actually represents in the minds of the majority of patients. In other words, the reaction to the discovery of cancer is far more than a simple clinical evaluation and psychiatric labeling process. Any health professional or family member who interacts with a cancer patient must understand the unique aspects of the psychological challenges of the disease state for that patient, which will depend on both the psychiatric diagnosis and the patient's unique biopsychosocial strengths and vulnerabilities.

The clinician needs to have a broad vision of the relationship between the concepts of illness and death to effectively work in the psychological world of the patient with neoplastic disease. Reviewing how the relationship between human illness and death evolved in Western culture demands discussion of some philosophical and existential considerations that provide a basis for comprehending the recent scientific psycho-oncological data.

Hundreds of publications since 1950 have suggested that the typical reaction to the diagnosis of cancer is the emotional equation in the mind of the patient that *cancer=death.* Even if the statistics about the possibilities of prevention, treatment, and survival from many types of cancer are well known, and in spite of the educational effort of the medical community to make clear that 10- and 15-year relative survival rates in some cancers are as high as 90%

TABLE 1–1. Universal fears and worries at time of cancer discovery

Fear of dying

Fear of becoming disabled and dependent

Worry about medical uncertainty

Worry over cancer's impact on life trajectory

Fear of suffering a painful death

or 100% (www.cancer.org), the first thought of those who receive a diagnosis of cancer continues to be, "Maybe I do not have much time left to live."

In everyday life most individuals do not think about death, tend to deny it, and believe that it can happen to others but not to themselves. Sigmund Freud (1915/1957) wrote that nobody really believes in his or her own death and that everybody is convinced of his or her own immortality because "our own death is irrepresentable; each time we try to represent it we notice that we are still present as observers" (p. 296), but that extreme experiences such as war sweep away the conventional way of thinking about personal mortality. Similarly, the fear of facing a cancer diagnosis can vanquish the conventional denial of death and force people to seriously consider the possibility of dying.

Disease and Death in a Historical Context

In Western culture, individuals have not typically viewed sickness and death as natural facts of life, to be accepted with peacefulness and without anguish; in fact, in the course of history, sickness and death have been attributed to different roles. In his essay "Death in the Western World," French historian Vovelle (1983) commented that in the fourteenth century, life expectancy in Europe was between 30 and 35 years. The great plague, leprosy, and famines attacked hundreds of thousands of people without defenses (McNeill 1976). Forty percent of men died before age 20, and the death of infants was often not even recorded.

In the sixteenth century, Montaigne thought, at the age of 39, that he had already exceeded the limits of common life (Montaigne 1580/1992); at that time in Italy, half the population of the city of Milan died of plague, and medical sciences to defend against epidemics were so lacking that King Henry IV of France used to protect himself from infections with a necklace of nuts filled with silver. The diseases of the seventeenth century were plague, small-pox, tuberculosis, typhoid fever, malaria, and "purpuric fever." In rural France, 45 out of 100 boys died by age 10 years. Death was so oppressive a presence that men and women tried to control it. The view of the afterlife in Christian theology gave hope to the dying. As a consequence, the powerful work of Christianization increased and manuals on *Ars Moriendi* (the art of dying) proliferated. The central theme of "how to die" was the consideration of life, and of disease, as an apprenticeship to death, which in turn was considered the realization and exaltation of the existential journey.

The real turning point in the attitude toward disease began in the seventeenth century. Although doctors still had insufficient knowledge and infant mortality was very high, disease and death in the Age of Enlightenment were considered natural facts that doctors and scientists could actively fight with the resources of reason and medicine. Talking to an older person about death, reported Diderot, became a "cruel rudeness." The process of secularization replaced prejudices, superstitions, and religious beliefs with a scientific view of disease. In the 1800s, the great offensive of medicine against the diseases began. During this century, some great discoveries were made: cell structure, "microbes," methods of antisepsis, X rays, vaccines, and anesthetics.

Progress continued into the twentieth century. Chemotherapy, insulin, penicillin, neurosurgery, organ transplants, resuscitation techniques, and gene therapies now allow long survivals. Life expectancy at birth is now, in the West, over 75 years for men and over 80 years for women. Men can aspire to a "long life ending without pain" (Morin 1951), and they can do it because death is no longer a daily presence; most people can easily exclude death from their minds.

Although modern medicine has triumphed over common infectious diseases, it has been less successful against some other forms of pathology, such as cancer. Cancer is the second leading cause of death in the West; it has occupied the place, in the collective imaginary, that was previously occupied by plague, tuberculosis, or cholera. The impact of a cancer diagnosis forces one to deal with the progress and limits of science in a cultural climate in which, more than in preceding periods of history, it is possible to deny the possibility of death and to attribute to the doctor the role of omnipotent healer. In the 1930s, only one person of five was alive 5 years after a cancer diagnosis. Today, according to the American Cancer Society (2012)—taking into consideration that survival statistics vary greatly by cancer type and stage at diagnosis—for all cancers diagnosed between 2001 and 2007, the 5-year relative survival rate is 67%, increased from 49% in 1975–1977. This increase mirrors progress in early-stage diagnosis of certain cancers as well as advances in treatment. The hope for a miracle drug has been fulfilled in some cases, but the "war against cancer" has not yet been won. Thus, for a patient whose cure is not possible, the difficult task at the time of cancer discovery is, as the German psychiatrist and philosopher Karl Jaspers wrote in his autobiography, "to react to the disabling effect of the condition of the sick," to include the disease in one's life, and to familiarize oneself with it in order to be able to accept it (Jaspers 1967/1993).

Existentialist philosophers argued that an existential experience that puts man in front of the reality of his own finality also allows the possibility of a more authentic life (Heidegger 1927/1964; Jaspers 1932/1981). This core concept is the theoretical background that has inspired many psychotherapists who work with cancer patients to view their work in a positive and exploratory manner and not just as an effort to mitigate pain and fear.

Reactions to Diagnosis

The impact of cancer on people's lives is related to four main factors (Razazi and Delvaux 1988): the existential threat of the disease, psychosocial consequences (e.g., suspension or loss of employment, changes in family role, significant changes in social life), consequences of the morbid disease process (e.g., pain, fatigue, dyspnea), and treatment and its effects (e.g., nausea, alopecia, surgical mutilation, loss of fertility).

The threat to physical existence has a disruptive effect on a patient's psychology and, in this sense, is comparable to a real physical trauma. The communication of a diagnosis of cancer has all the characteristics of what has been called a *shock trauma.* It gives rise to a reactive process involving the transition from the idea of *healthy* to the idea of *sick,* from a certain to an uncertain life, from a "reliable" body to a body that "may betray."

The diagnosis of cancer is a process with high psychic costs both for the patient and for family members, in whom unconscious mechanisms of defense against anguish, as well as personal cognitive and behavioral styles of managing stressful situations, are mobilized. It has been observed that the impact of the diagnosis creates a true existential crisis that manifests itself during the first 3 months in 70% of patients (Weisman and Worden 1984); the crisis is generally polarized on issues related to the dimension of time, personal identity, the theme of life and death, and the meaning of life. The crisis, as is well represented by the Chinese ideogram corresponding to the word *crisis,* contains in itself the concept of danger but also the concept of opportunity: facing a life-threatening disease creates the possibility of a reorganization of one's essential priorities, as well as the opportunity for change and for personal growth (Yalom 1980).

The idea that cancer may represent an opportunity for personal growth, as demonstrated in the following mentalization exercise, is the basis for many psychotherapies used specifically with cancer patients (e.g., existential cognitive psychotherapy, supportive-expressive psychotherapy, meaning-centered psychotherapy, dignity therapy; see Appendix 1–B):

> I told him to enjoy not having cancer; but I also told him that if he wanted to do an interesting exercise, he could imagine for a day that he had cancer, and then consider how not only life, but also people and things around us, suddenly appear in a different light. Perhaps a fairer light. (Tiziano Terzani 1984/2004, "One More Ride on the Merry-Go-Round," p. 9)

It is useful to consider the normal, nonpsychopathological coping responses to discovery of a cancer. There is typically an initial phase of shock or disbelief as the individual's psychological equilibrium is rocked by this unexpected news that can cause a fracture in the perception of one's own existential continuity. Often, a period of transient emotional turmoil follows, with signs and symptoms of anxiety, fear, and depressed or dysphoric mood (Petticrew et al. 2002). Alternatively, an irritable mood may predominate in this early response to cancer discovery. Sleep, appetite, and energy disruptions frequently occur, and concentration and attention often falter as newly diagnosed patients tend to be anxiously preoccupied with both coping with cancer discovery and needing to engage in prompt decision making.

It is common to observe, in cancer patients, mechanisms of defense against anguish that in other contexts are considered indicative of a psychotic or neurotic structure; they represent an attempt to manage a state of acute distress that exceeds the capacity of the psychic system to contain it. For example, rational and educated people may adopt behaviors of denial seemingly inexplicable in light of their educational level, or patients described as mild-mannered may show extreme reactions of anger and aggression toward doctors or nurses whom they judge guilty of continual diagnostic and therapeutic mistakes. Other patients may react with an almost manic-like hyperactivity in an attempt to exorcise the fear of weakness and dependence, or may regress to a liability that does not match with the behavioral style they previously had. Some patients may talk about their own situation with a kind of pseudo-indifference. Manic defenses, regression, projection, and isolation of emotions are just some ways in which patients, after diagnosis, try to stem their anguish about a life that suddenly seems to be acutely distorted.

The newly diagnosed patient may not be able to fully perform daily activities, especially in the context of the added challenge of an evolving medical workup and, often, early initiation of oncological therapy. During this initial period, patients may develop intrusive thoughts about their medical crisis; fearfulness about the future typically accompanies these intrusive ego-dystonic cognitions and can be debilitating (Breitbart and Alici 2009).

Case Vignette: A Revealing Dream

Joanna had a quadrantectomy (partial mastectomy) for a breast cancer and then began outpatient chemotherapy. The patient asked to have psychological support because chemotherapy fostered anxiety that she did not want to report to her family and friends. At the first consult, she had a positive affect; she was smiling, and she referred to feeling good and wanting to start back to work. She described herself as a strong woman who always bravely faced the difficulties of life. She did not modify her dietary habits after the chemotherapy, and she ate regular meals. On weekends she often took short and interesting trips to the countryside. In the hospital she was loved by the medical staff, and the other patients admired her for her vitality. During a psychological support session, she described a dream she had recently had: "I was in a boat with some friends on a sunny and peaceful day. Suddenly, the electrical system of the boat broke down, and the boat quit responding to commands. The sun went away, and everything became dark. I was in a panic, and I begged the others to go back to the dry land; we did not find the seaport and we hit a rock. We swam into a cavern; in the cavern there were an illuminated altar and some statues of angels."

After the surgical oncological intervention and/or the first months of chemotherapy treatment, patients are no longer as "resistant" to bearing the treatments and their side effects. They may enter a phase of psychological accommodation to a changed life situation in which they objectively reconsider their existential projects, and they look for a sense of what happened and try to integrate it into their representation of themselves. It is the time for them to review their priorities and to reflect on many of the lifestyle choices made before the disease (Culberg 1975). During this phase, the psycho-oncologist can "accompany" the patient in finding answers to these questions.

Case Vignette: Cancer as a New Form of Existence

Elizabeth, a 46-year-old woman working in a major governmental institution, was diagnosed with breast cancer and was treated with chemotherapy and radiotherapy + trastuzumab after quadrantectomy. After 1 year she reported to her therapist her initial reaction to the diagnosis: "I denied the illness. I had never thought before that I could get sick, and the diagnosis fell on me like a rock. On an emotional level, I felt fragile 'like a candle in the wind.' I have always actively avoided thinking about suffering in my life. During the first cycle of chemotherapy, I was in a state of semiconsciousness. I continued to deny the illness. When the nurse came with the vials of chemotherapy, I asked her to hide them under the bed. Those first months were all the same, only marked by chemotherapy infusions. When I had the surgical intervention, my colleagues sent me flowers. I said, writing them an e-mail, 'Yesterday we were all meeting together laughing at the table.... Today everything is changed: I have to turn terror into strength.'"

Determinants of the Reaction to the Diagnosis

The ability of an individual to manage and cope with the life-threatening discovery of a cancer depends on the interplay of biological, psychological, spiritual, and social factors (Grassi et al. 2010). Medical or biological factors that can influence coping include specific parameters related to the cancer itself. These include the site of origin (e.g., breast, lung, liver); the type of cancer and its presenting stage at discovery; the physical symptoms that the cancer is causing (e.g., pain, fatigue); the expected disease course; the treatment regimen planned, which may include combination of multimodalities such as surgery, systemic chemotherapy, radiation therapy, and increasingly immunotherapy; and the potential for rehabilitation from the cancer and treatment (Holland and Gooen-Piels 2003).

In addition to physical symptoms from the cancer and biological aspects of cancer treatment, patients may also develop psychological distress related to changes in body appearance and functioning. How patients incorporate bodily changes into their body image schema often derive from the site of tumor origin; this aspect of coping can be quite different for a lymphoma patient and for a breast cancer patient. The lymphoma patient may struggle with body image issues related to profound fatigue, alopecia, and decreased stamina, whereas the breast cancer postmastectomy patient feels a sense of loss and grief related to the loss of a breast. Thus, coping with surgical resection, such as mastectomy or lower-extremity amputation in the setting of an osteosarcoma, can lead to specific changes in body image assimilation and resultant distress. The individual's prior level of psychosocial adjustment, especially toward medical illness, is an important determinant in coping in this context, as are the potential threat and obstacles that cancer and treatment may pose in achieving developmentally appropriate life goals. Social factors reflect larger societal and cultural attitudes toward oncology care; these factors include a specific society's or culture's perceptions of cancer, as well as its state of knowledge. Evolving legal statutes mandating informed consent, while facilitating and improving doctor-patient dialogue regarding disease, therapeutic options, and prognosis, can also adversely affect some patients, who become overwhelmed and overburdened with complicated and often worrisome medical details related to treatment and disease course (Breitbart and Alici 2009).

Another important factor that can affect coping is social support, the perceived presence by the patient of emotionally supportive persons who play an active and ongoing role. The presence of social support can substantially help buffer the emotional impact of cancer discovery and subsequent medical care; conversely, the lack of necessary social support can have profound negative consequences for an individual dealing with a cancer diagnosis.

How well or how poorly a person copes with new cancer discovery relates to intrapersonal, interpersonal, and socioeconomic factors (Table 1–2). Intrapersonal factors consist of an individual's premorbid personality, coping traits, ego strength, and current developmental life phase (e.g., young adult vs. elderly). Interpersonal factors relate to social support, as described above. Socioeconomic factors include access to care, and lower socioeconomic status has been associated with inability to receive quality cancer care (Marmot 2005).

How effectively a cancer patient can be physically rehabilitated is also a significant factor in coping. Past psychiatric history of anxiety or mood disorder, as well as history of or active substance abuse or dependence, can significantly influence how and when a cancer is discovered, and at what stage, as well as how an individual copes and engages in intensive cancer care regimens. In this chapter, these specific points are illustrated through clinical cases presented in Appendix 1-A.

Coping Styles and Cancer

In the psycho-oncology literature, the concept of coping has assumed an increasingly significant role to individuate the subjective adaptation to stressful events in life and in particular to cancer. The importance of coping style in oncology is linked to the fact that coping has become one of the key factors in modulating the individual psychological reaction to disease and in influencing response and adherence to anticancer treatments.

Regarding the influence of coping on patients' survival and disease recurrence, some authors have observed an association between coping styles and biological course of the disease. We can currently affirm that there is little consistent evidence that psychological coping styles and personality traits play an important part in survival from or recurrence of cancer; however, a few studies seemed to support this possibility (positive findings tended to be confined to small or methodologically flawed studies) (Petticrew et al. 2002).

The coping process can be divided into two sequential stages: *evaluative* and *executive.* The evaluation phase is centered on the cognitive processes of attribution of meaning to the stimulus situation. In this regard, Lazarus (1993) identified two types of appraisal (evaluation): the primary appraisal is a cognitive process directed at the establishment of the significance or meaning of the event to the organism; the secondary appraisal is directed at

---

TABLE 1–2.   Characteristics of the patient at high risk for problematic coping with newly discovered cancer

---

Individual past history of psychiatric vulnerability of depression or anxiety disorder

Family psychiatric history of mood or anxiety disorder

Concurrent substance misuse, or past history of substance disorder

Poor social supports

Socioeconomically stressed family with patient as primary financial earner

---

the assessment of the ability to cope with the event (Scherer et al. 2001). The executive phase addresses the organization of responses and behaviors to cope with the disease.

Three different types of coping strategies have been identified: emotion-focused strategies, aimed at "affect regulation"; problem-focused strategies, directed at mitigating or solving the impact of the stressful event; and avoidant (e.g., escape) and approach (e.g., confrontive) strategies. Psychologists placed particular emphasis on the meaning attributed to the disease by the patients (Jenkins and Pargament 1988). For example, Lipowski (1970) listed eight possible meanings attributable to the disease by patients: challenge, enemy, punishment, weakness, relief, strategy, loss, and value. It is clear that different types of evaluation by the patient may lead to different types of emotional reactions and behaviors (for example, acceptance or rejection of the treatment).

Case Vignette: The Disease as Enemy

Oriana Fallaci, Italian journalist and writer, underwent surgical intervention for breast cancer. During an interview published in the journal *La Stampa* (13 March 1993), she said, "After the surgical operation I asked doctors to see what they had taken from my body. The cancer looked like a small, pretty and innocuous marble ball. After a few days, I examined the cancer under the microscope, and I realized what its reproduction was capable to do. I understood that I had an enemy inside me: an alien that invaded my body to destroy it. Now, we have a relation of war: I want to kill 'him,' 'he' wants to kill me."

Case Vignette: The Disease as Punishment

Rachel, a 25-year-old musician, was waiting for a surgical excision of a melanoma. Even before she was born, her mother had decided what kind of musical instrument the child had to play, according to family traditions. Rachel studied with the best teachers and won several prizes. However, she did not feel happy because the instrument she played did not enable her to really be a "protagonist," so she decided to become a singer. She dedicated all her time to studying and practicing, which led to important financial and personal sacrifices. Speaking about her cancer, she said, "There must be a reason for this disease. I heard about implications of the immune system. I recently experienced some very difficult moments. I also had herpes. But, why a skin cancer? Maybe I have an explanation: it is my obsession for perfection. I live the cancer as a punishment for the fact that I cannot accept the idea of not being perfect."

Case Vignette: The Disease as Loss

Denise, 47 years old, recently had a mastectomy and breast reconstruction for a breast cancer, and now she has to start chemotherapy and radiotherapy. At the psychological consult, she presented as an attractive and pleasant woman with long black hair and beautiful legs. She said that she was aware of the gravity of the disease, and that she considered the disease as a shame. She is a shopkeeper and is married with two children. Because she considers her marriage to be joyless and her husband to be "infantile and disturbed," she has found her serenity in extramarital relations. She had always felt young, but now she is feeling old. She is afraid of losing her hair because of the chemotherapy. Indicating the scars in her reconstructed breast, she said, "Who will court me with this disgusting stuff? It won't be possible any more for me to wear a lace brassiere! I was a real 'female.' For me the mastectomy is a tragedy, even more than the disease!"

Case Vignette: The Disease as Sense of Guilt

Patrick is a 51-year-old seaman, married with two children. He is undergoing chemotherapy because of lung cancer. He is markedly depressed: "They tell me that I should be stronger, but I am actually a pessimist. I grew up in an orphanage; my life has been a nonstop sacrifice. Being a seaman means to never see your own family. Now that I have a purpose for my life, now that I could start to enjoy my family, I get sick. I feel a sense of guilt. I do not know why. I have always been altruistic and a good believer. Why has Jesus Christ castigated me? It is not right."

Case Vignette: A Priest's View

Father David Maria Turoldo was born in Italy in 1916. He published two books of poems. He had pancreatic cancer in advanced stage when he was interviewed by a journalist. He said, "It is impossible that God is related to my disease. It is unthinkable that the God of Jesus, as we know Him through the Bible, may want cancer. If He is sending us cancer, might we be able to cure it? This discovery is terrible, but also comforting. When I pray, I ask God for the strength to accept, the strength to hope, I ask for help against the pain. But I do not attribute the disease to God. I understood, through the disease, that God loves His creatures so much that He respects the natural progress of life. Otherwise, there would not be freedom (*Corriere della Sera*, 25 September 1991).

A rich scientific literature exists on different strategies—both successful and maladaptive—to cope with cancer. Worden and Weisman (1984) described 15 ways to face the diagnosis of cancer: 1) rationalizing (e.g., searching for more information), 2) sharing concerns, 3) minimizing, 4) suppressing (trying not to think about the diagnosis), 5) moving (by engaging in other activities to distract), 6) dealing with the problem, 7) redefining (e.g., accepting the diagnosis but trying to find favorable aspects), 8) acting out, 9) being fatalistic or resigned, 10) thinking in a rational way (considering all the alternatives), 11) engaging in behaviors to reduce the tension (e.g., excessive drinking or eating), 12) engaging in behaviors to reduce the stimuli (isolating and withdrawing from social situations), 13) projecting (e.g., blaming someone else, such as relatives or doctors), 14) being compliant (following the directions of doctors), and 15) internalizing (blaming oneself). The authors noted that patients with high emotional distress mainly used repression, resignation, and fatalism and were not able to produce alternative strategies for adaptation; on the other hand, patients with low emotional distress had a way of coping more flexibly, characterized by confrontation, redefinition of problems, and compliance.

Watson et al. (1988) described five profiles of coping with cancer—fighting spirit, hopelessness/helplessness, fatalism, anxious preoccupation, and cognitive avoidance—and developed a questionnaire to assess the clinical utility of each profile. The data suggested that those patients who face a diagnosis with fighting spirit, using comparison responses that favor a more positive view of the event without reducing or underestimating its potential danger, and who adopt more flexible and differentiated cognitive and behavioral strategies, show less psychological morbidity and a greater sense of personal control of their health status.

In general, research findings on coping with cancer strongly indicate the supremacy of engagement-type coping strategies (e.g., maintaining a fighting spirit, engaging in problem solving, seeking social support, focusing on the positive) in improving psychosocial adaptation among survivors of cancer. In contrast, disengagement strategies (e.g., wishful thinking, blaming oneself, helplessness, hopelessness, resigning oneself to the disease impact) have been associated with poorer psychosocial outcomes among these survivors (Livneh 2000).

Understanding the types and effectiveness of the individual styles of coping with the disease assumes particular importance. If an individual's coping strategy is functional and adequate, adaptation to the disease may also turn into an opportunity for existential growth; each person, in fact, constantly builds himself or herself through life experiences, which are constantly changing. On the contrary, if an individual's situation is too stressful or skills to deal with it are inadequate, he or she may develop a psychopathological reaction and a state of intense subjective suffering.

Normal and Pathological Reactions

Anxiety, depression, or anger can represent a normal component of the emotional response of people to the experience they are living. Anxiety, depression, irritable mood, or hostile reactions are not necessarily expressions of a disease or a disorder. In normal conditions, the manifestation of emotions can have an adaptive significance for the individual in terms of relationships with others and can allow the release of internal feelings of tension and discomfort that are not otherwise manageable.

It is important for health professionals of various disciplines who treat patients with cancer to be able to differentiate between "normal" reactions and "psychopathological" reactions (Table 1–3), because psychopathological states that are not properly diagnosed and treated may increase and prolong subjective suffering, undermining the patient's ability to maintain hope. As a general rule, one can assume, for example, that anxiety and depression are subclinical when they are low or moderate, appear related to events or situations, and are episodic and of limited duration, when the person is aware of his or her status, and when subjective distress is transient.

Anxiety, depression, and anger move toward the pole of the pathological when their intensities are high and excessive, when the reactions are relatively independent from stimuli or situations, when the reactions are actually persistent conditions, when the episodes are repeated frequently, when the person's interpersonal relationships and capacity to interact with others are disturbed and altered, and when there is evident subjective suffering. In these cases, psychiatric assessment is clearly necessary.

Case Vignette: Pathological Anxiety

James, a 46-year-old patient with colon cancer, presented with a generalized anxiety disorder, emotional lability, and thoughts focused on the fear of death. He received the cancer diagnosis 3 months ago. His face is tense and has an expression of terror. He consulted the Internet and, despite the reassurances of doctors, is convinced that relapses are certain. He spends his time on the sofa, imagining how his life will end. He has asked to be reassured, but nothing seems to help him. For 3 months he has continued crying and has had persistent insomnia. He does not leave his house because the sight of healthy people is unbearable for him. He does not go to work because he thinks that his colleagues would view him as a walking dead man. He used to be a police detective who solved difficult cases. He always tried to do the best in his work, and life for him was "work and fun." He had never thought he could get sick. Now he says, "Life has no meaning. I will die. It is inevitable; no one can help me. Just tell me: what meaning does it have? Can you die at the age of 46? It is unfair. If I had known, I would not have been away from home so much for work…."

TABLE 1–3. **Criteria to differentiate normal and pathological reactions to cancer discovery**

Normal	Pathological
Low or moderate levels of reaction, related to specific situations	High levels of reaction, not related to specific situations
Time-limited episodes	Chronic or persistent episodes
Unaltered psychosocial functioning and interpersonal relations	Altered psychosocial functioning and interpersonal relations
Low subjective suffering	High subjective suffering

Discovery in Advanced Phase

In some cases the diagnosis of cancer occurs at an advanced stage, when the extension of the tumor and the development of metastases point toward an unfavorable prognosis and limited survival period. The reaction to the diagnosis of advanced cancer depends on many factors, including, not least in importance, whether and how medical doctors communicate the information. In many non–Anglo-Saxon countries, doctors tend to hide the truth from patients, aiming to protect them, and therefore the patient's awareness of the prognosis is very limited (Mystakidou et al. 2004).

In this section we discuss the mental condition of patients with a life expectancy ranging from a few months to about 2–3 years.

In studies that have tried to understand the different reactions to a diagnosis of early versus advanced cancer, results suggest that the fears and the coping modalities of patients with newly diagnosed cancer in its early stages (I and II) do not significantly differ from those of patients with cancer in more advanced stages (III and IV) of the neoplastic process. The authors of such studies hypothesize that the diagnosis of cancer has so disruptive an initial effect that successive differences related to the neoplastic process stage are mitigated (Gotay 1984). However, everyone with experience working with patients in advanced and terminal phases knows that medical, psychological, and spiritual problems can assume a complexity and an intensity unknown in other phases of the clinical course.

Patients with a diagnosis of advanced-stage cancer—whether they are fully aware of the seriousness of their condition or merely suspect it (despite the false reassurances of doctors and relatives)—do accept that dying is a certain event and recognize that the only uncertainties are when and how. The challenges for these patients are thus of two types: the first is deciding whether to accept or reject the reality of having to die (and acceptance does not necessarily mean giving up hope), and the second is finding sense and meaning in the situation—in other words, seeking answers to the questions "What do I value now?" and "What meaning does my life have if everything ends?" (Carey 1975).

Jean-Paul Sartre (1943/1964) wrote,

> Death is a boundary, and every boundary (whether it is final or initial) is a Janus Bifrons [i.e., it simultaneously looks in both directions]…The final chord of a melody is stretched out towards silence, toward the nothingness of the sound that follows the melody; and under this aspect it is made up of silence, because the silence that follows is already into the final chord, as a part of its meaning. But on the other side, the final chord adheres to the "plenum of being" which is the melody in itself: without it the melody would remain in the air and this final indecision would go backwards to the stream of musical notes, giving to each of them a character of incompleteness. Death becomes the sense of life as the final chord is the sense of the melody.

The philosophers Heidegger (1927/1964) and Jaspers (1932/1981) wrote that the confrontation with the reality of one's death offers a deeper sense of life and the possibility of a genuine and conscious existence.

Freud, who died of cancer in 1939 after having lived with this disease for about 20 years, emphasized the great impact that death has on all lives: the existence, deprived of the possibility of risking "the maximum," namely life itself, would be insipid; he compared it to an "American flirt, which states from the beginning that nothing can happen, in contrast to a love affair of the Old Continent, in which both partners are constantly aware of the serious consequences they handle" (Freud 1915/1957).

The clinical experience of psychotherapists who have worked with terminally ill patients demonstrates the validity of these philosophical considerations (Kübler-Ross 1969; LeShan 1990; Yalom 1980). In a study of 70 women with metastatic breast cancer, Yalom (1980) tried to systematically evaluate the personal changes subsequent to the disease. Most patients said that compared to before, they felt they had something valuable to teach others, they believed more in their personal rights, they better appreciated the beauty of nature, and they had moments of deep serenity. The crisis that stems from the threat of a deadly disease may, for some, become an opportunity for personal growth; the impact of limited life expectancy is often not a painless process and not free from contradictions.

As Jaspers (1932/1981) wrote, "The sweetness of being, because of the natural will to live, cannot disappear without fear"; a person who comes to know that his or her death might be imminent travels across a complex series of psychological stages. The identification of these psychological phases derives from the work, still relevant today, that Elisabeth Kübler-Ross conducted in the United States with hundreds of terminally ill people; she encouraged patients to talk about their clinical experiences in medical seminars, thus breaking the barrier between healthy and dying, and turning the patient from a "clinical case" to a "teacher" (Kübler-Ross 1974). The observed phases correspond to psychological defense mechanisms; simultaneously with or successively to each other, these phases can be implemented not only by cancer patients, but also by those who are facing serious events of loss or extremely dramatic life episodes.

The first reaction of someone who learns that he or she has an advanced disease is *denial:* "It is not possible, not me. There must be a mistake." The refusal is a temporary psychological defense that allows patients the opportunity to adapt to reality; sooner or later, denial will be replaced by partial acceptance. The need to deny the seriousness of the diagnosis is, however, not an exclusive characteristic of the first reaction step, but rather can occur at any time during the adaptive process. "Neither the sun nor death can be looked at steadily," said La Rochefoucauld; and indeed, according to Kübler-Ross, to maintain hope and continue to live, one cannot continually face the idea of death. It is important for those who assist the patient to respect these apparent contradictions and leave the patient at any time the possibility to protect himself or herself from anxiety and anguish. In the experience of Kübler-Ross, even those patients who more realistically accepted the fact of having a limited life expectancy hoped to be included in the trial of a new drug or in some scientific discovery of the last hour.

The stage of *anger,* rational or irrational, takes over when the patient is aware of reality: "So it's true. It's happening to me. Why me?" Taking the brunt of the anger, in some cases, is the doctor, who is blamed for not having understood the symptoms in time; in other cases, patients attack an "inhuman" nurse, or "disorganized and incompetent" trainee doctors, or some "insensitive" family member or friend. These reactions are difficult to tolerate for those who care for the patient, and often evoke discomfort and reactive aggression. It is important for the health care staff to avoid reacting defensively and to attribute these attitudes to the patient's suffering rather than consider them as personal attacks. Cassidy (1991) emphasized that anger is an important aspect to be recognized in managing the treatment of advanced stages of cancer. In this regard, she distinguished existential anger from anger against caregivers and from projected anger. The patient, full of resentment, may ask the physician the existential question, "Why did this happen to me, to me who has always been a good person?" Most often the question is rhetorical; nobody knows the answer, including the doctor, who can simply answer "I really don't know." The patient's anger against the health care staff, according to Cassidy, should never be ignored or underestimated. A patient must always have the opportunity to express feelings, both justified and unjustified. If anger is not justified, listening to the patient trying to reach a clarification of misunderstandings usually serves to resolve difficult situations in the best way. Very often, however, the impotence and frustration resulting from the awareness that the disease has irreversibly changed one's life, projects, and hopes provoke an uncontrollable rage, which requires finding an external object to discharge. Targets of this aggression are the people closest to the patient. It may be helpful, in these cases, to imagine being in the patient's shoes in an effort to understand his or her perspective. Allowing anger outbursts—without becoming a victim— and treating the patient with empathy will help him or her to ease mental tension and find some relief.

Case Vignette: Constant Anger

Christine is a 54-year-old woman who is married with three children. She has breast cancer with metastases at bone, uterus, bone marrow, and liver. She has a life expectancy of a few months. "I understand now that I will not heal. This is hell! Is this kind of life worth living? I don't laugh anymore, I don't cook anymore, I don't eat anymore. I feel far from everything. During these last days I did not care about my children, my mother, and my husband. I have always been proud of my children, and now I envy them because they can live. Is this me? Have I become so unfeeling? I rationally thought about suicide. I have so many drug prescriptions that I could easily reach 200 pills...." Her daughter reported, "I would like to know what we should do with Mum, how to interact with her. At first, it seemed that she didn't care about us at all; she didn't care about anything. But now, she is becoming more and more aggressive, angry, and dictatorial. It seems that she envies healthy people. She complains to her friends that she has three selfish children, but this is not true. I try to do whatever is possible for her, but it is all useless."

After the phase of incredulity and anger, the patient finds new forms of hope and enters into what has been defined as the *bargaining phase.* In most cases patients try to negotiate with "fate" or with their God. The patient requests a wish be granted (e.g., surviving until a child has graduated, or being free of pain) in exchange for something good that the patient promises in secret. The negotiation also implies accepting a limited time to live and not demanding more.

With the progression of the disease, the recurrent hospitalizations, and the full recognition of reality, the patient reaches the phase of *depression,* which has two forms: reactive and preparatory. *Reactive depression* is characterized by the perception of a loss of one's sense of integrity, physical beauty, independence, sexual intimacy, and social role. The task of psycho-oncologists and of the entire medical team is to support the patient in maintaining self-esteem by actively helping him or her in the transition to a more existential attitude, looking for meaning and purpose in the new condition of life. *Preparatory depression* relates to impending loss—that is, the pain of one's final separation from this world. Attachment to life gradually disappears in this phase; this process must be respected by others.

After the rejection of his or her fate, the envy for healthy people, the rage against the health carers, the attempts to bargain with fate, and the pain of preparation, the person finally reaches a stage of *acceptance.* The "war against cancer" ends in a calmness before the "long journey."

Case Vignette: Adaptation

Maestro Luciano Pavarotti, returning from New York to Italy after a surgical intervention for pancreatic cancer, answered to a reporter who asked him how he felt, "I take it philosophically. Life has given me everything. So if everything is taken from me, we are even with God." (*Adnkronos*, July 30, 2006)

Case Vignette: Acceptance Does Not Mean Being "Happy"

Lucy, a 59-year-old woman who is married with two children, lives in a small village in the countryside close to Rome. She knows that her cancer is so extensive that it is not useful for her to keep staying in a hospital. She said, "I am Catholic and I thank God for giving me the bravery to accept all this. My husband never accepted my disease. After my first surgical operation, I started to experience life more deeply. I became more tolerant; I changed for the better. I think that the disease colors the world: the air, the stars, the rain, the odor of spring. Certainly, the first relapse was hard. I did not have energy for doing anything, but the faith and the love of my children helped me to react. I live my life day by day. I am worried that my husband will suffer from his solitude and, as for me, I am quite worried about pain. So far, everything is still OK. I just do not move my legs, but I have accepted the idea of a wheelchair. I do not have regrets. Of course, I cannot say, 'Thank God for how things have gone,' but I think that I can keep on living for another while. And, moreover, not everything ends with 'this' life!"

Carey (1975) described a study in which patients with terminal illness were asked which factors were sources of major concern and anxiety and which factors were of major comfort in relation to the idea of having limited life expectancy. All the interviewed patients were aware of the fact that given the graveness of their clinical condition, death could arrive within a year. The results of the study indicated that three emotional factors were responsible for the patients' emotional adaptation: in descending order of importance, they were the level of physical discomfort, especially pain; the kinds of experiences the person previously had with people who were at the end of life; and the type of religious orientation.

In that same report, Carey (1975) listed the following factors as strongly related to negative emotional adjustment to cancer: high physical discomfort and pain; no previous experience of dialogue with people dying; no opportunity to meet people "in peace" when facing death; an egocentric lifestyle; the tendency to seek security, personal satisfaction, and improvement of social status; and an atheist orientation toward religion. Factors that indicated better adaptation were a moderate level of physical discomfort, a higher educational level, a lifestyle marked by strong faith and religious beliefs, a tendency to overcome a vision of life centered exclusively on personal needs, having had the opportunity to talk openly about possible consequences of the disease, and having been intimately close in the past to dying patients who accepted death with a sense of inner calm. A good adaptation to the diagnosis of cancer was also linked to the awareness of having lived fully, the affective presence of an important relationship, the support of a partner, the emotionally involved closeness of children and friends, having faced and coped well in the past with difficult events and crises of life, the hope of life after death, and a relationship with a doctor characterized by constant support and sensitive communication. The most intense fears and anxieties that were expressed during clinical interviews were centered on the process of dying rather than on concerns about life after death. Questions that troubled patients included these: "How much will I become dependent on others?" "Will I be a burden to people I love?" "Who will take care of them?" "How much will I suffer, and to what extent will the pain be controlled?" "What is the value of life since it is going to end?"

The results of Carey's (1975) study, in line with more recent scientific research, emphasize that several levels of assistance are necessary to take care of patients with advanced cancer who are facing death: a plan for symptom control, a plan to find meaning and significance of life in its new circumstances, a plan regarding religion and faith, maintenance of significant emotional relationships, a good relationship with the medical staff, and a plan for economic and practical aspects.

Conclusion

In this chapter, we have primarily discussed topics relevant to how a patient copes with the initial cancer diagnosis. The described results and considerations may be useful to health care professionals who have the responsibility of helping patients cope and manage at the time of their cancer discovery and as their treatment and evaluation proceed.

Philosophy and religion have always dealt with death. Hundreds of books have been written on the preparation for a "good death." Once, from

1300 to 1600, manuals on *Ars Moriendi* had a strong religious connotation. From 1700 to now they have taken an increasingly secular view.

A discussion about the end of life was not one of the objectives of this chapter. However, the considerations we have raised here do show the need to treat the sick person in all his or her human complexity: ignored or poorly controlled aspects tend to have a negative synergistic effect on quality of life and human dignity.

In relation to the positive influence of religious beliefs and faith in the survival of the soul, we refer to Immanuel Kant, who wrote: "Regarding the nature of the condition of the soul beyond the limits of life, we cannot say anything with confidence, because the edge of our reason extends up to that limit but not beyond it" (Kant 1986). As specialists of the human psyche, we do not deal with the afterlife. We simply take note of the important role of religion and spirituality, respecting the enormous importance they have in helping humans to cope with illnesses and death, as testified by psychoanalysts, historians, and anthropologists.

Key Clinical Points

- Assessment of psychosocial and psychiatric needs related to cancer and its treatment, as well as the formulation of appropriate treatment plans, is increasingly recognized as an essential and critical cornerstone of comprehensive cancer care.

- Universal concerns that patients face at the time of diagnosis include fear of death, fear of permanent disability, worry about life trajectory disruptions from cancer, and fears about effects from treatment that lead to dependence.

- The reaction to the discovery of cancer extends far beyond the clinical evaluation and psychiatric labeling process.

- The clinician needs to have a broad vision of the relationship between the concepts of illness and death to work effectively with the cancer patient.

- The impact of cancer on people's lives is related to four main factors: 1) the existential threat of the disease, 2) psychosocial consequences, 3) consequences of the morbid disease process, and 4) treatment and its effects.

- The diagnosis of cancer is a process with high psychic costs both for the patient and for family members, in whom unconscious mechanisms of defense against anguish, as well as personal cognitive and behavioral styles of managing stressful situations, are mobilized.

- It is important for health professionals to be able to differentiate between "normal" reactions and "psychopathological" reactions to cancer.

- The ability of an individual to manage and cope with the life-threatening discovery of a cancer depends on the interplay of biological, psychological, spiritual, and social factors.

References

Adler NE, Page AEK: Institute of Medicine Report: Cancer Care for the Whole Patient: Meeting Psychosocial Health Needs. Washington, DC, Institute of Medicine of the National Academies, 2007

American Cancer Society: Cancer Facts and Figures 2012. 2012. Available at: http://www.cancer.org. Accessed August 9, 2012.

Breitbart WS, Alici Y: Psycho-oncology. Harv Rev Psychiatry 17:361–376, 2009

Carey RG: Living until death: a program of service and research for the terminally ill, in Death: the Final Stage of Growth. Edited by Kübler-Ross E. New York, Simon & Schuster, 1975, pp 362–381

Cassidy S: Terminal care, in Cancer Patient Care. Edited by Watson M. Cambridge, UK, Cambridge University Press, 1991

Culberg J: Crisis and Development. Stockholm, Sweden, Bonniers, 1975

Freud S: Thoughts for the times on war and death (1915), in Standard Edition of the Complete Psychological Works of Sigmund Freud, Vol 14. Translated and edited by Strachey J. London, Hogarth Press, 1957, pp 273–300

GLOBOCAN 2008: Summary statistics, 2008. Available at: http://globocan.iarc.fr/factsheet.asp. Accessed July 20, 2012.

Gotay CC: The experience of cancer during early and advanced stages: the views of patients and their mates. Soc Sci Med 18:605–613, 1984

Grassi L, Travado L: The role of psychosocial oncology in cancer care, in Responding to the Challenge of Cancer in Europe. Edited by Coleman MP, Alexe DM, Albreht T, et al. Ljubljana, Slovenia, Institute of Public Health of the Republic of Slovenia, 2008, pp 209–229

Grassi L, Nanni MG, Caruso R: Emotional distress in cancer: screening policy, clinical limitations, and educational needs. Journal of Medicine and the Person 8:51–59, 2010

Heidegger M: Being and time (1927), in L'Esistenzialismo. Edited by Chiodi P. Turin, Italy, Loesher, 1964

Holland JC: History of psycho-oncology: overcoming attitudinal and conceptual barriers. Psychosom Med 64:206–221, 2002

Holland JC, Friedlander MM: Oncology, in Psychosomatic Medicine. Edited by Blumenfeld M, Strain JJ. Philadelphia, PA, Lippincott Williams & Wilkins, 2006, pp 21–144

Holland JC, Gooen-Piels J: Psycho-oncology, in Cancer Medicine, 6th Edition. Edited by Holland J, Frei E. Hamilton, ON, Canada, BC Decker, 2003, pp 1039–1053

Jaspers K: On My Philosophy (1932). Turin, Italy, Einaudi, 1981

Jaspers K: Schicksal und Wille: Autobiographische Schriften (1967). Genoa, Italy, Melangolo, 1993

Jenkins RA, Pargament KI: Cognitive appraisals in cancer patients. Soc Sci Med 26:625–633, 1988

Kant I: Lezioni di psicologia. Rome, Laterza, 1986

Kübler-Ross E: On Death and Dying. New York, Macmillan, 1969

Kübler-Ross E: Lessons from the Dying. Madrid, Spain, Sociología de la Muerte, 1974, pp 15–24

Lazarus RS: Coping theory and research: past, present, and future. Psychosom Med 55:234–247, 1993

LeShan L: Cancer as a Turning Point. New York, Penguin Books, 1990

Lipowski ZJ: Physical illness, the individual and the coping process. Psychiatry Med 1:91–102, 1970

Livneh H: Psychosocial adaptation to cancer: the role of coping strategies. Journal of Rehabilitation 66:40–49, 2000

Marmot M: Social determinants of health inequities. Lancet 365:1099–1104, 2005

Massie MJ, Holland JC: Overview of normal reactions and prevalence of psychiatric disorders, in Handbook of Psychooncology: Psychological Care of the Patient With Cancer. Edited by Holland JC, Rowland JH. New York, Oxford University Press, 1989, pp 273–282

McNeill W: Plagues and Peoples. New York, Doubleday, 1976

Mitchell AJ, Chan M, Bhatti H, et al: Prevalence of depression, anxiety, and adjustment disorder in oncological, haematological, and palliative-care settings: a meta-analysis of 94 interview-based studies. Lancet Oncol 12:160–174, 2011

Montaigne M: Essays (1580). Milan, Italy, Adelphi, 1992

Morin E: L'Homme et la Mort Dans l'Histoire. Paris, Correa, 1951

Mystakidou K, Parpa E, Tsilika E, et al: Cancer information disclosure in different cultural contexts. Support Care Cancer 12:147–154, 2004

Petticrew W, Bell R, Hunter D: Influence of psychological coping on survival and recurrence in people with cancer: a systematic review. BMJ 325:1066–1075, 2002

Razazi D, Delvaux N: Psychological aspects associated with the diagnosis and treatment of cancer [in French]. Acta Psychiatr Belg 88:60–79, 1988

Sartre JP: Being and nothingness: an essay on phenomenological ontology (1943), in L'Esistenzialismo. Edited by Chiodi P. Turin, Italy, Loesher, 1964

Scherer KR, Shorr A, Johnstone T: Appraisal Processes in Emotion: Theory, Methods, Research. Canary, UK, Oxford University Press, 2001

Sutherland AM, Orbach CE, Dyk RB, et al: The psychological impact of cancer and cancer surgery. Cancer 5:857–872, 1952

Terzani T: One More Ride on the Merry-Go-Round (1984). Milan, Italy, Longanesi, 2004

Vovelle M: Death in the Western World. Rome, Italy, Laterza, 1983

Watson MM, Greer S, Young J, et al: Development of a questionnaire measure of adjustment to cancer: the MAC scale. Psychol Med 18:203–209, 1988

Worden JW, Weisman AD: Preventive psychosocial intervention with newly diagnosed cancer patients. Gen Hosp Psychiatry 6:243–249, 1984

Yalom ID: Existential Psychotherapy. New York, Basic Books, 1980

Appendix 1-A

Consultation-Liaison Clinical Cases

To further illustrate the diverse emotional responses to new cancer discovery that physicians may encounter, we examine some case vignettes from clinical psycho-oncology and consultation-liaison psychiatry. These cases elucidate the diverse and variable ways in which cancer patients cope during the first stage of cancer discovery and as they engage in initial oncological evaluation and therapy.

Case Vignette 1

Lydia is a 46-year-old wife and mother of two teenage daughters who performs monthly breast examinations and has annual mammography screening. She receives a call from her internist who informs her that her recent mammogram was abnormal. Lydia, startled and anxious yet functional, shares this unexpected news with her spouse, who accompanies her for a stereotaxic breast biopsy from a radiologist the next day. She learns that the pathology is consistent with an invasive ductal carcinoma. Later that month, a breast surgeon performs a lumpectomy, revealing a stage II breast cancer, requiring further consultation with and eventual treatment from radiation and medical oncology specialists. Lydia also seeks formal consultation with a psycho-oncologist, who concludes with her that she is coping effectively. She begins attending a breast cancer support group, eliminates alcohol intake, makes healthy dietary change to lower her fat intake and lose weight, and increases weekly aerobic exercise.

In this vignette, Lydia is coping with a new, early-stage breast cancer diagnosis; she has a history of excellent adherence to breast health screening and copes well initially with this new life challenge of breast cancer discovery. She has intact social support from her spouse, family, and community; she does not have any past vulnerability to psychiatric disorders, such as anxiety or depression. With her healthy internal coping strategies and solid external social supports, she is able to manage effectively and to navigate with the help of her oncology team through this breast cancer discovery and diagnosis, as well as to embark on several months of multimodal treatment. She reaches out for further interpersonal support by joining and participating in a breast cancer support group. She also pursues psycho-oncological consultation to review and discuss her own coping strategies, her emotional resources and limitations, and positive ways for her family members to communicate and support one another in the context of this family medical crisis.

After recovering from left breast lumpectomy and sentinel lymph node biopsy, Lydia begins a chemotherapy course with doxorubicin and cyclophosphamide, with a course of paclitaxel to follow. Several weeks later, during her fourth cycle of doxorubicin and cyclophosphamide, she develops chemotherapy-induced neutropenia, fever to 103 degrees, and productive cough, and is admitted to the hospital for treatment of pneumonia. During this admission, she maintains positive with a buoyant spirit. She has ongoing support and care from her husband, daughters, and church community, as well as support from her breast cancer group members.

Five months later, during her radiation therapy course, Lydia's hemoglobin drops to 9.8 from radiation-induced hematological toxicity. She develops a clinically significant fatigue state, which triggers a major depression; she is treated with escitalopram titrated up to 10 mg/day and weekly interpersonal psychotherapy and has a robust response to this multimodal approach of psychiatric care. She completes her radiation therapy and starts hormonal therapy with tamoxifen and maintains euthymic mood.

Cancer patients such as Lydia who have healthy internal and external coping skills and resources nevertheless remain at risk for developing psychiatric complications over the course of their cancer treatment period, such as the development of an anxiety disorder or, as in this case, a major depression. Common anxiety syndromes encountered early in cancer treatment include adjustment disorder with anxious mood, generalized anxiety disorder, panic disorder, simple phobias, and posttraumatic stress disorder. The biological, or medical, factors relating to her intensive multimodal cancer treatment regimen (radiation-related fatigue after several months of dose-intensive chemotherapy) have placed Lydia at increased vulnerability to psychiatric complications.

Case Vignette 2

Anthony, a 66-year-old divorced man living alone, is seen in a local emergency room after experiencing acute pain in his throat and inability to swallow. He drinks a pint and a half of scotch daily and smokes two packs of cigarettes per day, habits that he has maintained for several decades. In the emergency room, he is noted to be clinically dehydrated, and this is medically corrected with fluids. An otolaryngologist performs laryngoscopy, and a large, friable laryngeal mass is visualized and biopsied. Upon further questioning, Anthony reports trouble swallowing for over 4 months, as well as several bouts of blood-tinged sputum which he had attributed to a persistent cold. This emergency room visit extends over several hours, his vital signs evolve, and he is noted to become tachycardic, hypertensive, and febrile. Social history further reveals that he has few social contacts and no longer maintains relations with his two adult children or his siblings. He becomes restless and expresses paranoid ideation, not noted on the initial hospital intake 10 hours earlier.

Anthony has had physical symptoms, dysphagia and hemoptysis, for many months yet had coped through avoidance and denial, and hence had adopted a passive stance toward his health status rather than actively seeking out medical care. Further complicating these impaired coping skills is his active substance dependence on both alcohol and tobacco. To add even more clinical complexity to this case, his vital signs have become unstable, which may be a manifestation of early signs of an impending alcohol withdrawal syndrome and perhaps a florid withdrawal-related delirium.

The discovery of Anthony's laryngeal cancer was significantly delayed by the maladaptive, passive coping style that he adopted when he first developed signs and symptoms. His chronic substance use and dependence with both alcohol and tobacco have also placed him at an especially high risk for developing a head and neck cancer, given that the combined chronic use of these two substances is known to be carcinogenic. Finally, as previously mentioned, the acute complication of an alcohol withdrawal syndrome now further jeopardizes, potentially delays, and further complicates his medical window of opportunity to access definite cancer evaluation and initiation of treatment for presumed laryngeal cancer.

Anthony is admitted to the hospital for further workup and management. He develops a fulminant alcohol-related withdrawal delirium, delirium tremens, and needs a critical care unit level of care to manage his acute state. In addition, he requires an ongoing staff aide at bedside to manage his agitation and ensure safety. Acute psychiatric consultation services are requested to expertly diagnose and assist in management of Anthony's acute and chronic psychiatric syndromes, as well as to help institute combination psychopharmacology treatment with a benzodiazepine and an antipsychotic.

After 10 days, the withdrawal syndrome is under improved control, although Anthony remains inattentive. He is unable to cognitively process the serious medical implication of his newly discovered laryngeal cancer and its recommended course of treatment. In this case, the neuropsychiatric complication of an acute alcohol withdrawal syndrome, with its own associated high morbidity and mortality, has delayed both his oncological evaluation and initiation of cancer treatment. His impaired internal coping skills, paucity of social supports, and active substance use disorders have adversely impacted the discovery of his laryngeal cancer, as well as further complicated and delayed the cancer evaluation and treatment trajectory. Anthony's behavior with a passive stance toward medical care is an example of abnormal illness behavior in the context of cancer discovery and its management (Grassi and Travado 2008). Anthony goes on to have laryngectomy for laryngeal cancer; develops a second, postoperative, delirium; and in the clinical context of lengthy inpatient admission and slow recovery, develops a major depressive complication requiring further hospital-based psychiatric care. He eventually needs placement at a rehabilitation center because he has been unable to master self-care for his laryngectomy and requires assisted feeds for nutritional support.

Case Vignette 3

A 71-year-old dentist, Thomas, is diagnosed with a low- to moderate-grade bladder cancer after presenting promptly for urological consultation when he noted gross hematuria while away on vacation. His urological oncologist has recommended that he begin therapy with intravesicular bacillus Calmette-Guérin (BCG) infusions, with a plan to perform serial cystoscopy over the next 18 months. When Thomas asks about his treatment options if BCG proves ineffective, his urologist communicates the potential surgical option of cystectomy and formation of a neobladder. Thomas has a history of recurrent moderate to severe unipolar major depressions, which have been in remission for several years. He has been maintained on fluoxetine

10 mg/day, prescribed by his internist, and has not been in formal mental health care for many years. Within 14 days of this bladder cancer discovery, Thomas becomes acutely withdrawn and spends most of his time in bed, although sleep is poor; he stops eating, and his self-care deteriorates. He cancels his dental office practice hours and misses his follow-up testing and uro-oncologist office visits; he does not start BCG intravesicular therapy. His spouse and family note that he is preoccupied, cries easily and often, and reports feeling hopeless and guilt-ridden. His urologist urgently refers him for psycho-oncological consultation and care.

Thomas's case elucidates how a preexisting Axis I mood disorder may complicate a patient's initial adaptation and ability to cope with cancer discovery, workup and staging, and the starting of treatment. Thomas exhibits abnormal illness behavior manifested with his profound withdrawal and negativism, passivity, and psychopathological regression. He is unable to function due to florid psychiatric symptoms from a recurrence of an acute major depression with melancholic features. This current mood disturbance recurs now in the context of the perceived stress of bladder cancer discovery and the perceived stress of understanding the potential cancer treatment trajectory, including the impact of major reconstructive surgery with major changes in bodily appearance and function.

Prompt psycho-oncological evaluation reveals a severe acute major depression with melancholic features and active suicidal ideation; Thomas is unable to care for himself. With the aid of his family and private internist, Thomas agrees to voluntary inpatient psychiatric admission to stabilize him in a psychotherapeutic milieu, titrate his antidepressant medicines, and institute and conduct a cognitive-behavioral therapy, and then to pursue further outpatient psychiatric resources. During his inpatient psychiatric stay, Thomas's fluoxetine dosage is increased to 20 mg/day, and he is also treated with oral lorazepam, 0.5 mg three times daily, for sleep and anxiety. His urologist visits as well and arranges a meeting between Thomas and a bladder cancer survivor who is 5 years postcystectomy to discuss quality of life issues related to urological functioning following cystectomy surgery. Thomas and his family become acquainted with outpatient psychosocial oncology resources, such as a support group for Thomas and another group for family members. His hospital-based psychotherapy is focused with a cognitive therapy schema to help address Thomas's negative cognitions and fears, which are concerned with living with bodily change and functioning if he were to need cystectomy in the future. When discharged from the inpatient psychiatric unit after 10 days, Thomas demonstrates clear clinical improvement and no longer feels hopeless or actively suicidal.

These three vignettes illustrate various key factors as to how individuals cope with and adapt to the discovery of a new cancer diagnosis and to the initiation of further medical workup and treatment. The ability of an individual to manage and cope with the life-threatening discovery of a cancer depends on the interplay of biological, psychological, spiritual, and social factors (Grassi and Travado 2008).

Appendix 1–B

Existential Psychotherapies

Supportive-Expressive Group Psychotherapy

Supportive-expressive group psychotherapy (SEGT) is the result of the original work by Yalom and Greaves (Yalom et al. 1977) and was subsequently refined by Spiegel and Classen, who introduced this form of therapy for oncology patients (Spiegel et al. 1978). SEGT utilizes themes from humanistic and existential psychology. Its aim is to provide support to improve the quality of life for patients in advanced stages of cancer in order to allow the person to live as authentic and full a life as possible. The analysis explores the meaning of the disease in the existential journey of the life of the patient. Patients in advanced stages of disease may relate to life with ambivalence. Sorrow at the loss of the future can be expressed through avoidance mechanisms, demoralization, or intolerance for those who live with a different condition. Sharing in a group setting offers support and the opportunity to explore and reformulate in a more adaptive way themes such as the meaning of the disease and its role in changing relationships, loneliness, death, and sense of self and of existence. This process encourages patients to plan new projects for their life, to regain assertiveness, altruism, and a sense of humor, and possibly to reach an acceptance of death. A further element of this process is the medicalization of the group culture, that is, the exploration of information and beliefs about the disease and treatments in order to promote compliance.

The role of the therapist, as in all therapy groups, is to maintain the cohesion of the group and an attitude of openness and acceptance to allow the exploration of issues and concerns expressed by the participants, without judging or steering the group. The ability to manage countertransference triggered by exposure to disease and death is a sensitive issue. Uncontrolled countertransference reactions, such as occurrence of the fear of death or defensive reactions of denial and emotional distancing in the relationship with the patient, are a barrier to the therapists' availability to question themselves on their existential position and then to establish the basis for an authentic relationship with patients (Costantini et al. 2012).

SEGT is an unstructured therapy, with weekly sessions lasting 90 minutes, developed in both short- and long-term versions, and has been set in a protocol so that it can be replicated. Observed data from both local and multicenter research have shown that group sharing of issues related to the disease has an important role in determining the development of more adaptive coping styles in patients both in early and advanced phases of the disease, thus improving quality of life, social and family support, and effective doctor-patient communication (Kissane et al. 2004; Spiegel et al. 1999). A German study reported a significant decrease in affective disorders in breast cancer patients treated with SEGT (Reuter et al. 2010).

Dignity Therapy

Dignity therapy (DT) is a recent and specific form of therapy developed by Chochinov and colleagues (Chochinov et al. 2005). DT addresses the existential needs of patients in palliative care. It is focused on the fundamental theme of dignity as the cornerstone of humanization in medicine. As a consequence of the hyperspecialization and technological transformation of medicine, in recent years, the concept of dignity has become very important in the context of defining the ethical limits of applicability of many medical practices and the need not to lose sight of the needs of the person as a whole (Thompson et al. 2008).

In the context of palliative care, the issue of dignity is particularly complex. The medical staff can deal with demands such as that of hastened death, which dying patients can desire when they perceive the latter part of their life as meaningless and with no value. Starting from the observations on the desire to die and suicidal ideation in the terminally ill patients, Chochinov and colleagues have investigated the concept of dignity from the patients' perspective by examining the role of a number of variables, such as pain, addiction, demoralization/depression, and lack of family and social support. Feelings of dependency and demoralization emerged as the crucial point of the patient's mental and physical suffering and the core reason for the loss of dignity experienced by patients in terminal illness (Chochinov et al. 2011). These results emphasize the important fact that the management of symptoms and pain is not the only task of palliative therapy and that methods that reduce demoralization, support hope, and restore a sense of value should be also included. In order to increase the patient's feeling that his or her life has had a purpose, the session of dignity therapy is first tape-recorded and then transcribed and printed to be returned to the patient, a family member, or a friend indicated for this purpose. The stability of sense of self and the possibility that the person can maintain the sense of identity regardless of the progression of the disease are attained by the therapist encouraging the person to speak of the central aspects of his or her life and personal history. Maintenance of roles related to the possibility of holding on to a sense of identification with the roles that one had played before the disease is another crucial aspect. During the meetings, the therapist uses questions to help the patient to discover and maintain a sense of identification with the role played in life. The patient's sense of pride is protected by having the opportunity to talk about results and achievements that have made him or her proud. The theme of hope is supported by the ability to maintain a sense of purpose of life and by helping the person to find a meaning to life that has been lived and life that is being lived. The fears and worries about the consequences of one's own death for loved ones is addressed by encouraging the patient to talk to loved ones about the future after his or her own death. Finally, the standards of care and the aspects of assistance are discussed with the patient to identify any issues that interfere with the maintenance of dignity.

DT is initiated via specific questions such as "Tell me a little of your personal history, the things you remember best; which do you think are most important?" "What would you like your family to know about you; are there things that you would like to be remembered for?" In DT, which has a narrative structure, the therapist uses an empathic, encouraging, and respectful style. In the individual sessions, which take place at the bedside of hospitalized patients or at home, the questions are structured so as to highlight aspects of life that have been meaningful for the person. In the last session the therapist, after having transcribed the tape and reedited it, reads the manuscript to the patient. From an emotional point of view, this is an intense moment. It also allows the therapist to make corrections before the final document is completed and delivered to the patient or to whomever the patient has elected. The aim is to draw up a document that represents the "legacy" of the person, something that is meaningful and will survive, thus helping to restore a sense of meaning, value, and dignity. A study comparing DT with standard palliative care and client-centered care showed that dignity therapy was significantly more likely to have been helpful, to improve quality of life, to increase sense of dignity, to change how patients' families saw and appreciated them, and to be helpful to the families. Furthermore, DT was significantly better than client-centered care in improving spiritual well-being and was significantly better than standard palliative care in terms of lessening sadness or depression.

Meaning-Centered Psychotherapy

Meaning-centered group psychotherapy (MCGP) is the result of an intense clinical and research program conducted by Breitbart at the Memorial Sloan-Kettering Cancer Center, spurred by the growing interest in the study of spirituality as a support tool for patients who face a terminal disease. The theoretical assumptions of MCGP are based on European and American existentialist psychology, in particular to Viktor E. Frankl's logotherapy

(Breitbart et al. 2002) The therapist's knowledge of existentialism and existential concepts is a key and a thread to refer to constantly in the course of therapy. As Frankl repeatedly emphasized:

> Life holds a meaning for each and every individual, and even more, it retains this meaning literally to his last breath..... The health care professional can show the patient that life never ceases to have a meaning..... We cannot show the patient what the meaning is, but we may well show him that there is a meaning, and that life retains it..... Even the tragic and negative aspects of life, such as unavoidable suffering, can be turned into a human achievement by the attitude which a man adopts toward his predicament." (Frankl 1959/2007)

Thus the goal of the MCGP is to provide a spiritual support tool for patients in advanced stages of disease, where the concept of spirituality does not necessarily correspond to religiosity but is considered in its broader meaning, connected to the need for sources of meaning and purpose of life present in every human being.

MCGP uses Frankl's experiences along with reading and discussion of his book *Will to Meaning* (Frankl 1969/1988) as an incentive and guide to the experiential work with patients. The concept of limitation of life, linked to the disease, is used in this perspective to promote the identification of the existential values that allow the patient to recover a sense of wholeness, meaning, coherence, and legacy with respect to his or her own life. The concept of legacy plays a particularly important role and is seen as building a sense of continuity between the life already lived, the life that is being lived, and what the patient hopes to leave. The aim is to create a bridge connecting past, present, and future in order to maintain a sense of continuity and meaning attributed to life.

The format of sessions is closed, either in individual (7 meetings) or group settings (8 meetings of 90 minutes), although it is specified that the MCGP is not a group psychotherapy, but a psychotherapy to do "as a group" where sharing with others is a source of learning. The meetings take place on a weekly basis and focus on the development of a specific issue. The therapist makes every attempt to find out the sources of meaning through which the patient's history can be explored. MCGP is not psychoeducational, but it is focused on the use of empathy and the co-construction of meaning, in which participants are encouraged to compare their experiences. Between sessions, exercises and homework are offered in order to stimulate creativity and the construction of a legacy project that represents the culmination of the therapeutic process. The first meeting is devoted to discussing the objective of the treatment. The therapist introduces Frankl's theory and discusses how the concepts presented will be considered as a means of inspiration and "sources of meaning." In the second meeting, the theme of "cancer and meaning" is examined from a subjective perspective: patients are asked to reflect on how the diagnosis of cancer has changed the perception of their own identity. In the following session, patients are encouraged to review their life's history, identifying "the historical sources of meaning." The themes of life as a legacy and of the relationship of continuity between past, present, and future are then introduced. Through guiding the patients, the therapist encourages them to regard the life they have lived, and are living, as a legacy that will remain when life itself ends. The purpose is to detect a life testimony that the patient wishes to pass on. During the final sessions, issues related to patients' attitudes when confronting life limitations such as loss, disease, and death are elaborated.

The focus of therapeutic work is aimed at emphasizing that when one is facing events that transcend one's choice, the remaining freedom is how one chooses to live these events, and this is the only possibility to transcend the limits of life. Exercises are offered that lead to the way in which participants would like to be remembered. One session is dedicated to reflecting on the experiences that still allow the person to connect with the meaning of life through the world of emotions, the contemplation of beauty, and irony. In the final meeting, the participants' legacy projects are delineated and feelings and emotions related to the end of the therapy are processed. The last session is focused on sharing legacy projects and hopes for the future. The theme of hope is used to reinforce the sense of value that belongs to life even in advanced stages of disease. The limited time structure makes this method particularly suitable for use in hospitals.

MCGP has been shown to be effective in improving quality of life, spiritual well-being, feelings of hopelessness, and the general coping style of patients with advanced and terminal cancer (Breitbart et al. 2010).

References

Breitbart W, Rosenfeld B, Gibson C, et al: Meaning-centered group psychotherapy for patients with advanced cancer: a pilot randomized controlled trial. Psychooncology 19:21–28, 2010

Chochinov HM, Hack T, Hassard T, et al: Dignity therapy: a novel psychotherapeutic interventions for patients near the end of life. J Clin Oncol 23:5520–25, 2005

Chochinov HM, Kristjanson LJ, Breitbart W, et al: Effect of dignity therapy on distress and end-of-life experience in terminally ill patients: a randomised controlled trial. Lancet Oncol 12:753–762, 2011

Costantini A, Navarra C, Brunetti S, et al: Psychotherapeutic interventions in psycho-oncology. Neuropathological Diseases 1:145–160, 2012

Frankl VE: The Will to Meaning: Foundations of Logotherapy (1969). New York, Penguin, 1988

Frankl VE: Man's Search for Meaning: An Introduction to Logotherapy (1959). Boston, Beacon Press, 2007

Kissane DW, Grabsch B, Clarke DM, et al: Supportive-expressive group therapy: the transformation of existential ambivalence into creative living while enhancing adherence to anti-cancer therapies. Psycho-oncology 13:755–768, 2004

Reuter K, Scholl I, Sillem M, et al: Implementation and benefits of psychooncological group interventions in german breast centers: a pilot study on supportive-expressive group therapy for women with primary breast cancer. Breast Care (Basel) 5:91–96, 2010

Spiegel D, Yalom ID: A support group for dying patients. Int J Group Psychother 28:233–245, 1978

Spiegel D, Morrow GR, Classen C, et al: Group psychotherapy for recently diagnosed breast cancer patients: a multicenter feasibility study. Psycho-oncology 8:482–493, 1999

Thompson GN, Chochinov HM: Dignity-based approaches in the care of terminally ill patients. Curr Opin Support Palliat Care 2:49–53, 2008

Yalom ID, Greaves C: Group therapy with the terminally ill. Am J Psychiatry 134:396–400, 1977

CHAPTER 2

Cancer

A Family Affair

Lea Baider, Ph.D.

The Patient's Illness
Within the Family

Feeling real is more than existing. It is finding a way to exist and grow as one-self and to be able to relate to the "other" as oneself.... [to] be part of the family in which to retreat and feel secure and accepted.... By becoming real to them, we become real to ourselves.

D.W. Winnicott (1971)

Crises occur naturally throughout the family life cycle, and most families cope effectively, generating novel abilities for adaptively negotiating their private world. Before a major disease is diagnosed, a family may never have had to negotiate a situation that is perceived as threatening not only to the normal life of a family member but also to the integrity of the family as a system of growth, development, and stability.

Families matter. They matter because they provide the context of adjustment in which the person diagnosed with cancer responds to his or her disease. When a person develops cancer, it is family members who endure this experience. However, the family itself is often profoundly affected by the intrusive presence of the disease and the unpredictable outcome.

Family adaptation to cancer diagnosis is a continuous process, with many critical cycles. It is a tapestry of hope and desperation. Stressors caused by the disease are not simply short-term single events, but rather a complex set of changing conditions with a history of previous events and an unpredictable future course. The illness is often so intangible that family members are generally unaware of the intricate impact it has on shaping the psychological and emotional dynamic of this new reality within the family milieu.

The family's appraisal of the illness is an integral part of living and interacting together. Their constructed meanings of illness include understanding how members are expected to behave with one another when someone begins the long trajectory of cancer. They invoke a family legacy of sharing a specific intrapersonal language, learned from one event to the next and from one member to the next. A clear understanding of what to ask and what actions to take, in essence, leads to a greater ability for each individual to develop appropriate responses and comprehensible rules regarding new roles within the family during times of highly stressful events such as cancer and death (Hill et al. 2003).

Along this path, individual families may be led into a maze of alternative behaviors as "victims of a bad spell," "warriors and heroes of resilience," "survivors of many other losses," and/or "objects of anger and helplessness." These behaviors are not sequential and are affected by the need for inquiry, exploration, and social expectations that guide the family through illness circumstances (Anderson and Martin 2003).

Families with the insight and capacity to resolve normative and non-normative situations arising from the illness will be challenged to function more effectively and may be more able to confront conflict and disappointments. Moreover, they may cope better with new alternatives, reorganize life priorities, and share and respect their own private meanings of illness, survivorship, or death as individual members and as a family system of mutual care (McLean et al. 2008).

The study of possible influences exerted by the family unit on its members has been strengthened by the quality of evidence-based theory and corresponding measures that will enable links between family features and the individual member diagnosed with cancer. Based on theory and research on family stress, coping, and adaptation to the cancer process, the concept of family resilience entails more than managing stressful conditions, shouldering a burden, or surviving an ordeal. It involves the potential for personal and relational transformation and growth that can be forged out of adversity (Patterson 2003). Family resilience focuses on strengths under stress, in the midst of crisis, and in overcoming adversity. Resilience involves dynamic processes fostering positive adaptation within the context of significant adversity. These strengths and resources enable patients and families to respond successfully to crises and persistent challenges and to recover and grow from those experiences (Walsh 2003). Table 2–1 lists low- and high-resilience variables that can have negative and positive influences, respectively, on the family's coping in crisis situations.

TABLE 2–1.   Family resilience variables

Low-resilience variables	High-resilience variables
Lack of emotional support	Common values
Withdrawing	Meaning
Rigidity	Flexibility
Helplessness	Openness
Resentment	Problem-solving
Loneliness	Growth
Blaming	Open communication
Covert communication	
Isolation	

Low Family Resilience: Shattering Voices

Four years after being diagnosed with metastatic breast cancer, a 50-year-old patient described her family: "We struggle…without purpose…. We did not nor do we now know how to be together. Each of us is in our own corner, protected by the cancer 'relocation' within the family space. Anger, frustration, silences are the language created by despair and helplessness…. Nothing is the same nor will be the same…." (Translated from Hebrew)

High Family Resilience: Restoring Strength

Three years after a diagnosis of metastatic colon cancer, a 55-year-old patient described his family: "We all know the reality…my time reality. We weave our faith and hope together at every moment. We support our common pain, learning how to live jointly with my dying…. It is our responsibility as a family to build dreams in the immense sea of possibilities…and we are learning to make choices with voices of love…." (Translated from Hebrew)

Family, as a dynamic system, is assessed relative to each family's values, structure, resources, and life challenges. Processes for optimal functioning and the well-being of members are seen to vary over time, as challenges unfold and families evolve across the life and illness cycles. Although no single model of family fits all, a family resilience perspective is grounded in a deep conviction in the potential for family recovery and growth out of adversity (Thomas et al. 2002).

No psychological and physiological data favor one particular family cycle (patient age or role) over another with regard to where cancer intrudes into family life (Erikson 1963). Thus, the cancer population comprises a heterogeneous group when it comes to diagnosis, survival, treatments, quality of life, and quality of death. Although all families face the undeniable realities of chronological age and declining biological functions, families manifest different individual coping styles based on their sociocultural backgrounds (Goldzweig et al. 2009).

In cancer treatment, concerns for patients' survival have been expanded to include the ongoing adjustment of patients and their families (Shields et al. 2000). Adjustment to cancer by both younger and older adults "may be compromised within the family and the social environments—with respect to marriage and intimate ties, social participation, socio-economic status and mental and physical health" (Watson 2007). Notwithstanding the fact that cancer is the leading cause of death among women ages 40–70 and among men ages 60–79, and one of the three leading causes of death in those over age 70, many cancer patients are living and surviving long after their initial cancer diagnosis and treatments (Ershler 2003; Wedding et al. 2007).

According to Rolland (2002), the challenges confronting families experiencing cancer are strongly shaped by medical factors, such as type of cancer, extent of disease, type of treatment, and phase of illness. The family's reactions are also influenced by qualities of the family and its environment, such as developmental stage, coping resources, social support, and concurrent stressors. The family's social background and the personal meanings ascribed to cancer may also color the experience of confronting the illness phases. The phase of the illness—initial diagnosis, treatment, recovery, survival, recurrence, or terminal illness—has a particularly important effect on the type of demands families encounter and the dilemmas they bring to treatment. The capacity of the family to accommodate each of these phase-specific difficulties is influenced by several aspects of family functioning: 1) openness of communication, 2) flexibility of family structure and mutuality, 3) adaptiveness of personal meanings associated with illness, and 4) response to existential/mortality issues (Rolland 2009).

Although some families are shattered by crisis due to the chronicity and severity of the illness, many others emerge strengthened through resilience and the resourcefulness of family mutuality (Wynne et al. 1968). "Potentially spaced" mutuality is the relational counterpart to self-esteem. Within the family, members search to find other members with whom they can commiserate and create a common space (Winnicott 1971). In a mutual exchange, there is an active awareness of the other, an understanding of how one's actions affect the other, and an ability to emotionally move the other. Striving to enhance mutuality in a family helps the patient regain what has been "lost" and helps validate each family member's pursuit of authentic connection (Skerrett 1996).

Mutuality means emotionally being with another—joining in. It always occurs in the space between people and the family as a unit of interaction. To know that family members can share emotionally the experience of one member's illness and of being together with that person means that the individual is not alone. Laing (1972) calls it "the family inside me." Surrey (1987) describes mutuality as an experience of "being with" and sensing one another's feelings in a conjoining communion. It is this connection that enables family members to respond accurately to the illness event, to enjoy being together, and to provide each other with new information about each individual's emotional needs in the illness process. This does not lead simply to the idea that emotional support and sharing, on the one hand, and the patient, on the other, are competing demands on family life. Rather, the two are complementary conditions of the same process within the family relationship (Reiss and Neiderhiser 2000).

Families should not strive for a single view or collective appraisal of their emotional needs—or promote a single style of behavior. Rather, there is a need to learn to accept and respect individual differences through mutual understanding and cooperation.

The Triad: The Couple and the Illness

These are ties which though light as air, are as strong as links of iron.

Edmund Burke (speech on conciliation with America, 1775)

She is concerned in part with privacy and the limits of compassion, but at the heart of her life-death dilemma lies recognition of the constraints of verbal relatedness. The intimacy that I had with being as sick as I was when I was sick, I just cannot give it to you in words…. Intimacy and intensity…lie at the heart of our intrinsic silence. (L. Baider, private diary of patient cases, translated from Hebrew, 2010)

Following diagnosis of a life-threatening illness, patients often cite their spouses as their primary sources of support. The illness experience and associated treatment regimens are potent enough, however, to provoke various forms of emotional disorders in patients' partners, including anxiety, depression, and fear of recurrence and losing one's partner to death. As many as 29% of sampled couples who had been receiving cancer treatment reported clinically significant levels of emotional distress (Weihs et al. 2002).

Marital and family relationships are affected by the constant threat of cancer. The emotional support provided by an intimate partner can have a profound buffering effect on the patient's and family members' quality of life and on the stress levels experienced by the cancer patient as he or she contends with both the psychological and the physiological sequelae of the illness (Acitelli and Badr 2005; Shields et al. 2000). Accordingly, patient and healthy partner may treat illness differently depending on the extent to which they see the disease as a "relational" and "mutual" problem.

The effect of cancer on marital quality is largely undetermined (Northouse et al. 2001). Some researchers argue that there is no change in quality or that if there is a change, it is a positive association between illness and the spousal relationship because the cancer brings spouses closer together. Others point to negative impacts on the spousal relationship. It has been suggested that a worsening of marital quality can be explained by a multiplicity of variables, such as the financial implications of illness; the unpredictable behavior of the sick person; a changed division of the couple's roles, including the loss of shared activities; and isolation and restricted social life (Boehmer and Clark 2002).

Studies addressing the couple unit in particular found that in the face of a cancer diagnosis, spouses experienced levels of distress either similar to or even greater than those of their affected partners (Manne et al. 2006). This close association between partners' distress levels implies a strong mutuality in their response: that is, if one partner becomes distressed, the other partner more than likely will also. The caregiver is as likely to experience psychological distress as the cancer patient—again lending weight to the assertion that both members of the dyad experience similar levels of distress. Clinical attention should consider the patient-caregiver dyad as the "mutuality of support of care" (Baider et al. 2004; Hodges et al. 2005).

Emotional support is conceptualized in the literature as communication of care, concern, empathy, and comfort and reassurance, given both verbally and nonverbally (e.g., through facial expressions and gestures). Specifically, emotional support provided by husbands has been linked to lower emotional distress, fewer depressive symptoms, and better role adjustment in their wives who were experiencing breast cancer. In fact, cancer patients—particularly those who experienced greater impairment from their illness and treatment course—cited emotional support, as opposed to informational or instrumental support (i.e., problem solving), as the most enduring and beneficial form of support. This is consistent with observations from other studies in which increasing feelings of vulnerability in the cancer patient were assuaged by intimate exchanges characterized by high empathy and low withdrawal from the spouse (Hagedoorn et al. 2006; Naaman et al. 2009).

Indeed, many patients turn to their partners for increased involvement during the course of illness and treatment. However, partners are also experiencing extreme distress, and this may impair their ability to provide the expected psychological support to the patient. The shared or dyadic stressors can affect both partners' well-being as well as the quality of their relationship, and thus innovative coping skills are required (Berg and Upchurch 2007).

In a study of 191 couples who completed surveys at baseline and at 3 and 6 months after beginning treatment, Badr et al. (2010) found that mutual coping differentially impacted patient and spouse distress. They also found that taking a team approach to managing cancer-related stress (by engaging in positive mutual coping) may generalize to other marital domains by improving or maintaining shared adjustment for both persons. Positive coping, however, may not affect patients and partners in the same way. Whereas patients experienced slight increases in distress, partners experienced slight decreases in distress. Because the decrease as a function of positive mutual coping was not significant, results should be interpreted with caution. In any event, they are consistent with other research. For example, in a study of couples coping with chronic illness, Badr et al. (2008) described that viewing one's relationship as an extension of oneself (or having a high level of "couple identity") minimized the negative and maximized the positive effects of the caregiving experience on caregiver mental health.

Braun et al. (2007) indicated, in a study on patient-partner attachment, that problems in the marital relationship were an important contributor to the spouse caregiver's depression. Furthermore, marital dissatisfaction was found to be an even more important contributor to depression than objective caregiving burden. Giving care to a cancer patient not only demands that the spouse be attuned to the partner's needs but also requires the couple to interact in intimate and difficult situations.

In a review of the literature dealing with elderly cancer patients within the marital context, Manne et al. (1999) found only 20 studies that included both patients and partners—half comprising breast cancer patients and their husbands. However, the available data on psychological factors affecting distress levels of the spouse within the marital context of elderly couples have yielded inclusive, contradictory, and controversial results (Baider et al. 2004). Moreover, marriage does not appear to protect elderly people from symptoms of psychological distress (Hagedoorn et al. 2006).

Illness highlights the significance of an open exchange of thoughts and feelings for patients and their spouses to achieve better adjustment. To the extent that couples' ability to communicate varies, many avoid truthful and open communication with each other, with the extended family, and with others outside the family (Watson 2007).

Bodenmann (2005) and Bodenmann and Shantinath (2004) reported that couples who displayed avoidance, self-blaming, lack of active problem solving, and covert communication at the beginning of the illness process were significantly more likely at the 5-year follow-up to be among those who were in a stressful and unsatisfying relationship. These findings indicate that the chronic stress of the illness figures as an important negative predictor of marital intimacy and stability.

Denial, avoidance, negative self-verbalization, and withdrawal are often clear symptoms of the negative quality of marital relationships. Consequently, the chronicity of cancer will impede the ability of couples to support each other emotionally and psychologically and to engage in mutual intimacy. It is hard for an individual in the dyad to reach out to the partner when psychological resources are mostly depleted. Intimacy and trust become null and void as a natural mode of interaction. On the other hand, active engagement, constructive problem solving, optimism, positive communication, and reframing of the illness situation are among the more functional behaviors and adaptations during and after the pivotal point of the illness dimension.

Even when partners are trying to support each other, stylistic differences in coping and in appraisal of the situation may lead to entanglements. Men and women within the dyad often have dissimilar approaches to how to behave and communicate under duress. Variations can range from a total sharing of information to feelings of loneliness and isolation. Women perceive that there are, generally, no verbal exchanges with their male partners about feelings and admit that questioning this could open up new problems. Any modality of intervention should acknowledge the couple's distorted communication, loud silences, and unspoken need for binding together (Ballard-Reisch and Letner 2003).

Most couples want clear, complete, and accurate information about their disease, prognosis, and possible treatment options. Through a process of shared inquiry, providers, patients, and partners exchange information about the disease, prognosis, and treatment options, thereby formulating health care conclusions. Shared decision making can facilitate a greater sense of participatory involvement in the patient's outcome, thus promoting a higher degree of empowerment and development of effective coping strategies.

Cancer illness can erode support and intimacy through its negative effect on relationships. It can decrease warmth and increase hostility, criticism, and negativity during marital relations. Couples who can maintain open and enduring lines of verbal and nonverbal communication in times of stress will experience less distress and enhanced marital quality and intimacy.

A couple's intimacy—as a system of mutual trust and support—should provide a reliable network for their relationship, in which each partner is able to feel free and intimate, to accept and be accepted, and to turn effectively to the other at any time and in any place during the trajectory of their life (Hann et al. 2002). Intimacy means feeling secure within a "supported vulnerability," making innermost thoughts known, and sharing core truths, excitements, longings, fears, and neediness—as well as responding to these in the other person. It means being able to negotiate closeness and balance autonomy and relatedness—to feel comfortable with closeness while accepting separateness and building a space for the "I" together with the "we" (Cassidy 2001). A patient of mine captured this dynamic:

> "And I was alone...and he was alone.... The agonizing truth made the depths of the cliff an infinite abysmal silence of tears...tears of death....We were side by side touching and embracing the love that was disappearing through his skin.... How can I take away his death and encapsulate it in my own private death?...How can our souls embrace in a symbiotic and intimate dance of life?...But we are singled out by death, within our own universal space together.... We are dying together...part of my being will die with him.... His death will be mine forever within my soul, my eyes, my bones...within the permanency of our shared memories.... My soul will only embrace memories...."
> (L. Baider, private diary of patient cases translated from Hebrew, 2010)

The prognosis of chronic and terminal illness reverses the illusion of immortality and takes away the fantasy of an infinite tomorrow for the intensity of a today. Intimacy addresses one's deepest nature and innermost self, the core of one's being, the truth about who one really is. A couple's intimacy is sharing one's essence and truth, one's heart, with another, and accepting, tolerating, and giving to another person in moments of loss and impending death (Candib 2002).

A Glance at Psychological Family Intervention

For whom should interventions be designed and addressed—for the family, the couple, the children, the care recipient, or all of them? The professional's responsibility to every individual and system is not necessarily diverse or unidirectional, and helping one may result in a disservice to the other (Jacobsen and Heather 2008; Stefanek et al. 2009). The challenge for the health care professional should be to integrate and tailor interventions suitable to the specific needs of the care recipient and to relate directly to the family as the basic and enduring unit of care (Northouse et al. 2010).

Evidence-based data indicate that patient adaptation to the process of illness, or the proximity of loss, is facilitated by family trust, communication, and involvement of professional empathy and compassionate care (Coyne et al. 2006; Moorey and Greer 2002).

What interventions might facilitate communication, emotional support, and compassionate language? The health care professional should begin by normalizing the disruptive effect of cancer on family life and its tendency to foster chaotic, paralyzing, and bewildering behavior. Heightened stress should be reframed as a function of and reaction to illness rather than family inadequacy. The professional's attitude of respectful understanding and empathy may help engage the family in meaningful dialogue about how the illness has affected each member's roles, relationships, work, mood, energy level, social life, and dreams for the future. If necessary, a broad range of learning processes, drawn from various theoretical family therapy models, should be employed to help families share their experiences, explore changes in relationships, and raise awareness of cancer as a family rather than an individual illness.

Family interventions with patients diagnosed with cancer (Berman et al. 2008) should be focused on basic variables:

- Family structure and dynamics
- Gender, age, education, socioeconomic status, culture, and religious beliefs
- Medical status, perception of the illness, and treatment consequences
- Communication between patient-family health care team
- Degree of objective and subjective burden experienced by family members
- Extent to which the disease is perceived as a threat or as a life challenge
- Past meaningful events and coping styles
- Locus of attributions made for the disease and cancer-related outcomes, and the meaning made of personal experience
- Availability of a network of friends and family members who can provide tangible emotional and instrumental support

Empathic Listening

Carl Rogers (1951) built his whole system of client-centered therapy on unconditional positive regard and empathic listening to promote psychological and emotional growth in the individual and the family. Today, health care professionals might recommend that family members participate in tailored interventions to learn a new language of care, enhance quality of life, regain control and autonomy, and accept and incorporate the subjective meanings of illness and death (Baider et al. 2003; Hodges et al. 2005).

The following dialogue, from a Hebrew transcription of a social worker's visit to a family, is an example of how a mental health professional can listen, be silent, and accept that, at times, he or she should simply observe a transient family drama. The social worker is visiting two boys, ages 11 and 15, and their 41-year-old mother, whose husband is in the terminal stage of lung cancer and has been hospitalized for more than 2 months in a palliative care unit.

YOUNGER BOY: Why are we here? I want to watch my TV program.

OLDER BOY: Shut up! You're always such a crybaby!

YOUNGER BOY: No, you shut up!

MOTHER: We need to talk about Daddy, and I want both of you to listen for once.

OLDER BOY: But Mom, we know that Dad does feel OK and is in another hospital,…but I want to watch my TV program. Please, Mom, let's talk about it later…

MOTHER: Don't you love Daddy enough to hear how he feels? By the way, there's a lady here who knows Daddy and would like to talk with both of you.

OLDER BOY: About what? She can't tell us more about Dad that we don't already know. I spoke with Dad by phone last week, and he told me that he feels OK and will be coming home soon.

YOUNGER BOY: I also talked with him, and he promised that we would go on a special trip for my birthday, and…Mom, you always let me watch my program, and then I want to meet with my friends to go to the shopping mall. I also want to watch the program in my room, but I don't want Danny coming in…

MOTHER (*screaming*): You both will not watch any TV today. Go to your room, do your homework, and also write a letter to your father saying that you love him!

OLDER BOY: Mom, not now! Anyway, Dad knows that I love him, and he'll be home soon.

(*Both boys go to their rooms.*)

MOTHER (*begins to cry*): I can never talk to them. They spend all day watching TV or fighting with each other or with friends. They don't know that their father will never come home, and…I am very frightened to talk to them…. We don't talk…. My husband always says that people who have time to talk don't work. He always says that there is nothing to talk about, and if he needs something, he'll ask. I don't have the patience to sit with my children and talk. It won't do any good. Maybe it's better that we don't talk…and, in any case, they'll find out. It is better that way.

The distancing behavior of the two adolescent boys in this drama reflects their emotional reaction of anger and helplessness to their father's illness and their anxiety about the inevitably terminal outcome. The dialogue depicts a withdrawn, impotent, and painfully frustrated family. The mother/wife's unrequited need to express her sense of powerlessness, loneliness, and grief leads her to impose harsh rules and mete out punishment to her two sons.

Family Narrative

People speak to each other as a means of packaging experiences in cognitively and emotionally coherent—and at times incoherent—ways. The family narrative, as a therapeutic approach, accounts simultaneously for storytelling as an interactive event and as a unique portrait of illness events. However, family members are not always ready to listen to any narrative—whether it comes from inside or outside the family circle. Narrative events are defined broadly as conversations that recapitulate past and present events. Because the perception of what constitutes a narrative may differ from one family member to another, Lindenmeyer et al. (2008) avoided imposing any structural criteria on tales of illness or death. Analysis of the texts proceeded through a set of quantifiable coding categories designed to capture variations on each dimension of narrativity, voices, and behavior (Table 2–2).

Families have the capability to construe illness narratives in ways that can promote or inhibit healthy responses. Families can mediate the context by 1) integrating multiple perspectives generated within and beyond the interactive family, 2) providing or rejecting conditions that reframe or ease illness experience and behavior, and 3) coordinating key players to co-construct congruent themes aimed at accepting the perception of the illness.

Sample Intervention

The following is an eight-session outline from a protocol I use in family interventions. The intervention techniques used in each session incorporate psychodynamic interactions, systems theory, communication skills, reframing (cognitive skills), problem solving, and perceptual guided imagery. Modeling and sharing are based on a dynamic framework of Mann (1973) and on Hoffman's (1982) group process. Following some sessions, families are given specific tasks and exercises to accomplish during the week. After the outline, I briefly describe four of the sessions.

Thematic Time-Limited Group Dynamic: Family Trajectory Through Illness[1]

1. I—We
   - Presentation of self
   - Name: Meaning
   - Presentation of "we"

---

[1]From Hebrew protocol of family couple intervention, property of L. Baider.

TABLE 2–2. Narrative analysis

What values, beliefs, and conflicts are revealed in this story?

How does the couple view life (as a romance, tragedy, comedy)?

What life themes emerge?

What parts of the story are given more importance?

How does their past influence their present?

What unresolved conflicts are surfacing?

With what style is the story told?

How distant or close to their reality is the story?

Are the protagonists (the couple) portrayed as martyrs, warriors, victims, or heroes?

---

2. Coping
   - Story of "A Fence, a Sheep, a Man and a Problem" (Biran 1994)
   - How we choose the common coping mechanism for us
   - Homework: Find a common style for the story "The Taken House" (Cortázar-Bestiario 2003)

3. Emotional Turbulence
   - Denial—anger—guilt
   - Story of "The Old Man and His Leaf" (Ever-Hadani 1988)
   - The need to cover and protect
   - Victim
   - Homework: New experience

4. Normalcy
   - Exercise between the couple
   - What is different? Story by H.G. Wells (1998)
   - Homework: Relate to the experience of being different

5. Social Support
   - Exercise with photos
   - During the illness—disappointments—surprises
   - Expectations of each other
   - Homework: Redefine each family member

6. Perception of the "I" and the "We"
   - Body image—how we see each other—others
   - How we would like to be seen before—after
   - Homework: Experience the "we" as complementary

7. Family Communication
   - How we talk: About what? When? To whom?
   - Silences—family taboos—secrecy
   - Pictures: René Magritte (Belgian surrealist painter, 1898–1967) (Calvocoressi 1998; Meuris 1992)
   - Homework: Discover something new

8. Hope—Meaning—Spirituality
   - What provides security?
   - Sharing individual gifts

Outline of Four Sessions

Session 1.   How does the family as a system present itself—as each individual person; as "I"; as "we" referring to just the couple; as "we" involving all those present in the room (common space); or as "we" also integrating the absent members? It is relevant to understand the subtext of how families reveal and view themselves. The vocal and silent members will serve as guides for the therapist for behavioral clarification, but not for interpretation (refer to concepts of *family distality* in Bakan 1968 and in Laing 1972).

Session 2.   Sharing a story is an effective way of creating a shared family identity. "A Fence, a Sheep, a Man and a Problem" is an illustrative children's story relating how sheep cope when confronted with an obstacle that hinders their movement. It helps families reflect on their own coping styles when confronted with illness and adversity.

Session 6.   This intervention can be done with the entire family, with an individual patient, or within family groups. The therapist presents these items for verbal discussion:

   - I.
   - My name. Meaning.
   - How I see myself.
   - How I describe myself.
   - How I describe my family.
   - How I think my family sees me.
   - How I think my friends see me.
   - Any difference?

Session 7.   Pictures such as those by Magritte arouse diverging meanings for different viewers. When choosing artwork, the clinician needs to understand his or her reason for presenting a specific picture (e.g., know what reaction is intended within the group). A figurative picture allows a more direct identification with the illness situation. Family members may express emotions through creating a story from the picture, thereby revealing inner conflicts projected to external situations.

The degree of participation by family members in the intervention sessions raises the issue of how access to the information contained in the self-disclosure—that is, open narrative—is related to the "entitlement" to tell a private story. Whose stories in the family are told by whom and to whom? In discussing narratives that call for family response, some families experience the "illness event" of the narrative as a mutual family interaction rather than an isolated informative situation (Garro 2003). A multiplicity of voices at the level of telling can also transform relations between the family members. It is an issue of involvement—an internal, even emotional connection individuals feel that binds them together in the family and within the illness experience (Zinn 2005).

Pinnegar and Daynes (2007) distinguished between high-involvement and low-involvement narrative response strategies, particularly regarding illness information. High-involvement response strategies focus on the tale and the teller. They include devices such as requests for information, confirmations of information, and listener contributions to the narrative. Low-involvement response strategies focus on the telling.

Ecker and Hulley's (2000) depth-oriented brief therapy offers a linguistic-based assessment strategy that can be used at the beginning of and throughout therapy to generate discourse based on three essential clinical variables: 1) the multiple interpretations of illness appearance and behavior that promote or hinder psychological distress, 2) available collective cognitive-developmental resources, and 3) the recursive dimensions of the interactive family that support or inhibit psychological adaptation to illness.

Rigazio-DiGilio (1997) presents a constructivist intervention in which the theoretical and clinical aspects of systemic-cognitive developmental therapy emphasize the systemic and relational dimensions of the illness narrative within a family context. Beginning with the family unit, and working internally with its members and externally with the wider social environment, systemic-cognitive developmental therapy operationalizes developmental constructs that can be applied and studied in a therapeutic context of family illness.

Intervention: Family Process of Terminal Illness

Is he waiting for a friend's visit, for family...? In a deeper sense, he is not waiting for something outside of himself. What he is waiting for is already happening inside of himself. His body is a room, a bed—he is in it. The family is silenced by mystery, plenitude...waiting....

R. Charon (2006)

Grief is a family affair. Family members struggle to make sense of their illness and immediate loss. They attach meaning as a cognitive representation in search of venues of illusion or overtures of hope. The ebb and flow of affection within the family's interpersonal relationships involves a continual process of disengagement and reengagement, which does not suddenly stop when a family member dies. In fact, it continues as an illusory process of the past as if the person were still among the living (Kissane and Bloch 2002).

Symbolic interaction and family systems theories may help in understanding the need for family meaning during terminal illness. Both theories are useful in family meaning research and grief therapy. Symbolic interaction theory provides a way of thinking about how meaning is jointly created by every family member. It includes the assumption that humans live in a symbolic environment and acquire a complex set of subjective meanings. If the patient or members of the family define situations as real, they behave according to their subjective belief. It is less important to validate whether a specific circumstance actually happened than whether it was perceived to happen in a particular way, knowing that interaction emerges from the meanings that family members give to such events (Neimeyer 2002).

Not all thematic meanings that arise during a psychological intervention may bring comfort. Some actually bring distress. Family themes of death and dying may cause pain and anger, a sense of failure for not having acted on time or searched for new options, and a sense of blame and disbelief. The complexity of feelings may be expressed by deep regret and remorse. Negative emotions may steer family members into rebelling against any passive acceptance of the death and dying process.

The following are basic themes of acceptance that might be topics during family intervention:[2]

- Presence—family spiritual meaning
- The gift of "being"
- "We" as joint family memories
- Separation as a process of "attachment"
- Loneliness—our internal space
- Grief—time, silence, acceptance

Working with grieving families consists, first of all, of hearing their stories expressed in the most obfuscated, diffuse, and intricate language. A genuine helper listens for meanings, accepting those that are not coherent or

---

[2]Translated from Hebrew protocol of family intervention within palliative care, property of L. Baider.

logical without the urgent need to verify their significance. Support for emotional loss needs to be congruent with what the imminent death means to each family member. It is important to hear the family's stories again and again, looking each time for subtle differences as previously held meanings evolve into new ones—as changes in meaning mark the complex introjection of each individual's personal experiences into the family process (Pinsof and Wynne 2001).

Family intervention should be seen as an educational approach in which the therapist respectfully accepts each member's thoughts and feelings, regardless of differences among them. Change and willingness to accept involve a collaborative learning process in which the therapist only facilitates new patterns of thinking, feeling, accepting, and renewing family continuity in being alive.

As professionals, we should allow the family to learn how to grieve in their own private and personal way, just as they had to accept the challenge of a future that carried with it all the meanings from the past. For us, as caring professionals, the essence is our presence—just being there for them and honoring everything we have learned from them in their enigmatic journey through illness and death.

Family Communication: Unspoken Words

> But still the heart do need a language....
>
> Friedrich von Schiller, *The Aesthetic Letters*

This was a "normal family life"...a working couple, mid-sixties, three married children, eight grandchildren. Nothing unusual in their daily routine.

Only an intrusion of a sudden pain...a constant unwelcome pain. From then on, the days and hours became a means of either relief or agony. One sunny, blue-skied day, all the test results arrived—advanced pancreatic carcinoma, metastases in the liver and spleen....

And in a split second, the bright-colored day turned to ominous black. B acquired an unwanted role—an unwelcome label of "'patient" diagnosed with a terminal illness called pancreatic cancer. B called her family—one by one—and presented the information, the options and the irreversibly inevitable outcome. From then on, nothing was as "a normal family life." No more lights of the day or shadows of the night. Life became an abysmal hole with no point of return...no language, no piercing sound of crying...only the intensity of enduring silence....

> With the naiveté of a toddler, the family began to stumble along the path
> of a new language whose lexicon was filled with words of fear, sadness, pain,
> anxiety, separation, love, death, hope.… Could it be possible to learn to com-
> municate with this new complexity of metaphors?
> (L. Baider, private diary of patient cases translated from Hebrew, 2010)

Until recently, there has been a notable lack of attention to the presence of adaptive models of communication patterns within the family system that coexist with the chronicity of cancer (Baider 2008a). Family members find themselves catapulted into an unfamiliar environment in which they have little or no time emotionally and psychologically to incorporate the diagnosis of a life-threatening illness into their lives (Vangelisti 2004).

Communication is often constrained by a lack of knowledge and conditioned by the time of diagnosis of one's life span, leading to a constant reassessment and transformation of the affected family members. Communication with the cancer patient and the family unit should be constantly revised, redefined, negotiated, and renegotiated during the entire journey along the illness trajectory (Nussbaum et al. 2003).

The ability to communicate effectively is a critical aspect of healthy functioning for all families during all stages of life development. When chronic illness is present, it becomes even more important. The family needs to make crucial decisions, solve problems, and consider complex medical information that is often ambiguous or contradictory (Badr et al. 2008).

The growing rate of cancer diagnosis, the complexity and diversity of treatment options, and the likelihood of long-term relations with health professionals may increase families' needs for effective and appropriate family-patient health care communication. Moreover, effective family communication hinges on the exchange of information among all members about feelings regarding self and others, allowing permissiveness, acceptance of independent and diverse thoughts, and silences that do not necessarily represent denial. When patients verbally avoid or deny the reality of the illness or indicate that they are unwilling to discuss any treatment details, it is important for the family to respect this protective shell of denial, to be supportive of this "conspiracy of silence," and to wait for a signal of readiness and openness to share the familial quandaries concerning the frightening cancer experience (Porter et al. 2005).

Several threats emerge as barriers to open discussion of cancer in the family. The assumption that family members should be optimistic as they interact with the patient and the belief that the patient should sublimate negative thoughts about the situation may lead the family to avoid discussing topics related to cancer. Patients may assume that family members already have a lot on their minds because of the illness and not want to worry them further. These issues may manifest themselves in a tense relationship between patients and family members that does not stimulate open communication (Fitzpatrick 2004).

Blum (1997) presented a view of communication as a collective family relationship that involves a level of shared intentionality and interrelationship as "we." Family conversations create contextual frames, each bounding a set of interactive messages and sharing a common premise of mutual relevance within the illness process.

In a cross-sectional cohort study on family caregiver–patient communication, Fried et al. (2005) reported that 39.9% of family caregivers said they desired more communication, 37.3% reported that communication was quite difficult, and 22% said that patients refused any open dialogue. Although family caregivers' desire for increased communication may be a modifiable determinant of caregiver burden, this desire was independently associated with increased caregiver burden, measured in terms of emotional distress. Burden was associated with patients' covert and detached communication.

Mesters et al. (1998) reported that openness of discussion in families is related to a theoretical model of coping with cancer stress. This model is based on the assumption that harm and threat caused by cancer may lead to stress through a process of primary and secondary appraisal (Lazarus and Folkman 1984). Primary appraisal is the assessment of harm and threat by the disease; secondary appraisal is the assessment of one's coping abilities and resources (e.g., social support) and the patient's estimation of adequacy of resources to meet the harm and threat. The four main psychological responses to cancer stress are 1) uncertainty, 2) negative feelings, 3) loss of control, and 4) threatened self-esteem.

Family members decide to whom they will or will not reveal news about the illness. Some individuals engage in coalitions, others need the alliance of silence, and others may find solace in sharing their intimate experiences. Nonetheless, family members may be psychologically unprepared to hear and communicate the diagnosis or prognosis at one specific moment. Silence may be the natural consequence of not being able to accept and assimilate the explicit truth about the illness, accompanied by responses of overwhelming grief, despair, and avoidance (Baider 2008b; Zhang and Siminoff 2003).

One of the most compelling and confounding features of family relations is the tendency for the individual members to develop distinct interpretations of the illness event. These differences seem to increase as antagonism and disagreements over causation, responsibility, and blame obscure choices for suitable patient care. Family members may provide varying interpretations for rational explanations, according to each individual's subjective knowledge and needs for positive reassurance, as they assign emotional meaning to each message about the pivotal steps on the unknown journey of cancer (Wilmot and Hocker 2001).

Each patient's story, as shared within the family, provides insight into the power of the spoken word or the silent monologue; both are the language of the family unit. It is an opportunity for mutual family healing, hope, and meaning. The patient's story brings the family system of care one step closer to understanding the impact that cancer diagnosis has on family life (Andersen and Martin 2003). It both elucidates the difficult and enlightening moments during the journey and indicates how these moments affect the family's resilience as they walk along the path of illness, survival, and death. The voices of the stories, the words of lamentation, and the silent language allow for a reconstructed and broadened resumption of a "normal family life."

Key Clinical Points

- The family is a dynamic system that incorporates each member's identity and integrates that identity into its own internal and external resources.

- It is important to understand that there are diverse theoretical definitions and eclectic concepts of family as a dynamic system, particularly when families are confronted with a diagnosis of cancer.

- Clinicians should avoid focusing on family weaknesses and dysfunctions, and instead should consider the resilience and capacity of families to withstand crises, to learn new adaptive coping behaviors, and to enhance their quality of life.

- Marital relationships are interconnected systems of unconditional emotional support with the capacity to provide pragmatic responses to illness and to absorb psychological distresses of the patient and/or the healthy caregiver spouse.

- Intimacy, open communication, and mutual trust between partners allow for more adaptive coping during the chronic trajectory of the cancer illness.

- Health care professionals should carefully assess family needs and internal resources—by means of evidence-based diagnoses of ability to function—before offering any kind of intervention.

- Clinicians should focus on specific problems or conflicts arising from the illness and have a clear, objective outcome for any appropriate intervention.

- The family may have the capacity and ability to communicate with each member while respecting silences, withdrawal, hidden emotions, and angry outbursts.

- There is no universal appraisal for family illness. Individual family members need to search for their own explanations and subjective meanings of "Why me?" and "Why us?"

- Cancer has an unpredictable trajectory. When faced with cancer, the family has its own process of interjecting and absorbing the truth and of assimilating unwanted outcomes; its own internal resources for learning a different language of loss, pain, and suffering; and its own way of pursuing a meaning of life and death.

References

Acitelli LK, Badr HJ: My illness or our illness? Attending to the relationship when one partner is ill, in Couples Coping With Stress: Emerging Perspectives on Dyadic Coping. Edited by Revenson TA, Kayser K, Bodenmann G. Washington, DC, American Psychological Association, 2005, pp 121–136

Anderson JO, Martin PG: Narratives and healing: exploring one family's stories of cancer survivorship. Health Commun 15:133–143, 2003

Badr H, Acitelli LK, Carmack CL: Does talking about their relationship affect couples' marital and psychological adjustment to lung cancer? J Cancer Surviv 2:53–64, 2008

Badr H, Carmack CL, Kashy DA, et al: Dyadic coping in metastatic breast cancer. Health Psychol 29:169–180, 2010

Baider L: Communication about illness. Supp Care Cancer 16:607–611, 2008a

Baider L: Will you still care for me? J Med Person 6:55–59, 2008b

Baider L, Ever-Hadani P, Goldzweig G, et al: Is perceived family support a relevant variable in psychological distress? A sample of prostate and breast cancer couples. J Psychosom Res 55:1–8, 2003

Baider L, Andritsch E, Goldzweig G, et al: Changes in psychological distress of women with breast cancer in long-term remission and their husbands. Psychosomatics 45:58–68, 2004

Bakan D: Disease, Pain, and Sacrifice. Chicago, IL, University of Chicago Press, 1968

Ballard-Reisch DS, Letner JA: Centering families in cancer communication research. Patient Educ Couns 50:61–66, 2003

Berg CA, Upchurch R: A developmental-contextual model of couples coping with chronic illness across the adult life span. Psychol Bull 133:920–954, 2007

Berman EM, Heru A, Grunebaum H, et al: Family-oriented patient care through the residency training cycle. Acad Psychiatry 32:111–118, 2008

Biran Y: Ways of Solving a Fence (in Hebrew). Tel-Aviv, Israel, Saar Publishing House, 1994

Blum KS: Dinner Talk: Cultural Patterns of Sociability and Socialization in Family Discourse. Mahwah, NJ, Erlbaum, 1997

Bodenmann G: Dyadic coping and its significance for marital function, in Couples Coping With Stress: Emerging Perspectives on Dyadic Coping. Washington, DC, American Psychological Association, 2005, pp 33–50

Bodenmann G, Shantinath SD: The Couples Coping Enhancement Training (CCET): a new approach to prevention of marital distress based upon stress and coping. Family Relations 53:477–484, 2004

Boehmer U, Clark JA: Communication about prostate cancer between men and their wives. J Fam Pract 50:226–231, 2002

Braun M, Mikulincer M, Rydall A, et al: Hidden morbidity in cancer: spouse caregivers. J Clin Oncol 25:4829–4834, 2007

Calvocoressi R: Magritte. London, UK, Phaidon Press, 1998

Candib LM: Truth telling and advanced planning at the end of life. Fam Syst Health 20:213–228, 2002

Cassidy J: Truth, lies and intimacy: attachment perspective. Attach Hum Dev 3:121–155, 2001

Charon R: Narrative Medicine, XII. London, UK, Oxford University Press, 2006

Cortázar-Bestiario J: The Taken House [translated from the Spanish, La casa tomada 11–21]. Buenos Aires, Argentina, Punto de Lectura, 2003

Coyne JC, Lepare SJ, Palmer SC: Efficacy of psychological interventions in cancer care. Ann Behav Med 32:104–110, 2006

Ecker B, Hulley L: The order in clinical "disorder": symptom coherence in depth-oriented brief therapy, in Constructions of Disorder: Meaning-Making Frameworks for Psychotherapy. Edited by Neimeyer RA, Raskin JD. Washington, DC, American Psychological Association, 2000, pp 63–90

Erikson EH: Childhood and Society. New York, WW Norton, 1963

Ershler WB: Cancer: a disease of the elderly. Support Care Cancer 1:5–10, 2003

Ever-Hadani Y: The Shaklat [The Old Man and His Leaf, adapted from the Hebrew book Hashalkat]. Tel Aviv, Israel, Sifrayat Paolim, 1988

Fitzpatrick MA: Family communication pattern theory: observations on its development and application. J Fam Commun 4:167–179, 2004

Fried TR, Bardley EH, O'Leary JR, et al: Unmet desire for caregiver-patient communication and increased caregiver burden. J Am Geriatr Soc 53:59–65, 2005

Garro LC: Narrative troubling experiences. Transcult Psychiatry 40:5–43, 2003

Goldzweig G, Hubert A, Walach N, et al: Gender and psychological distress among middle- and older-aged colorectal cancer patients and their spouses: an unexpected outcome. Crit Rev Oncol Hematol 70:71–82, 2009

Hagedoorn M, Van Yperen NW, Coyne JC, et al: Does marriage protect older people from distress? The role of equity and recency of bereavement. Psychol Aging 21:611–620, 2006

Hann D, Baker F, Denniston M, et al: The influence of social support on symptoms in cancer patients. Psychosom Res 52:279–283, 2002

Hill J, Fonagy P, Safier E, et al: The ecology of attachment in the family. Process 42:205–221, 2003

Hodges LJ, Humphris GM, Macfarlane G: A meta-analytic investigation of the relationship between psychological distress of cancer patients and their carers. Soc Sci Med 60:1–12, 2005

Hoffman L: Foundation of Family Therapy. New York, Basic Books, 1982

Jacobsen PB, Heather SJ: Psychosocial interventions in adult cancer patients: achievements and challenges. CA Cancer J Clin 58:214–230, 2008

Kissane DW, Bloch S: Family Focused Grief Therapy. Buckingham, UK, Open University Press, 2002

Laing RD: The Politic of the Family. London, Vintage Books, Tavistock Publishers, 1972

Lazarus RS, Folkman S: Stress, Appraisal, and Coping. New York, Springer, 1984

Lindenmeyer A, Griffiths F, Green E, et al: Family health narratives: midlife women's concepts of vulnerability to illness. Health 12:275–293, 2008

Mann J: Time-Limited Psychotherapy. Cambridge, MA, Harvard University Press, 1973

Manne S, Alfieri T, Taylor K, et al: Preferences for spousal support among individuals with cancer. Journal of Applied Social Psychology 29: 722–749, 1999

Manne SL, Ostroff JS, Norton TR, et al: Cancer-related relationship communication in couples coping with early stage breast cancer. Psychooncology 15:234–247, 2006

McLean LM, Jones JM, Rydall AC, et al: A couples intervention for patients facing advanced cancer and their spouse caregivers. Psychooncology 17:1152–1156, 2008

Mesters I, van den Borne H, McCormick L, et al: Openness to discuss cancer in the nuclear family: scale, development, and validation. Psychosom Med 59:269–279, 1998

Meuris J: Magritte 1898–1967. Cologne, Germany, Taschen Verlag, 1992

Moorey S, Greer S: Cognitive Behaviour Therapy for People With Cancer. London, UK, Oxford University Press, 2002

Naaman S, Radwan K, Johnson S: Coping with early breast cancer: couple adjustment process. Psychiatry 72:321–342, 2009

Neimeyer RA: Meaning of Reconstruction and the Experience of Loss. Washington, DC, American Psychological Association, 2002

Northouse LL, Templin T, Mood D: Couples' adjustment to breast disease during the first year following diagnosis. J Behav Med 24:115–136, 2001

Northouse LL, Katapodi MC, Song L, et al: Interventions with family caregivers of cancer patients. CA Cancer J Clin 60:317–339, 2010

Nussbaum JF, Baringer D, Kundrat A: Health communication and aging: cancer and older adults. Health Commun 15:185–192, 2003

Patterson J: Integrating family resilience and family stress theory. J Marriage Fam 64:349–360, 2003

Pinnegar S, Daynes JG: Locating narrative inquiry historically: thematics in the turn to narrative. In Handbook of Narrative Inquiry: Mapping a Methodology. Edited by Clandinin DJ. Thousand Oaks, CA, Sage, 2007, pp 3–34

Pinsof WM, Wynne LC: Toward progress research: closing the gap between family therapy and research. J Marital Fam Ther 27:1–8, 2001

Porter L, Keefe F, Hurwitz H, et al: Disclosure between patients with cancer and their spouses. Psychooncology 14:1030–1042, 2005

Reiss D, Neiderhiser JM: The interplay of genetic influences and social processes in developmental theory: specific mechanisms are coming into view. Dev Psychopathol 12:357–374, 2000

Rigazio-DiGilio SA: Systemic-cognitive-development therapy: a counseling model. Int J Adv Couns 19:143–165, 1997

Rogers C: Client-Centered Therapy. Boston, MA, Houghton Mifflin, 1951

Rolland JS: Cancer and the family: an integrative model. Cancer 104:2584–2595, 2002

Rolland JS: Chronic illness and the family life cycle, in The Expanded Family Life Cycle: Individual, Family, and Social Perspectives, 4th Edition. Edited by Carter E, McGoldrick M, Garcia-Preto N. Boston, MA, Allyn & Bacon, 2009, pp 348–367

Shields CG, Travis LA, Rousseau SL: Marital attachment and adjustment in older couples coping with cancer. Aging Ment Health 4:223–233, 2000

Skerrett K: From isolation to mutuality: a feminist collaborative model for couples therapy. Women Ther 19:93–106, 1996

Stefanek ME, Palmer SC, Thombs BD, et al: Finding what is not there. Cancer 115:5612–5616, 2009

Surrey J: Relationship and Empowerment, Work in Progress, Working Paper, Series No. 13. Wellesley, MA, Stone Center, 1987

Thomas C, Morris SM, Harman JC: Companions through cancer: the care given by informal carers in cancer contexts. Soc Sci Med 54:529–544, 2002

Vangelisti AL (ed): Handbook of Family Communication. Mahwah, NJ, Erlbaum, 2004

Walsh F: Family resilience: a framework for clinical practice. Fam Process 42:1–18, 2003

Watson M: Cancer in the elderly: the influence of life stage on psychosocial, supportive and informational needs and patient perceived ageism. Project grant application March 2008. Population and Behavioural Sciences Committee, 2007

Wedding U, Pientka L, Hoffken K: Quality-of-life in elderly patients with cancer: a short review. Eur J Cancer 43:2203–2210, 2007

Weihs KL, Enright T, Simmens S: High quality spousal or long-term partner relationships predict time to recurrence of breast cancer, after control for disease severity. Psychosom Med 64:107, 2002

Wells HG: The country of the blind, in The Complete Short Stories of HG Wells. Edited by Hammond J. London, UK, Butler & Tanner, 1998, pp 629–648

Wilmot WW, Hocker JL: Interpersonal Conflict, 6th Edition. New York, McGraw-Hill, 2001

Winnicott DW: Playing and Reality. New York, Basic Books, 1971

Wynne L, Ryckoff I, Day J, et al: Pseudo-mutuality in the family relations of schizophrenics, in A Modern Introduction to the Family. Edited by Bell N, Vogel E. Toronto, Ontario, Canada, Free Press, 1968, pp 628–650

Zhang AY, Siminoff LA: Silence and cancer: why do families and patients fail to communicate? Health Commun 15:415–429, 2003

Zinn JO: The biographical approach: a better way to understand behavior in health and illness. Health Risk Soc 71:1–9, 2005

CHAPTER 3

Communicating With Cancer Patients and Their Families

Walter F. Baile, M.D.
Anna Costantini, Ph.D.

MOST PEOPLE RECOGNIZE the tremendous importance of communication in everyday life. However, they often regard communication skills as being inherent, assuming that everybody knows intuitively how to communicate effectively. Nothing could be further from the truth. Communication is a skill that needs to be cultivated. Although not all clinicians will be engaged in public speaking, clinicians are "on stage" every time they interact with patients and their families who rely on professionals for information, advice, encouragement, and support. Philibert (2005) reminded doctors about the importance of communication as a skill to be learned for various professionals: "Musicians, actors, lawyers giving closing arguments, clergy preparing sermons would not consider engaging in these activities without some form of rehearsal, either as an explicit trial of the activity in a 'low-stakes' setting, or at least as a deliberate 'mental walk-through' of all the steps that will go into the actual performance" (p. 1).

The model of relationship-centered oncology (Epstein and Street 2007) has emerged as an important guide to help cancer practitioners treat the whole patient. (Table 3–1 contrasts this model with the traditional medical model.) This model requires that cancer practitioners adopt an approach consistent with the idea that patients have a right to be informed about their illnesses and to participate in decision making. To deliver this type of cancer care, clinicians must be competent in a number of communication and interpersonal skills (Table 3–2).

Being conscious of both the verbal and nonverbal behavior that we use in all of these tasks is the essence of the art and skill of communication. Delivered poorly, information and advice can take a patient down the wrong path. Unless clinicians are able to show empathy, patients will view them as aloof and unsupportive. A clinician's skill at communicating can make a difference between a patient's wanting to give up and marshaling the strength to go through with treatments. In this chapter, we explore effective communication in the oncology setting, focusing on practical skills that are needed to meet the challenges of patient-centered medicine.

The Value of Communication

Communicating is the essential way that we as humans both transmit information to others and receive it. It is a given that we cannot "not communicate." Studies have shown that in the process of communicating, we pick up on the most subtle of cues from both verbal and nonverbal behaviors of others. Our brain is always processing the input that we receive from the signals that others give us.

What we as clinicians say to patients and how we say it can profoundly affect their mood and coping. Consider the difference between the following two statements in which a diagnosis of advanced cancer is disclosed to a patient:

1. You have a terminal disease and have six months to live. I suggest you go home and get your affairs in order.
2. I'm afraid I have to tell you that you have advanced cancer, but we are going to give you the best treatment available.

Although both statements are factually correct, the messages to the patient are entirely different. The first could be interpreted as a dismissal and the second as an encouragement. Obviously, the impact on patient morale could be substantial. Consider also the following ways of explaining information to a patient:

1. You have a Philadelphia chromosome positive AML and are likely going to need a transplant in the future.
2. You have a serious disease of the blood called leukemia. There are many ways to treat it, and you are likely going to need intensive treatment, which I can explain more in detail.

TABLE 3–1. Approaches to medical care	
"Traditional" or medical model	Relationship-focused model
Goal of provider is only to diagnose disease.	Goal of provider is both to diagnose disease *and* to understand impact of disease on patient and family.
Focus of provider is on signs and symptoms.	Focus of provider is on signs and symptoms, as well as patient information (needs, expectations, concerns).
Directive: provider tells patient what to do.	Participatory: provider provides a plan, which patient affirms.
Provider chooses treatment.	Provider explains treatment options.
Patient autonomy = patient listens and agrees.	Patient autonomy = patient asks questions and decides.
Support = reassurance that things will be okay.	Support includes addressing emotions and concerns.

The second statement is much more likely to be understood by most patients.

Communication as a Skill To Be Learned and Taught

The notion that communication is a skill is central to the discussion of how clinicians learn to become competent in these skills and then to teach these skills. Fundamentally, communication is a set of defined verbal and nonverbal behaviors that can be observed, recorded, coded, measured, and taught. Take, for example, the simple behavior of asking patients about their understanding of their medical situation before giving them bad news. The purpose of this simple question is for the clinician to assess the information patients already have about their illness so as to correct misperceptions and to understand when patients and families are in denial. This question is particularly useful when patients have been seen by several practitioners who may have given them incorrect information.

TABLE 3–2.   Exhibiting valued physician behaviors

Valued physician behaviors	How clinician might show these behaviors or attitudes
Imparts confidence	Greets patient with warmth
	Makes eye contact
	Assures patient he or she will get the best treatment available
	States experience in treating specific medical conditions or performing procedures
	Encourages patient's queries about medical information acquired from other sources (regardless of accuracy or inaccuracy)
	Makes recommendations
Empathetic	Elicits patient concerns
	Is sensitive to emotions
	Acknowledges distress
Humane	Uses appropriate physical contact
	Is attentive, and is present to patient and situation
	Sits down when appropriate
	Identifies appropriate resources to assist patient
	Gives bad news compassionately
Personal	Asks patient about his or her life
	Uses appropriate humor
	Acknowledges patient's family
	Remembers details about patient's life from previous visits
Forthright	Doesn't sugarcoat or withhold information
	Avoids medical jargon
	Explains choices when these are available
	Asks patient to recap conversation to ensure understanding

TABLE 3–2. Exhibiting valued physician behaviors *(continued)*

Valued physician behaviors	How clinician might show these behaviors or attitudes
Respectful	Offers explanation or apology if patient is kept waiting
	Listens carefully and does not interrupt when patient is describing medical concern
	Provides choices to patient as appropriate but is also willing to recommend specific course of treatment
	Solicits patient's input in treatment options and scheduling
	Takes care to maintain patient's modesty during physical examination
Thorough	Provides detailed explanations
	Gives instructions in writing
	Follows up in a timely manner
	Expresses to patient desire to consult other clinicians or research literature on a difficult case

Note. Specific physician behaviors will affect patients differently. Although many patients are likely to appreciate a physician's empathy in sharing a relevant personal story, this can be a neutral or even a negative experience for some patients. There is no substitute for physicians knowing their patients and responding accordingly.

Source. Adapted from Benaputi, *Mayo Clinic Proceedings.*

Case Vignette

John is a young man with widely metastatic pancreatic cancer. He had a surgical consult, which showed that he had inoperable cancer, and was referred to the medical oncologist for chemotherapy. When Dr. Kirk asked the patient to explain what he had been told about his disease, John responded, "The surgeon told me that right now he could not operate, but if you could shrink down the tumors, he might be able to take it out." This put Dr. Kirk in the awkward and uncomfortable situation of having to give John the bad news about his disease. Whether John had correctly interpreted what the surgeon had told him is less important than the fact that the medical oncologist, although hoping for a chemotherapy response, must tell the patient that it is unlikely that he will be able to accomplish what the surgeon had led him to believe. Otherwise, John may entertain unrealistic expectations of being operated on in the future.

Although asking patients about their understanding of their medical situation is a communication skill that is commonly left out of bad news discussions, this question is recommended by most guidelines on breaking bad news. However, this skill can be easily learned, and once clinicians understand the usefulness of having the information and the impact on patient satisfaction, they can find the correct way of asking and make a conscious effort to practice it. With enough practice, the behavior can become part of a clinician's armamentarium. The same is true for other complex behaviors, such as responding to patient and family emotions.

A number of studies have shown that communication skills, especially the more complex ones, must be learned and practiced in order for clinicians to be effective in using them. This becomes strikingly evident when even experienced clinicians stumble when trying to explain the diagnosis or prognosis of cancer to a patient. Phrases such as "You have a widespread cancer and have six months to live" can devastate a patient (Bedell et al. 2004). Sentences such as "I wouldn't touch your problem with a ten-foot pole" can frighten patients unnecessarily, but expressions similar to this one are not uncommon in medical practice. Even attempts to reassure patients with expressions such as "Everything is going to be all right," although aimed at comforting the patient, can be experienced as false reassurance, and rightly so, because a clinician cannot really know the outcome of treatment for any patient. Confirmation of this fact was shown in an educational intervention called Oncotalk (www.depts.washington.edu/oncotalk). In an Oncotalk retreat for medical oncology fellows, a baseline assessment was done of their pre-intervention communication skills using the breaking bad news interview in standardized patient encounters. Of 150 medical oncology fellows, 44% struggled with rapport-building skills, such as asking open-ended question or greeting the patient; 45% neglected to ask patients what they understood about their cancer; only 51% used the word *cancer* in breaking bad news; 0% responded empathically to the expression "I'm scared" by the patient; and 53% summarized the follow-up plan. Moreover, other studies by Drs. James Tulsky and Peter Maguire and their groups have found significant gaps in communication skills even among seasoned practitioners (Maguire and Pitceathly 2002; Pollack et al. 2007; Table 3–3).

Other studies have shown that communication skills do not necessarily improve with experience. Even senior clinicians may be at a relatively novice level of communication when having difficult conversations with patients and families. For this reason, communication training workshops that allow practitioners to learn the how-tos of communicating and then to practice them in standardized patient situations have been initiated and been shown to be effective. For example, Fallowfield et al. (2003) reported that workshop participants demonstrated more expression of empathy (69% increase),

TABLE 3–3.   Results of observational studies of communication skills

Typical behavior of oncologists	Impact on patient
Engage in long explanations and monologues	Patients have little time to ask questions
Neglect to ask open-ended questions such as "Do you have any concerns?"	Patients do not have opportunities to feel what is worrying them
Respond to emotions with logic instead of empathy	Emotions are not addressed satisfactorily
Use too much jargon and technical language	Patients fail to understand explanations
Use euphemisms for cancer	Patients are misinformed
Are vague or fail to discuss sensitive issues such as prognosis	Patients fail to understand the purpose of cancer treatment
Underestimate how much information patients want	Patients leave the encounter with unmet information needs

Source. Adapted from Maguire P, Pitceathly C: "Key Communication Skills and How to Acquire Them." *British Medical Journal* 325:697–700, 2002; Pollack KI, Arnold RM, Jeffreys AS, et al.: "Oncologist Communication About Emotion During Visits With Patients With Advanced Cancer." *Journal of Clinical Oncology* 25:5748–5752, 2007.

more focused and open questions (27% increase), and more appropriate responses to patient cues (38% more). According to Razavi et al. (2002, 2003), those trained in workshops were more "in control" of the interview and used less emotionally neutral utterances and more words associated with "distress." In another study, Back et al. (2007) reported that participants acquired a mean of 5.4 "giving bad news" skills ($P<0.001$) and a mean of 4.4 "transition to palliative care" skills ($P<0.001$). Most changes in individual skills were substantial.

Dynamics of Patient Care in Oncology: Why Communication Is Particularly Important

Cancer carries a social stigma unlike that of any other disease. Despite the enhanced efficacy of modern treatments, it often evokes fears of death, suffering, and disability. The American Institute for Cancer Research (2007) reported that cancer is the disease Americans fear most. The following findings were reported in the institute's "Facts and Fears" survey of 1,022 cancer patients ages 18 and older: 48% feared it more than any other disease, 32% feared it more than any other catastrophe in their lives, 28% ranked curing cancer higher than any other public goal except providing health care to all children, and 32% had experienced an acute stress disorder.

Cancer patients face many crises, as noted in Table 3–4. In times of crisis, patients and families often go through a phase of confusion about what to do. Their fear and helplessness increase, and they are more likely to reach out for help and form strong emotional bonds with caregivers, on whom they become dependent for expertise and support. Patients and families ward off hopelessness and fear by looking for optimism in the words and actions of their cancer providers. However, they also can be easily discouraged by excessive bluntness and expressions such as "There is nothing more we can do" that take away their hope. In some cultures and countries, where attempts to protect the patient from psychological "damage" result in bad news being given in vague, ambiguous, and overtechnical ways or with the use of words such as *tumor* or *inflammation* instead of the word *cancer,* patients can become confused and discouraged. Moreover, failure to tell the truth to the patient can set a tone of mistrust that can ripple through the treatment team and color the nature of subsequent relationships between doctor, patient, and the family. For example, the staff in such instances must remain careful not to divulge the "forbidden" information. In research with several hundred oncology nurses, Sivesind et al. (2003) reported that nurses often found themselves in the compromised situation of avoiding patients' rooms or even lying to them to maintain an illusory prognosis.

Clinical Vignette

Dr. Tan is a kind and compassionate oncologist who makes it a practice never to discuss a prognosis with a patient, even when asked about the possible outcome of the disease. He is famous for the phrase "Let's not worry about that, and focus on the treatment we have for you." This often puts his staff in an awkward position when patients and families ask about their future. Often, after referring them back to Dr. Tan, staff members have to deal with the frustration in the response, "We can't get him to tell us anything." Because of what they perceived as his poor communication skills, many of the staff wished that they didn't have to work with Dr. Tan even though they thought he was a pleasant person.

In the complex jumble of patient and family emotions, there is significant opportunity for cancer providers to be therapeutic through their communications. The purpose of these communications, which we call "support," is discussed later (see "Purposes of Communication" section), but basically such communications can be powerful tools in restoring and helping maintain morale in the face of devastating illness. In other words, the relationship with

TABLE 3–4. The crises of cancer
Hearing the diagnosis
Having a poor prognosis
Treatment failure
Disease recurrence
Losing body parts
Estrangement from family and friends
Financial setbacks
Irreversible side effects
Transition to palliative care

the patient can be therapeutic in itself (Table 3–5). As Gerretsen and Myers (2008) put it, the oncology team can be the patient's "secure base" by providing reassurance that the patient will have a helping hand from the professional care provider during the cancer experience. Providing this secure base may require, for example, being available to answer questions for the patient; helping the patient understand the nature of cancer treatments and the choices for care; responding empathically to emotions and expressing understanding at times when the patient confronts a crisis in care, such as disease recurrence; giving reassurance that the care provider will not abandon the patient even when the disease takes a turn for the worse; and guiding the family in how they can best support the patient during the illness.

Long-Term Challenges to the Individual in Cancer Care

Dealing With Uncertainty

For a person with a life-threatening disease, not knowing what is going to happen is a major source of anxiety. For those individuals who highly value the ability to plan and know what is coming around the corner, this may be a particularly vexing problem. For example, those with compulsive personality characteristics may desire a level of detail about treatment that other patients might find excessive. Identifying patients' personality types and understanding how they deal with disease can help clinicians communicate more effectively.

Patients who shun information

Often described as being "in denial," patients who shun information typically do not want to know details and may even leave decision making to others. This behavior is felt to be a coping mechanism to help ward off the anxiety of uncertainty. In working with these patients, the clinician should try adopting a nonconfrontational approach to exploring patients' anxiety.

Compulsive and in-control personalities

Individuals who are compulsive and who like to be in control often want to have lots of information or even to be involved in decisions on a minute level. They will have a hard time with a role of dependency and often clash with staff over being "told what to do." The clinician should use an empathic approach, demonstrating patience and acknowledging with these patients the challenge of not having exact answers to all of their questions.

Borderline personalities

Patients with borderline personalities have a fragile identity and difficulty trusting. They often can be angry for no apparent reason and may complain to different staff members about other staff (splitting). Working with these patients requires a consistent approach to limit setting and bringing in professional help, such as a psychologist, to deal with patient challenges around issues of trust.

Case Vignette

Joan was admitted with sepsis during her third course of chemotherapy for colon cancer. She had unexplained bouts of depression, and when hospitalized she challenged many of the decisions made by staff about her care. Only when a history was taken did the psycho-oncologist discover that beginning at age 9, she had been both physically and sexually abused by her stepfather. She had learned not to trust anyone, especially those on whom she was dependent.

Dependent patients

Dependent patients often make staff angry because they are difficult to mobilize. They may cling to staff and be passive about rehabilitating. Recognizing the patient's underlying need for attention may prevent staff from reacting to their own frustration with anger toward the patient. To help in devising some practical approaches to the care of the dependent patient, the clinician can begin by taking a thorough psychosocial history, including asking questions such as these: "Have you been sick before?" "What has that been like for you?" "What would help you most in coping with your illness?"

Dealing With Side Effects and Disabilities Caused by Cancer and Cancer Drugs

Physical pain and discomfort are major stressors for patients. Often, patients do not want to complain about pain until it causes physical dysfunction.

TABLE 3–5. Therapeutic communication

Technique	Impact on patient	Example
Listening to the patient's story without interrupting; eliciting the patient's concerns	Feels regarded as a person	"Tell me about your cancer." "What are you most worried about?"
Providing information	Decreases uncertainty	"Here's the plan for the next three months…"
Using praise	Feels effort has been acknowledged	"I know the chemo was tough and I appreciate your hanging in there."
Encouraging the patient	Bolsters optimism	"I have seen some good results with this treatment."
Providing absolution	Relieves guilt	"You did not do anything to bring on the cancer."
Being empathic	Acknowledges feelings	"I can see you weren't expecting this news."
Negotiating	Feels views are respected	"Yes, we can put off the treatment until after your daughter's wedding."

Some side effects of treatment, such as peripheral neuropathy, can be crippling and destroy mobility. When pain or other symptoms are chronic, they can erode morale. Therefore, symptoms of treatment need to be taken seriously and not trivialized by cancer practitioners.

Dealing With Dependence on Others

Being a master of one's own life and self-directive is often taken for granted. Having to depend on others for simple tasks such as bathing can be experienced as humiliating. For people who are hyperindependent, this dependence can be even more challenging.

Maintaining Self-Esteem

A person's identity is often tied up with the ability to self-direct, have choices, and be productive, either at work or home. When an individual has cancer, however, independence or the ability to engage in an important source of self-esteem such as productive work may be eroded. For patients in times of distress, the experience of having a clinician take a personal interest in them can be a lifeline. This may be especially important for individuals whose self-esteem had been fragile prior to cancer onset and who are at risk for developing a psychological disorder such as increased anxiety or depression.

Maintaining Important Connections

Friends, family, and work colleagues are often important sources of support and satisfaction. Undergoing cancer treatments or being disabled from the disease may suddenly change these connections and relationships. In many cases, these changes develop and evolve over many months. The psychological impact of the disease is often greater in countries where the population is highly mobile and family members are geographically scattered. In contrast, greater support for both the patient and other family members can be more easily offered when the members of the nuclear family live within short distances of one another. Although some of these challenges have been mitigated by modern communication technology, such as Internet video, there is no substitute for a smiling face or a gentle touch on the part of the professional caregiver. Patient-to-patient support services also play an important role in helping the patient establish a new network of connections. For example, the Anderson Network, at MD Anderson Cancer Center (www.mdanderson.org), connects newly diagnosed cancer patients with so-called veterans who have successfully gone through treatment and can serve as a source of information and inspiration for patients and families.

Financial Challenges

Patients whose unemployment or medical benefits for illness are limited can suffer significant financial setbacks due to cancer. Cancer treatments can also be very expensive; certain drugs such as bevacizumab (Avastin) cost thousands of dollars per dose, and treatments such as bone marrow transplant cost in the hundreds of thousands of dollars. Including financial considerations in discussions with patients as to whether to continue therapy with expensive anticancer drugs or to forgo treatment is still very controversial but is becoming increasingly important as the quality of life of cancer patients receives more emphasis and attempts at containing the cost of cancer care move to the forefront (McFarlane et al. 2008).

Family Entanglements

Sometimes families, in their desire to protect the member who is ill, infantilize the person and limit his or her information about the disease; this may deprive the patient of important information needed to cope. Family disagreements regarding the patient or the treatment may erupt when families have been living in conflict or disagreement.

Case Vignette

Dana is a 45-year-old woman with breast cancer who had a poor relationship with her sister Alma, whom Dana felt inappropriately intruded in her life, commenting frequently on the men she dated, her clothes, and her choice of job. When Dana was diagnosed with breast cancer, Alma flew unexpectedly to Dana's home and began accompanying her to doctors' visits. The oncologist noted that Alma often spoke for Dana during the visits and that Dana often looked frustrated. Only after the social worker spent some time alone with Dana did the relationship between her and her sister become apparent. Although it made Alma angry, Dana's oncology team decided that meeting alone with Dana at her visits would give her the kind of autonomy she needed.

Cancer and Mood Disturbance

There is a mistaken belief that depression is a normal part of the cancer experience or that most cancer patients are depressed. This mistaken attitude results from the failure to differentiate the normal grieving process from demoralization and clinical depression (see Chapter 4, "Demoralization and Depression in Cancer"). Clinical depression is a syndrome characterized by discrete symptoms including loss of interest in usual activities, social withdrawal, pervasive hopelessness, inability to experience the normal pleasures of life, and sometimes suicidal ideation. Demoralization, however, can happen when one receives bad news or has a setback from cancer treatment, such as the onset of peripheral neuropathy. It is characterized by frustration, sometimes anger and irritability, and discouragement. Patients sometimes feel hopeless about the future, but not in the pervasive way that characterizes clinical depression. Grief often occurs as a result of the losses that accompany cancer. There is often a sense of not being the same person one used to be, as well as sadness about the many things that may have happened or been taken away, such as the ability to work, ambulate, and even pay one's bills.

These syndromes may be hard to distinguish from one another because sadness may be present in all of them. Patients with clinical depression often have a history of previous depression, and their mood problem is often debilitating and can last months. Patients with demoralization often experience a temporary setback, which responds to encouragement (whereas clinical depression often responds to antidepressants). Patients with grief often have an existential experience of loss, which can respond to counseling. The important point is that the clinician should not consider sadness in a cancer patient to be "normal" but rather should explore why the person is sad. In the case of loss and demoralization, there are often clear-cut antecedents. Either of these problems may also progress to clinical depression, but when they do not, patients often benefit from careful listening and empathy.

Purposes of Communication

As discussed in the preceding section, "Communication as a Skill To Be Learned and Taught," communication is a way to convey information, and the way that this information is conveyed can profoundly affect patients' emotional status and the way that they cope. However, communication also has a number of other purposes that are crucial in the treatment of cancer patients and their families. Table 3–6 lists some of the positive outcomes associated with improved clinician communication.

Establishing Rapport With Patient and Family

Trust on the part of the patient and family is essential in allowing the patient to feel comfortable with the care provided by health practitioners. Trust also can inspire hope at a time when optimism may be in short supply. In oncology, establishing rapport is particularly important because of the invasive procedures often necessary to make a diagnosis or assessment; the prolonged nature of treatment, which can often be very harsh; and the dependence that patients have on doctors, especially at the end of life. Patients and families need to be sure that cancer practitioners care about them, have their best interests at heart, and will not abandon them when the disease progresses. Patients can often be very sensitive regarding the latter issue. Clini-

TABLE 3–6.   Outcomes associated with communication skills

Outcome	References
Increased satisfaction with medical care and improved information retention	(Coleman et al. 2002; Haskard et al. 2008; Shilling et al. 2003)
Reduced malpractice litigation	(Ambady et al. 2002; Levinson et al. 1997; Meruelo 2008)
Improved clinical trial accrual	(Albrecht 1999; Ruckdeschel 1996)
Decreased likelihood that patients may receive unnecessary medical treatment toward the end of life	(Emanuel 2002; Jirillo 2002; Wright 2008)
Reduced provider burnout under the stress of diminished resources	(Girgis 2009; Ramirez 1995)
Increased physician competence in discussing difficult topics such as transitioning patient to noncurative treatments	(Back and Arnold 2006a, 2006b; Baile et al. 1998; Fallowfield et al. 2002; Lenzi et al. 2010)
Enhanced teamwork among members of oncology patient care teams	(Catt et al. 2005)
Improved feeling of support by patients in times of crises caused by cancer	(Baile 2008; Zachariae et al. 2003)

cians sometimes underestimate the importance of patients' desires for a personal but professional relationship with their doctor.

Communication studies (Greisinger et al. 1997; Morse et al. 2008; National Cancer Institute 2012) demonstrate that cancer clinicians unfortunately spend most patient visits dominating the time with a discussion of the technical aspects of care rather than eliciting patient concerns and preoccupations. Therefore, patients often hold back from discussing important aspects of their care, such as the experience of side effects, worries about the impact of the disease on family members, and concerns about how to talk to their children about their disease. There is a strongly held belief on the part of cancer providers, which in our opinion is a myth, that asking patients about their concerns will open a Pandora's box of complaints on the part of the patient. Although this may be true in rare cases, most patients understand that their doctors and health care providers are busy and make an effort to respect their time. Having a personal relationship with a patient is often misconstrued as giving hugs or being friends with a patient. The doctor's emotions play an important part in the relationship with the patient and family, especially at the time when bad news is given. At such moments, a provider may feel sad, helpless, or even a failure. Avoidance of these feelings can be a major source of burnout and can affect the patient negatively.

Case Vignette

Gloria, age 24, had been fighting acute leukemia for several years. Over the past 3 months, she had done quite poorly and was admitted to the hospital several times with sepsis and other complications. It was now apparent that she had little time left to live. She had become quite attached to her clinic doctor, Dr. Mays, and although she had asked to see him several times, he had avoided coming to see her, always creating an excuse. Underneath this façade of disinterest and insensitivity, however, were feelings of helplessness and ineffectiveness on his part. In fact, Dr. Mays almost never went to see his patients near the end of life because he felt so bad. In a moment of frankness, he confessed to a nurse, "I just wouldn't know what to say."

For the patient, having a guiding hand at times during the illness is crucial. For the clinician, being able to allay patient and family fears via behaviors such as asking patients or family members what they are most worried about will often provide information that the provider can address with additional information or, for individuals with spiritual concerns, referral to chaplaincy services. Table 3–2, earlier in the chapter, provides some guidance as to those interpersonal skills that patients most value in their doctor.

Gathering and Transmitting Information

Taking a medical history is important not only in helping to diagnose a disease but also for putting the disease in the context of the patient's life. Cancer in a young woman without children may evoke a very different kind of reaction than in an older woman who has already borne children. Important information can be gathered about the patient's current coping, previous coping, and concerns about treatment.

Dealing With Emotions That Come Up During Cancer Treatments

Cancer evokes fear of death and suffering and is an illness in which losses are common. In addition to the potential for loss of life, patients may face loss of security about the future, loss of body parts, loss of connections with friends and family, and economic losses. Responding to patients' and families' emotions is a challenge for many practitioners, but demonstrating empathy for the patients' feelings can be a powerful source of support. The concept of empathy, however, is often a confusing one for health care providers, who often assume that empathy means to put oneself in the shoes of the other person and to actually experience the emotions that the other person is experiencing. This level of empathy is not possible because it would require the clinician to actually *become* the other person.

Perhaps it is more useful to think of empathy as a process that involves several different steps. The first is to recognize when another person is experiencing an emotion. This requires a certain vigilance and acceptance of the primacy of addressing emotions in the clinical encounter. The clinician not only must believe that acknowledging emotions can deepen the relationship with the patient by helping him or her to feel supported, but also must understand that emotions represent a roadblock to patient comprehension in that when a patient is in an emotional state, he or she will have difficulty hearing what the clinician has to say. For example, a common observation is that when clinicians give bad news to patients, many patients fail to grasp much of the dialogue or explanation that ensues. One reason for this is that because the patient's emotional brain is so activated, the area of the brain that is involved in processing information, the executive area in the prefrontal and frontal cortex, is shut down. By acknowledging emotions, the clinician helps to decrease their intensity, and then the executive area of the brain can begin to process information.

We mentioned that the first step in acknowledging emotion is to detect that an emotion is present. If, after hearing bad news, a patient puts head in hands and says, "Oh no," the cancer practitioner can be pretty sure that the patient's emotional brain is lit up. The second step is for the clinician to acknowledge to the patient that he or she has seen that the patient is upset. This is usually done with what is called an empathic response, such as "I can see that this really took you by surprise" (Table 3–7).

The purpose of the empathic response is to provide patients with support by "aligning" with them, which allows them to feel less isolated and alone. When going through an emotional experience, a person is likely to feel more comforted when someone acknowledges that what the person is going through is awful, rather than claim to understand (one can never completely understand another's feelings, and saying one does sounds condescending). Other, often ineffective ways of responding to emotions include using phrases or communication strategies such as saying, "Things are going to get better" (because nobody can know that for a fact), immediately offering advice (because most people want compassion first, and then perhaps advice), or telling about a similar experience (because the patient who is suffering likely does not want to hear about someone else). In fact, these are ways that clinicians often do ineffectively respond to patient emotions.

TABLE 3–7. Making empathic responses to emotion

Objectives: to acknowledge feelings and to prevent them from escalating; to demonstrate being "tuned into" patient or family

---

Family member (feels) says:	Clinician can say:
(Defeated) "I just don't know how I'm going to do this alone."	"It sounds like it's been pretty rough."
(Sad) "We were expecting a better result…"	"So was I. I know this comes as a shock…"
(Stunned) "You mean he needs more surgery?"	"I know you weren't expecting to hear this…"
(Angry) "No one told us that he'd be so tired!"	"It can be very frustrating."
(Happy) "It's so great to have a normal scan."	"I can see I've made your day."

Tables 3–8 and 3–9 describe several other, potentially more effective, ways that clinicians can use to respond to patients' and families' emotions.

TABLE 3–8. Responding to emotions: exploring the emotional "subtext" behind the question or statement

---

Objective: to clarify what patient or family is implying, feeling, or asking when it is not obviously clear

---

Family member says:	Clinician can say:
"Tell me, what will the end be like for her?"	"What has been worrying you?"
"I feel like I'm not doing enough for her…"	"Enough?"
"He's just not going to take any more chemo…"	"Tell me more about it…"
"Don't tell my father about the recurrence. He can't take it."	"Can you tell me what you think might happen?"

TABLE 3–9.　Making validating responses to emotion

Objective: to legitimize the patient's thoughts or feeling

Patient says:	Clinician can say:
"I'm really undecided whether to risk another surgery."	"A lot of patients struggle with the same decision…"
"I feel guilty about putting my family through this again."	"That's something I often hear from patients."
"Those steroids can really make me feel wired."	"They are known to do that."

Helping Patients Make Decisions About Treatment

The diagnosis of cancer places an enormous challenge on patients to understand complex treatments that may or may not be successful, to learn a new vocabulary having to do with their cancer and its treatment, and to understand the prognosis of the illness and the probability that any treatment will be successful. Cancer treatments all come with a cost. Patients who understand what these consequences are may be in a better position to make care-related choices that are consistent with their values and beliefs.

Helping Patients and Families Cope With Disease

Communication can be therapeutic in helping the family adapt to the illness and feel supported during the illness crisis. A study by Zachariae et al. (2003) illustrates the importance of two simple communication tasks—listening to the patient without interrupting, and expressing empathy—on patient perception of support. In this study, both behaviors were correlated with patient satisfaction about the interpersonal aspects of care, and patients were more satisfied with the medical management, more confident in their ability to manage their disease, and more likely to perceive their practitioner as caring. A study by Parle and colleagues (1996), on the other hand, illustrates how patient concerns that are not addressed can be a prelude to subsequent anxiety and depression.

Key Communication Skills for Routine Encounters With Patients and Families

Recognizing That a Little Bit of Caring Can Go a Long Way

As mentioned in the earlier section "Communication Skills," cancer patients are often vulnerable due to the loss of self-esteem, uncertainty about the future, and anxiety. Treating the patient with positive regard can acknowledge the fact that there is a person behind the disease. Taking a personal history can give a message to the patient that he or she is valued as an individual, as well as establish a unique connection with the clinician on a human rather than a medical level. Patients often have fascinating stories about their lives that can serve as humanistic bridges in the caregiving process. Being polite, respectful, and receptive to questions can enhance rapport and convey a sense of caring.

Realizing That First Impressions Count

When patients are filled with anxiety and uncertainty, certain clinician behaviors may have an untoward effect on first impressions. If a clinician is multitasking or ignoring the patient while typing on the computer, is not giving him or her space to ask questions, or is blunt in communicating bad news, the clinician may be taking a poor initial step in gaining the patient's trust. A good way of launching a collaborative relationship is to be friendly and listen carefully.

Asking Before Telling

Before giving information, it is important for the clinician to understand what the patient already knows or understands about his or her disease. This is particularly true if the patient has previously seen other practitioners about the cancer. Having this knowledge will allow the clinician to correct misperceptions or deal with patient or family denial or unrealistic expectations.

Dealing With Emotions Before Facts

As mentioned previously, attempting to provide information to a patient who is tearful, angry, or confused is usually fruitless. The executive functions of the frontal lobe, which process information and are involved in decision making, are effectively excluded when the limbic lobe/amygdala part of the brain is activated. The concept of "amygdala hijacking," based on the work of LeDoux (1996) and applied to interpersonal relationships by Goleman (1995), helps explain this phenomenon. Thus, when patients do not remember what they have been told, it is not merely a question of psychological "denial" or not wanting to hear the facts but a true neuroanatomical barrier by which the presence of emotion impedes the processing of new information. Therefore addressing emotions to lower their intensity can restore the patient's ability to reason and make decisions.

Watching Out for "Amygdala Hijacking"

Clinicians need to pay attention to their own emotional activation to be able to more effectively respond to the patient and family. For the clinician, speaking when upset, angry, or experiencing great sympathy for the patient can often cause regret later. A good example of this is when the provider attempts to "undo" a patient's emotional reaction to bad news by reassuring the patient that the situation is not all that bad.

Making "Wish" Statements

Wish statements allow practitioners to align with the patient while still promoting a realistic assessment of the situation. For example, after hearing that there is no further chemotherapy that can be helpful, a patient may respond, "Isn't there anything more you can do?" By responding "I wish there were," the clinician aligns with the patient's desire but simultaneously defines reality.

Reflecting on Intention

Communication often has a subtext, and the clinician is often faced with determining whether there is a question behind the question or a reason (that may be unclear) why a patient might be upset. Attention to a deeper meaning of communication is required to understand, for example, that a patient who asks, "How long do I have to live?" really means, "Will I get to see my daughter marry?"

Giving the Patient Time to Absorb Information Before Intervening Verbally

When patients get upset, clinicians do not need to respond right away. Sometimes, being quietly present is sufficient to allow the emotion to pass. Although clinicians often find this silence difficult because they experience an urgency to help patients by making them feel better, waiting for patients to respond will allow them to take the lead in asking for information that means most to them instead of the clinician imposing an agenda on the subsequent discussion. Thus, when a patient is emotional, using an empathic response or just waiting until they finish emoting will usually result in their asking for additional information.

Communication Challenges in the Clinical Setting

Communicating Bad News

SPIKES is an acronym given to a series of steps for giving bad news (Table 3–10). It was originally developed by Dr. Robert Buckman and was elaborated on for cancer patients by the present chapter's first author, Dr. Walter Baile. SPIKES is widely accepted as a useful guide for getting through a conversation in which a clinician needs to discuss a cancer diagnosis, prognosis, disease recurrence, or end-of-life issues. Although it has not been empirically tested in a clinical trial, SPIKES also reflects the general wishes of patients as to how they would want bad news given to them if they were diagnosed with cancer (Parker et al. 2001).

Dealing With Families Who Want to Block Provision of Information to the Patient

Some families want to "protect" the patient from knowledge of the illness. Though more common in some cultures than others, this desire can be seen in any culture. In these situations, the best advice for clinicians is to 1) ask family members to explain their concerns and 2) ask them what they think the loved one already knows.

In many instances, when asked to explain their concerns, the family will report fear that their loved one might not be able to handle the news. Some patients have a preexisting coping problem or emotional illness, and some families are afraid that they will not know how to handle the patient's distress (which may or may not materialize). In any case, the clinician should listen carefully to the family and empathize with their fears.

In many cases, asking what the loved one already knows will reveal what the family believes the patient knows. Asking this question often leads to a proposal to ask the patient (with the family present) what the patient already knows and wants to know. In fact, the clinician can propose to the family that if the patient does not want to know, then his or her wishes will be respected. This type of approach—to ask, listen, tell, and negotiate—often is successful in getting the family on the clinician's side.

TABLE 3–10. The SPIKES protocol

S	Get the Setting right. Try not to have conversations in the hallway but ensure privacy and give yourself enough time. Have a plan of action, especially reviewing how to deal with emotional reactions to the bad news. Bring someone with you for support if necessary (e.g., nurse or social worker).
P	Perception. Inquire as to what the patient already knows about the disease, and the reason you did testing (e.g., if you were suspecting disease progression).
I	Invitation. Ask if the patient is ready to hear bad news. Set goals for the interview (e.g., "I'd like to go over the results of your CT. Is this OK?").
K	Knowledge. Give the information in small chunks, checking periodically for patient understanding. Try to avoid medical jargon. Do not initiate a 5-minute monologue.
E	Emotions. Respond to all emotions before giving any further facts.
S	Strategy and summary. Make a plan with the patient. Ask the patient to repeat back to you what he or she understood. If you can, dictate a note that the patient can use to know what is next.

Source: Adapted from Baile WF, Buckman R, Lenzi R, et al.: "SPIKES—A Six-Step Protocol for Delivering Bad News: Application to the Patient With Cancer." *Oncologist* 5:302–311, 2000.

Responding to Difficult Questions

Patients often do not directly express their worries and concerns because they have not formulated them clearly to themselves or because they may expect to be told their concerns are foolish or trivial. They may not want to bother doctors or take up their time or are afraid that a concern, especially about a side effect, may lead to further testing or the stopping of treatment. Although it may be tempting to respond to a question such as "How long do I have to live?" by giving statistics or saying, "No one knows," it is more useful to use an exploratory question, such as "I would be happy to try and give you an answer, but could you first let me know what makes you bring that up at this point?" Often, behind the question lies a concern, such as whether the patient will be able to attend a grandson's wedding or whether the individual should be thinking about making a will. Understanding the patient's concern can help the provider frame the response according to the patient's concern. "Tell me more" is a powerful phrase to have available when a patient asks a vague or difficult question.

Case Vignette

Bob was a 56-year-old man with a diagnosis of Stage IIIb non–small cell lung cancer. He had completed four courses of chemotherapy with some reduction in the size of his tumor, but his prognosis was very guarded. On a visit to his oncologist, Bob asked, "Doc, am I going to make it?" Dr. Walker was about to offer some words of encouragement, such as "Let's try and be hopeful." However, he stopped himself and decided that he needed to know more about what Bob meant, so instead he said, "I'd be happy to talk more about that, but first let me ask why you bring that question up now." Bob then went on to explain that he and his wife had an option to buy a condominium in a ski area. They would have to take out a mortgage, which would mean that Bob would have to go back to work. Given the grave prognosis, Dr. Walker explained that Bob had a serious disease and it was not clear if he would respond to treatment and be able to go back to work. He advised Bob that it might be wise for him to put off the purchase of the condo until it was clear whether he would be able to go back to work.

Responding to Demoralization

When patients appear down, they may be demoralized rather than depressed. Often, they have a concern they are not discussing, have received bad news about their illness, or are frustrated about the course of their treatment. Making a simple observation, such as "You look a bit down today," may provide very useful information about a patient's concern. Just listening to concerns can be a powerful source of support for patients.

Dealing With Emotions

Although the topic of dealing with emotions has been covered in several previous sections of this chapter, it bears repeating. Patients who are under stress and who are faced with losses, anxiety about the future, and feelings of loss of control are often prone to emotions such as anger, sadness, and denial. In most cases, emotions are due to underlying concerns. Providers often miss emotional cues or to try to "fix" emotions with expressions of reassurance. However, responding to a worried patient who asks, "How am I going to tell my children?" with advice such as "Just give it some time" is not effective. Instead, exploring patient concerns by using the phrase "Tell me more about what you are concerned about" will often provide the clinician with more specific and useful information.

Case Vignette

Henry's wife was hospitalized for graft versus host disease affecting her small intestine. She was ill and vomiting and could not eat. After 10 days she became demoralized and withdrawn. Henry became upset at the lack of progress, and when the primary care team came around, he expressed his anger, stating, "Maybe I should just take her to another hospital." The attending physician, recognizing Henry's frustration, responded empathically, "It has been really hard for us to get this under control, and I know for you it has been difficult to stand on the sidelines and watch her not get better." Henry was able to acknowledge his helplessness and fear for his wife's life.

For the clinician, it is important to resist the desire to try and fix the patient's emotion by prematurely offering reassurance that "things are going to go fine," which may be totally untrue. Instead, acknowledging (empathizing), validating, and exploring emotions will tend to lower them and allow the patient to talk about what is truly on his or her mind. Some good examples of appropriate responses are given in Tables 3–7 to 3–9. To develop competency at responding to emotions, the clinician must make an effort not to respond emotionally to a patient's or family's emotions (see earlier subsection "Watching Out for 'Amygdala Hijacking'").

Advocating for the Patient

Mental health clinicians, nurses, social workers, or other caregivers often end up "picking up the pieces" after a patient receives bad news from a physician. Sometimes, these professionals must provide emotional support to the patient. At other times, the patient has important questions or is lacking information that the attending physician did not provide. In this case, the supportive caregiver may not be able to answer a question about the prognosis or other important piece of medical information and may need to advocate for the patient with the primary team. One useful way of approaching an attending physician in such a case is to use SPIKES RN (Table 3–11).

Recognizing Communication Issues

Very often, what appear to be ethical issues are actually issues of communication. For example, family members who demand that "everything be done" may not have accurate information about the patient's illness. Families who request that a patient not be told about the disease may be fearful of their loved one's emotional response. Patients who want to pick and choose their own treatments may have had friends, relatives, and loved ones who responded poorly to a treatment offered them. In any case, exploring the situation with the patient (e.g., by saying, "Tell me more about why you want treatment A over treatment B") can go a long way toward resolving this type of dilemma.

Assessing Patient Preferences About Family Involvement

Patients should be consulted about which family members or friends they would like to have involved in their care. This will help prevent confusion

TABLE 3–11.   SPIKES RN

S   Setting. Approach the physician and ask for permission to discuss a patient's concern. Select a time when the attending physician does not seem overwhelmed by other tasks. Be friendly but serious. Indicate that you have something serious to talk about. "Do you have a minute? I have something important that I'd like to let you know about Mr. Brown."

P   Perception. Find out if the physician was aware that the patient had important questions. This line of questioning lets the physician off the hook by allowing him or her to be surprised that the patient has questions instead of implying that the physician neglected to inform the patient. "Were you aware that Mr. Brown had some important questions about his treatment?"

I   Invitation. Extend an invitation to discuss a plan for interaction. "Would it be OK if I discussed these with you for a minute?"

K   Knowledge. Explain the interaction. "Well, Mr. Brown is really worried about his wife, who is home sick, and he wonders how long he is going to have to stay here for treatment."

E   Emotions. Respond to the doctor's emotions. "I'm sure you already discussed that with Mr. Brown; however, I don't think he heard anything after the bad news."

S   Strategy. Present a strategy for meeting together with the patient. "When you have time, could we go in together so I could reinforce what you have to say when I talk to him later?"

Source: Adapted from Baile WF: "S-P-I-K-E-S RN: A Quick Reference Guide for Nurses." Houston, University of Texas MD Anderson Cancer Center, February 19, 2013; and Orlovsky G: "Workshops Train Providers to Deliver Bad News, Difficult Discussions." 2006. Available at: http://www.nursezone.com. Accessed August 16, 2012.

when other people arrive on the scene and attempt to take over patient care. Because many visitors may arrive at the hospital or clinic during the initial phase of treatment, having discussed this issue with the patient helps providers understand with whom they may share information about the patient's condition as well as which individuals should be excluded.

Giving Hope

Practitioners are often reluctant to talk about bad news, especially when the prognosis is poor. This attitude can lead to incomplete information being given to patients and can have a negative impact on their coping. Most patients and families desire complete information about the cancer even if the news is negative; however, some patients may shun information or want family members but not themselves to be provided with details. Balancing the patient's right to know with providing hope can be very tricky at times. If a patient has a poor prognosis at the time of diagnosis, it may be misleading to be overly optimistic about the chances of a cure. One way of addressing this issue is with a "hope for the best and prepare for the worst" approach. In other words, the clinician assures the patient that he or she is going to get the best treatment available but that the cancer is a very difficult one to treat. Although this sort of "warning shot" approach may not work for every patient, the literature suggests that it meets the information needs of most patients (Back et al. 2003). A second strategy may be to let the patient know that the cancer is not curable but that the goal of care is to contain the cancer. When cure is not possible, the clinician can also explore the patient's other hopes and expectations, such as by asking, "If we cannot cure your cancer, what else is important to you?" This is a particularly useful strategy near the end of life when a number of cancer treatments have not worked. When a clinician decides to discuss prognosis, the patient has a good idea about the probability of the treatment's success. Then the patient can share in the decision-making process, balancing his or her values and desire for a quality life against the side effects of the treatments, which can sometimes be considerable. Maintaining the attitude of "preparing for the worst while hoping for the best" and providing reassurance that the patient will get the best treatment available and not be abandoned, no matter how severe the disease, are excellent ways of encouraging hope (Sardell and Trierweiller 1993).

Considering Cultural Issues

Understanding the impact of culture on treatment choice, decision making, and coping is an important component in today's pluralistic society. A cultural history might include the topics outlined in Table 3–12.

Working With the Oncology Team

Teamwork has become more and more important as cancer care becomes more complex, hospital stays decrease, and patient safety issues evolve. Particularly in specialties such as palliative care, teamwork serves to address the complex psychosocial issues that can emerge in advanced disease. The following are some important considerations about teams in medicine:

- Teams function better when each member knows the roles of other members.
- The attitude that "no one can do it alone" helps cultivate a culture of shared responsibility for patient problems.

TABLE 3–12.	BALANCE: seven areas to cover in taking a cultural history
B	Beliefs and values that influence perceptions of illness and the patient's and family's definition of a life worth living. For example, patients/ families may have different ideas about the causes of cancer.
A	Ambiance (living situation and family structure)
L	Language and health literacy (role of interpreters, accuracy of translation, metaphoric meanings, as well as understanding of the medical condition and treatment protocols)
A	Affiliations (community ties, religious and spiritual beliefs)
N	Network (social support system)
C	Challenges (of work environment)
E	Economy (socioeconomic status and community resources)

Source. Adapted from Surbone A, Kawaga-Singer M, Baile WF: "BALANCE: A Guide for Addressing Cultural Sensitivity." Unpublished manuscript, September 2011.

- Teams must focus on communication among team members to be effective.
- Disagreement among team members is not necessarily a sign of dysfunction but instead is a healthy questioning of decisions.

Teaching and Learning Communications Skills

Good communicators are made and not born. Many clinicians and providers have good "bedside manners"—that is, they have good basic or first-order skills, such as listening without interrupting and being polite with the patient and family; however, good communication requires much more. Higher-order skills—including the ability to give bad news, discuss prognosis, and respond to difficult questions such as "Are you going to give up on me?"—are best learned through skills practice. As mentioned earlier in "Communication Skills," studies show that learning and then practicing skills in standardized patient encounters lead to significant change in the communication behaviors of those attending workshops (Fallowfield et al. 2003). Other modalities, such as virtual reality, videotaping clinical encounters and reviewing them with a coach, and sociodrama have been used to improve communication skills (Baile and Walters 2012).

Conclusion

Communication is both an art and a science. Sensitivity to the patients' and family members' attitudes, feelings, and concerns needs to be balanced with the use of key skills, such as listening effectively, being empathic, and managing one's own emotions. In all our years of working in the field of oncology, we have observed that when physicians are caring and skillful in their interactions with patients and family members, they are rarely blamed for therapeutic failure. On the other hand, poor communication can rob the clinician of a relationship that can otherwise be the "icing on the cake" of a successful medical outcome.

Key Clinical Points

- Clinicians' manner of communicating with cancer patients can have profound effects on the patients' mood and coping.

- Good communication requires more than just a "bedside manner." It is a set of defined verbal and nonverbal behaviors that can be taught and learned.

- Effective communication helps to establish rapport, helps patients and families cope with the disease, and assists them with making informed decisions.

- Eliciting patients' and families' concerns is supportive and can be therapeutic. It is also an aid to truthful communication, which in turn can establish trust.

- The many communications challenges in a clinical setting include communicating bad news, responding to difficult questions, dealing with patients' and families' emotions such as fear and discouragement, considering cultural issues, working with the oncology team, and giving patients and families hope.

Suggested Readings

Back A, Arnold R, Tulsky J: Mastering Communication With Seriously Ill Patients: Balancing Honesty With Empathy and Hope. New York, Cambridge University Press, 2009

Clayton JM, Hancock KM, Butow PN, et al: Clinical practice guidelines for communicating prognosis and end-of-life issues with adults in the advanced stages of a life-limiting illness, and their caregivers. Med J

Aust 186(suppl):S77–S108. Available at: http://www.mja.com.au/public/issues/186_12_180607/cla11246_fm.html. Accessed August 16, 2012.

Kissane DW, Bultz BD, Butow PM, et al (eds): Handbook of Communication in Oncology and Palliative Care. New York, Oxford University Press, 2010

Loprinzi CL (ed): Art of Oncology: Honest and Compassionate Responses to the Daily Struggles of People Living With Cancer, Vols 1 and 2. Alexandria, VA, American Society of Clinical Oncology, 2010

Rodin G, Zimmermann C, Mayer C, et al: Clinician-patient communication: evidence-based recommendations to guide practice in cancer. Curr Oncol 16:42–49, 2009. Available at: http://ukpmc.ac.uk/articles/PMC2794681. Accessed August 16, 2012.

Web-Based Resources for Effective Communication

Australian Government, National Health and Medical Research Council: Psychosocial Clinical Practice Guidelines: Information, Support and Counselling for Women with Breast Cancer. A toolkit of essential communication skills to help patients make informed decisions about their cancer care.
    http://www.nhmrc.gov.au/_files_nhmrc/publications/attachments/hpr25_0.pdf

Cancer Australia: Communication Skills. Specific communication modules for how to give bad news and other topics.
    http://canceraustralia.gov.au/clinical-best-practice/cancer-learning/communication-skills-training-0

Cancer Care Ontario: Joint Nursing, Palliative, and Psychosocial (NPPS) Collaborations Evidence-Based Series. Provider-patient communication guidelines for effective communication.
    http://www.cancercare.on.ca/toolbox/qualityguidelines/clin-program/jointcollab-ebs

Institute of Medicine of the National Academies: Assessing and Improving Value in Cancer Care: Workshop Summary. Summarizes 2009 workshop discussions and presentations, which focused on the goal of describing value in oncology.
    http://iom.edu/Reports/2009/Assessing-Improving-Value-Cancer-Care.aspx

Institute of Medicine of the National Academies: Ensuring Quality Cancer Care. The National Cancer Policy Board defines quality care and recommends how to monitor, measure, and extend quality care to all people with cancer. Approaches to accountability in health care are reviewed. http://iom.edu/Reports/1999/Ensuring-Quality-Cancer-Care.aspx

Institute of Medicine of the National Academies: From Cancer Patient to Cancer Survivor: Lost in Transition Recommends that each cancer patient receive a "survivorship care plan" that summarizes information critical to the individual's long-term care, such as the cancer diagnosis, treatment, and potential consequences; the timing and content of follow-up visits; tips on maintaining a healthy lifestyle and preventing recurrent or new cancers; legal rights affecting employment and insurance; and the availability of psychological and support services. http://iom.edu/Reports/2005/From-Cancer-Patient-to-Cancer-Survivor-Lost-in-Transition.aspx.

Institute of Medicine of the National Academies: Improving Palliative Care for Cancer. Examines the barriers—economic, policy, social, and scientific—that keep people from getting good palliative care, and proposes a series of steps that could improve this situation. http://iom.edu/Reports/2003/Improving-Palliative-Care-for-Cancer.aspx

Institute of Medicine of the National Academies: National Cancer Policy Forum. Summarizes 2011 workshop held to discuss ways to create a more coordinated, patient-centered cancer treatment planning process. http://www.iom.edu/Reports/2011/Patient-Centered-Cancer-Treatment-Planning-Improving-the-Quality-of-Oncology-Care.aspx. Accessed February 19, 2013.

International Confederation of Childhood Cancer Parent Organizations: Guidelines for the Communication of the Diagnosis, and Guidelines for Valid Informed Consent and Participative Decision Making http://icccpo.org

Journal of Clinical Oncology: Patient Communication. Displays list of articles about the topic of patient communication. http://jco.ascopubs.org/cgi/collection/aoo6

National Cancer Institute: Communication in Cancer Care (PDQ) http://www.cancer.gov/cancertopics/pdq/supportivecare/communication/patient/page1

National Cancer Institute: Patient-Centered Communication in Cancer Care: Promoting Healing and Reducing Suffering http://www.outcomes.cancer.gov/areas/pcc/communication/pcc_monograph.pdf

Oncotalk Teach. Videos illustrating approaches to difficult conversations in 11tients with serious illnesses. http://depts.washington.edu/oncotalk/videos

Palliative Care Curriculum for Undergraduates (PCC4U): Communication Skills in Palliative Care. A communication learning resource funded by the Australian Government. Covers topics of communication with people with life-threatening illnesses, including self-care strategies. http://www.pcc4u.org

The University of Texas MD Anderson Cancer Center: Interpersonal Communication And Relationship Enhancement: I*CARE. A compendium of videos illustrating skills for basic and difficult communications. http://www.mdanderson.org/icare

References

Albrecht TL, Blanchard C, Ruckdeschel JC, et al: Strategic physician communication and oncology clinical trials. J Clin Oncol 17:3324–3332, 1999

Ambady N, Laplante D, Nguyen T, et al: Surgeons' tone of voice: a clue to malpractice history. Surgery 132:5–9, 2002

American Institute for Cancer Research: Food, Nutrition, Physical Activity, and the Prevention of Cancer: A Global Perspective (Second Expert Report). 2007. Available at: http://www.dietandcancerreport.org/expert_report. Accessed February 19, 2013.

Back AL, Arnold RM: Discussing prognosis: "How much do you want to know?" Talking to patients who are prepared for explicit information. J Clin Oncol 24:4209–4213, 2006a

Back AL, Arnold RM: Discussing prognosis: "How much do you want to know?" Talking to patients who do not want information or who are ambivalent. J Clin Oncol 24:4214–4217, 2006

Back AL, Arnold RM, Quill TE: Hope for the best and prepare for the worst. Ann Intern Med 138:439–443, 2003

Back AL, Arnold RM, Baile WF, et al: Efficacy of communication skills training for giving bad news and discussing transitions to palliative care. Arch Intern Med 167:453–460, 2007

Baile WF: Alcohol and nicotine dependency in patients with head and neck cancer. J Support Oncol 6:165–166, 2008

Baile WF, Walters R: Applying sociodramatic methods in teaching transition to palliative care. J Pain Symptom Manage Aug 11, 2012 [Epub ahead of print]

Baile WF, Beale E, Baumbaugh M, et al: Communicating with cancer patients: format and outcomes of workshops for oncologists and oncology fellows. Patient Education and Counseling 34(suppl):S43–S44, 1998

Bedell SE, Graboys TB, Bedell E, et al: Words that harm, words that heal. Arch Intern Med 164:1365–1368, 2004

Catt S, Fallowfield L, Jenkins V, et al: The informational roles and psychological health of members of 10 oncology multidisciplinary teams in the UK. B J Cancer 93:1092–1097, 2005

Coleman EA, Hardin SM, Lord JE, et al: General characteristics and experiences of specialized standardized patients: breast teaching associate professionals. J Cancer Educ 17:121–123, 2002

Emanuel EJ, Ash A, Yu W, et al: Managed care, hospice use, site of death, and medical expenditures in the last year of life. Arch Intern Med 162:1722–1728, 2002

Epstein RM, Street RL: A framework for patient-centered communication in cancer care, in Patient-Centered Communication in Cancer Care (NIH Publ No 07-6225). Bethesda MD, National Cancer Institute, 2007, pp 17–38

Fallowfield L, Jenkins V, Farewell V, et al: Efficacy of a Cancer Research UK communication skills training model for oncologists: a randomised controlled trial. Lancet 359:650–656, 2002

Fallowfield L, Jenkins V, Farewell V, et al: Enduring impact of communication skills training: results of a 12-month follow-up. Br J Cancer 89:1445–1449, 2003

Gerretsen P, Myers J: The physician: a secure base. J Clin Oncol 26:5294–5296, 2008

Girgis A, Hansen V, Goldstein D: Are Australian oncology health professionals burning out? A view from the trenches. Eur J Cancer 45:393–399, 2009

Goleman D: Emotional Intelligence. New York, Bantam Books, 1995

Greisinger AJ, Lorimor RJ, Aday LA, et al: Terminally ill cancer patients: their most important concerns. Cancer Pract 5:147–154, 1997

Haskard KB, Williams SL, DiMatteo MR, et al: Physician and patient communication training in primary care: effects on participation and satisfaction. Health Psychol 27:513–522, 2008

Jirillo A, Boscaro M, Pasetto LM, et al: Chemotherapy at the end of life: an open question. Tumori 91:104–105, 2005

LeDoux J: The Emotional Brain. New York, Simon & Schuster, 1996

Lenzi R, Baile WF, Costantini A, et al: Communication training in oncology: results of intensive communication workshops for Italian oncologists. Eur J Cancer Care (Engl) 20:196–203, 2011

Levinson W, Roter DL, Mullooly JP, et al: Physician-patient communication: the relationship with malpractice claims among primary care physicians and surgeons. JAMA 277:553–559, 1997

McFarlane JJ, Riggins J, Smith TJ: SPIKE$: A six-step protocol for delivering bad news about the cost of medical care. J Clin Oncol 26:4200–4204, 2008

Meruelo NC: Mediation and medical malpractice: the need to understand why patients sue and a proposal for a specific model of mediation. J Legal Med 29:285–306, 2008

Morse DS, Edwardson EA, Gordon HS: Missed opportunities for interval empathy in lung cancer communication. Arch Intern Med 168:1853–1858, 2008

National Cancer Institute: PDQ Communications in Cancer Care. 2012. Available at: http://www.cancer.gov.cancertopics/pdq/supportivecare/communication/healthprofessional. Accessed February 12, 2013.

Parker PA, Baile WF, de Moor C, et al: Breaking bad news about cancer: patients' preferences for communication. J Clin Oncol 19:2049–2056, 2001

Parle M, Jones B, Maguire P: Maladaptive coping and affective disorders among cancer patients. Psychol Med 26:735–744, 1996

Philibert I: Simulation and rehearsal: practice makes perfect. ACGME Bulletin, December 2005. Available at: http://www.acgme.org/acwebsite/bulletin/bulletin12_05.pdf. Accessed July 22, 2012.

Ramirez AJ, Graham J, Richards MA, et al: Burnout and psychiatric disorder among cancer clinicians. Br J Cancer 71:1263–1269, 1995

Razavi D, Delvaux N, Marchal S, et al: Does training increase the use of more emotionally laden words by nurses when talking with cancer patients? A randomised study. Br J Cancer 87:1–7, 2002

Razavi D, Merckaert I, Marchal S, et al: How to optimize physicians' communication skills in cancer care: results of a randomized study assessing the usefulness of posttraining consolidation workshops. J Clin Oncol 21:3141–3149, 2003

Ruckdeschel JC, Albrecht TL, Blanchard C, et al: Communication, accrual to clinical trials, and the physician-patient relationship: implications for training programs. J Cancer Educ 11(2)73–79, 1996

Sardell AN, Trierweiller SJ: Disclosing the cancer diagnosis: procedures that influence patient hopefulness. Cancer 72:3355–3365, 1993

Shilling V, Jenkins V, Fallowfield L: Factors affecting patient and clinician satisfaction with the clinical consultation: can communication skills training for clinicians improve satisfaction? Psychooncology 12:599–611, 2003

Sivesind D, Parker PA, Cohen L, et al: Communicating with patients in cancer care: what areas do nurses find most challenging? J Cancer Educ 18:202–209, 2003

Wright AA, Zhang B, Ray A, et al: Associations between end-of-life discussions, patient mental health, medical care near death, and caregiver bereavement adjustment. JAMA 300:1665–1673, 2008

Zachariae CG, Pedersen AB, Jensen E, et al: Association of perceived physician communication style with patient satisfaction, distress, cancer-related self-efficacy, and perceived control over the disease. Br J Cancer 88:658–665, 2003

CHAPTER 4

Demoralization and Depression in Cancer

David W. Kissane, M.D.
Matthew Doolittle, M.D.

PSYCHIATRISTS SEEM to have little to say about existential distress, based on the relative dearth of psychological literature on the phenomenon of loss of meaning and its resolution at various phases of the life cycle, including the end of life. A typology of existential distress, such as that shown in Table 4–1, is much needed to better understand the diverse coping responses found in the clinical settings of oncology and palliative care. In this chapter, we focus on two intertwined but distinguishable phenomena: depression and demoralization. Depression is an identifiable set of perceptions and experiences subject to screening and management. The discussion of depression is instrumental: what actions to take or not to take and what strategies to deploy or not to deploy in the interest of solving a problem that has already emerged. The discussion of demoralization is observational: what stories to hear and what morals to perceive so that the ruptured threads of the sufferer's life can be woven back together in a pattern that is coherent even if the mend is highly conspicuous.

Depression

Cancer is never planned. Even patients who have been aware of family risk, or have taken care of loved ones with cancer, or have been convinced for weeks that surely their symptoms represent cancer, are nonetheless shocked by the diagnosis. Every diagnosis begins with a set of unexpected demands.

TABLE 4–1.   Typology of existential distress

Challenge	Features of adaptation	Type of distress	Common symptoms	Related disorders
Death	Courage and awareness of dying	Death anxiety	Fear of process of dying or state of being dead; panic and dread; struggle with uncertainty	Anxiety disorder Panic disorder Agoraphobia Generalized anxiety Acute stress disorder Adjustment with anxiety
Loss and change	Adaptive grief	Sense of unfairness; nonacceptance of disability and disfigurement; chronic sadness and distress	Intense tearfulness, sadness, anger, waves of emotionality; potential to progress into depressed mood, anhedonia, insomnia, social withdrawal; chronic sadness and discontent	Adjustment disorders Complicated grief Depressive disorders
Meaning	Sense of fulfillment and accomplishment in life; contentment	Loss of purpose and meaning	Pointlessness, meaninglessness, and hopelessness about the futility of the future; loss of role; helplessness; pessimism; desire to die	Demoralization syndrome Depressive disorders

TABLE 4–1.	Typology of existential distress *(continued)*			
Challenge	Features of adaptation	Type of distress	Common symptoms	Related disorders
Aloneness	Secure attachments, supported by family and friends	Existential aloneness	Isolated, alienated, and sense of complete aloneness in life; family conflict, separations	Dysfunctional family Marital or relationship problems Absence of social support
Freedom	Acceptance of frailty and reduced independence	Loss of control; fear of being a burden	Angst at loss of control over life; need for obsessional mastery; trouble with decision making; unrealistic choices and treatment compliance problems; fear of dependency on others	Obsessive-compulsive disorder Substance use disorders
Personhood	Sense of dignity and worth	Loss of self-worth	Horrified, angered, or distressed by illness or handicap; shame; body image concerns; worthlessness	Adjustment disorders Depressive disorders
Mystery	Awe, wonderment, and reverence for nature and life; transcendent spiritual peace	Spiritual doubt and distress	Loss of faith; fear of future and punishment by higher power; guilt and shame; distress	Anxiety disorders Adjustment disorders Depressive disorders

The first is that the patient remembers the details of the diagnosis and starts to think about a medical plan, even though most patients retain very little in the moments after the word *cancer* is first used. Subsequent demands include telling the family, scheduling visits, arranging time away from work or children, arranging transportation, signing forms, and acknowledging receipt and understanding, over and over, of things patients never wished to receive or understand. Later, the patient may be expected to tolerate pain, nausea or vomiting, fatigue, and treatments that are damaging to the healthy body as well as the cancer. The burden of cancer becomes clear.

For much of the time, most patients are able to adapt, and to negotiate a new way of living and a new set of relationships with family or friends and with doctors who are intimate strangers. Mostly, patients start living with expectations for a life that is different in visible and invisible ways from whatever came before. Grief, fear, sleep deprivation, loneliness, boredom, pain in the body, and medications that alter neurotransmitters or hormones can all affect the patient until the person's emotional and physical ability to negotiate the ongoing shock of cancer is no longer adequate to the task. Patients can develop a profound sadness or pervasive guilt, accompanied by less ability to take in new and complex information, less ability to manage a schedule or tolerate the symptoms or humiliations of serious disease, less ability to take pleasure even when free of the symptoms of disease, less interest in people around them, and less belief in the things of life they used to cherish. A significant proportion of cancer patients have these experiences during their treatment or recovery, and when they interfere with the patient's ability to function, they are known as depression.

Depression is associated not only with loss of quality of life, but also with decreased ability and desire to adhere to treatment, with increased length of hospital stay, with thoughts of suicide, and even with worsened outcome of cancer treatment (Grassi et al. 2005). Those individuals with a personal or family history of depression are at even greater risk.

Depression as a Cause of Cancer

The stresses of cancer are so great that it is not difficult to understand why depression is common among cancer patients, regardless of previous risk; however, the direction of causality was not always so well established. A number of studies explored the relationship between depression and onset of cancer. Older and methodologically limited studies, such as a 20-year follow-up on Minnesota Multiphasic Personality Inventory (MMPI) testing, suggested a twofold increase in cancer development for people who were depressed (Persky et al. 1987). A series of subsequent studies with solid epidemiological methodology refuted this report (Hahn and Petitti 1988;

Kaplan and Reynolds 1988; Zonderman et al. 1989) and showed that depression is not associated with an increased rate of cancer in the general population (Sihvo et al. 2010). Similarly, life events such as bereavement do not cause cancer (Ewertz 1986), and stress itself is no longer considered a cause of cancer (Li et al. 2002).

Depression, however, is associated with a higher risk for obesity in women, exemplified in the third National Health and Nutrition Examination Survey with an odds ratio of 1.82 (95% CI, 1.01–3.3) (Onyike et al. 2003), and obesity in turn has a clear relationship with increases in endometrial and breast cancer through estrogenic mechanisms (Kulie et al. 2011). This association between depression, obesity, and cancer is less consistent in men. Similarly, depression is associated with smoking and alcoholism (Azevedo et al. 2010; Graham et al. 2007), both of which, especially heavy smoking (Murphy et al. 2010), have in turn been associated with increased incidence of cancer. Thus, comorbidities associated with depression, including obesity, smoking, physical inactivity (Chwastiak et al. 2011), and alcohol use, do increase risk for malignancies.

Depression as a Consequence of Cancer

There are many comprehensible reasons why depression develops as a consequence of cancer, including the biology of cancer and its treatment, the psychological impact with its existential threat, and the social changes altering lifestyle and opportunity. Evidence also indicates that untreated depression is associated with shorter cancer survival, particularly once cancer has recurred. Patients who are helpless, hopeless, depressed (Temoshok et al. 1985; Watson et al. 1999, 2005), socially alienated (Goodkin et al. 1986), and socially deprived (Boesen et al. 2007) have all been shown to have shorter cancer survival times. Some work also suggests that fatalistic and stoic attitudes may handicap survival (Pettingale et al. 1985; Temoshok et al. 1985). It is clear that psycho-oncology has a role in promoting coping, treating depression, and ensuring that cancer patients are connected to supports. Whether group therapy is able to improve survival substantially remains contentious, but in one study it was shown to prevent the development of depression (Kissane et al. 2007).

An important consequence of untreated depression is its impact on cancer treatment adherence (DiMatteo et al. 2000). In a meta-analytic study by DiMatteo and colleagues, the odds were reported to be three times greater that depressed patients would be nonadherent to their medical treatment recommendations than nondepressed patients (DiMatteo and Hanskard-Zolnierek 2011). Depression can interfere with adherence via cognitive, motivational, and resource-related pathways (see Table 4–2).

TABLE 4–2.   Associations between depression and adherence

Reduced capacity to understand diagnosis and treatment

Difficulty planning attendance for anticancer treatments

Decreased motivation for self-care and healthy behaviors

Pessimism about treatment and its benefits

Greater difficulty tolerating treatment side effects

Social isolation and withdrawal; poorer family support

Limited use of community resources

Prevalence of Depressive Disorders

Prevalence rates for major depression in studies of cancer patients have ranged up to 38%, whereas rates for depression spectrum disorders have been as high as 58%, compared with rates of 6.6% for 12-month prevalence and 16.6% for lifetime prevalence in the general community (Massie 2004). In the classic Psychosocial Collaborative Oncology Group (PSYCOG) study, randomly sampled inpatient and outpatient oncology patients were shown to have a 47% rate of DSM-III psychiatric disorder, of which 13% demonstrated major depression and 68% an adjustment disorder (Derogatis et al. 1983; Mitchell et al. 2011; Wilson et al. 2007). Because only 11% of these patients had evidence of prior psychiatric diagnoses, most cases were considered a response to the cancer diagnosis. A more recent meta-analysis of 94 studies suggests that prevalence of depression spectrum disorders in the cancer care setting may be 38%, which seems to be comparable to rates found in a general palliative care setting (Mitchell et al. 2011). Perhaps even more important than the numbers is the evidence that depression is associated with greater physical, social, and existential distress, and with measurable reductions in the quality of life of cancer patients (Wilson et al. 2007).

Contributory Factors to Depression in Cancer

Gender may be among the most important risk factors contributing to the development of depressive syndromes in cancer. In one study of breast cancer, for instance, patients were found to have double the rate of depression compared with women in the general community (Kissane et al. 2004). On the other hand, predominantly male groups of patients with cancer, including prostate cancer, have been shown to have rates of depression that are mildly elevated but closer to those among men in the general population (Couper et al. 2006). The wives of men with prostate cancer can approach twice the rates of depression found in the general female population, suggesting that women bear the burden of emotional distress in the cancer setting (Couper et al. 2006).

Other factors that contribute to depression in cancer patients include advanced disease with pain and poor symptom control, comorbid neurological disorders, and a range of other metabolic and endocrine disorders. Medications that may have a direct effect on depression or its treatment include those used in cancer treatments—interferon, interleukin-2, steroids, certain chemotherapy agents (vincristine, vinblastine, procarbazine, L-asparaginase, vinorelbine, paclitaxel, docetaxel), hormonal agents (tamoxifen, cyproterone, leuprolide)—and other medications such as antihypertensives (propranolol, reserpine, methyldopa) and antibiotics (amphotericin). Specific cancers that have been linked with depression include pancreas cancers, which may increase proinflammatory cytokines (interleukin-1, interleukin-6, tumor necrosis factor-alpha) (Ebrahimi et al. 2004; Musselman et al. 2001), as can lymphomas, lung cancers, and a range of other cancers associated with paraneoplastic syndromes that also contribute to mood disturbance.

Diagnosis of Depression in Cancer

Cancer itself and its treatment effects may contribute to somatic symptoms that might be attributed to depression, including changes in appetite, weight, energy, and concentration, as well as sleep disturbance and fatigue. Debate has existed about whether diagnosis of depression in the medically ill should include or exclude such symptoms, with Endicott (1984) suggesting four substitutive symptoms: depressed appearance instead of appetite or weight changes; social withdrawal or decreased talkativeness instead of sleep disturbance; brooding, self-pity, or pessimism in place of fatigue; and lack of reactivity in situations that would normally be pleasurable instead of reduced concentration. Regression-tree analysis showed DSM-IV major depression to be highly associated with combinations of either 1) pessimism and worthlessness, or 2) pessimism, loss of interest, and thoughts of death (McKenzie et al. 2010).

Barriers to Recognition of Depression

The potentially confounding effect of medical symptoms is only one of several barriers to the recognition of depression in cancer patients. The most basic is perhaps time. In a busy oncology clinic, or even in the hospital setting, patients may have to wait to see their doctors, and the time with the oncologist may be seen as too precious to discuss anything that does not seem directly related to cancer. Even when time is not limited, the general social stigma attached to any psychiatric diagnosis is accentuated in a subtle way in the oncology setting. For family members and even for medical staff, the acknowledgment of depression may seem like a denial of the reality or distress of cancer, or a criticism of the sufferer's coping. "Isn't this normal?" or "Wouldn't you be depressed?" are questions that simultaneously reflect an awareness of the emotional suffering of the patient and an expression of indignation that it should be observed. In fact, responding to such complicated emotions, or acting in accord with cultural beliefs, family members, who in the case of cancer are often more engaged with the care of their loved ones than is true in many other illnesses, may deliberately or inadvertently conceal the patient's psychological distress from treating physicians. Even if such concealing does not occur, physicians themselves are more accustomed to focusing on physical symptoms, and proper diagnosis may require a more active approach on the part of physicians.

Screening for Depression

To assist physicians in taking a more active approach, the standard of care developed in 2003 by the National Comprehensive Cancer Network Distress Management Panel includes periodic screening for depression in all cancer patients (National Comprehensive Cancer Network 2003). Brief self-report instruments have proven most practical in the clinical setting, although they may return more false-positive results than long structured interviews that are the gold standard for psychiatric diagnosis (Passik and Lowery 2011). A systematic review of screening instruments suggests that the Beck Depression Inventory (BDI), General Health Questionnaire–28 (GHQ-28), and Center for Epidemiological Studies Depression Scale (CES-D) are reliable and valid in the cancer setting (Vodermaier et al. 2009). The Patient Health Questionnaire–9 (PHQ-9) is briefer than any of these measures, freely available, highly reliable, and widely used, although it has not yet been fully validated for cancer patients (Passik and Lowery 2011). The Distress Thermometer is a single unitary measure that has less reliability but offers a simple way of identifying patients who may need further assessment (Roth et al. 1998). Even asking the single question "Are you depressed?" can identify a majority of patients who should have further evaluation (Miller et al. 2006).

Suicide and Cancer

Some of the complex factors contributing to a desire for hastened death are summarized in Figure 4–1. Studies have generally suggested an increased rate of suicide in the cancer setting, especially for older men (Allebeck and Bolund 1991; Fox et al. 1982; Hem et al. 2004; Louhivuori and Hakama 1979). Risks for completed suicide include pain and poor symptom control, debility, social isolation, delirium, depression, demoralization, alcohol abuse, and past history of psychiatric disorder. Some cancers, such as lung

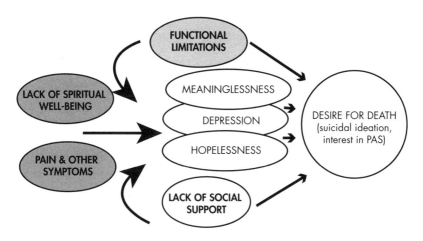

FIGURE 4–1. Factors associated with desire for hastened death, including physician-assisted suicide (PAS).

and head and neck cancers, are associated with greater physical morbidity and therefore increased suicide rates.

Differentiation of acceptance of dying from a desire for hastened death is crucial. Some patients close to death develop an adaptive conservation-withdrawal syndrome, in which they accept their frailty and the pending closure of their life, and which needs to be differentiated from depression (Ironside 1980). Some patients develop fleeting, passive thoughts of suicide, whereas others develop active plans with intent (Chochinov et al. 1995). Admission, close observation, and active treatment of depression, hopelessness, and demoralization are needed for the actively suicidal patient.

Dutch studies have shown that the rate of request for euthanasia is four times higher by patients with depression than by those without (van der Lee et al. 2005). A series of studies has explored the change that can be seen in patients' interest in life-sustaining treatment when depression is actively treated (Breitbart et al. 1996; Ganzini et al. 1994; Hooper et al. 1996). In these studies, people with depression tended to select only 6 of 14 potential medical therapies, such as the use of oxygen, blood transfusion, or being treated with antibiotics, whereas they selected 10 out of 14 therapies when the depression had cleared.

Demoralization

Old constructs such as acedia (the tedious meaninglessness of life), spiritual torpor, Engel's giving up–given up complex (Engel 1967), Gruenberg's social breakdown syndrome (Gruenberg 1967) in the institutionalized mentally ill, and Seligman's learned helplessness (Miller et al. 1975) have all represented demoralization (Kissane et al. 2001). Demoralization was found empirically as a nonspecific form of distress in the community (Dohrenwend et al. 1980), and Frank (1974) saw its correction as the vital step in all psychotherapies. De Figueiredo and Frank (1982) suggested that the development of a state of subjective incompetence was the hallmark of demoralization.

Folkman's studies of coping by the caregivers of men dying from AIDS in San Francisco in the early 1990s highlighted meaning-based coping as the key source of positive affective states (Folkman 1997). She recognized the omission of meaning-based coping from earlier approaches to coping— emotion-based and problem-based coping—proposed in 1985 by Lazarus and Folkman. New importance was placed on recognizing the role of lost hope and meaning in the development of psychiatric disorders, especially in medically ill patients. Loss of morale spans a spectrum of mental states, ranging from disheartenment (a mild loss of confidence) through despondency (starting to lose hope and sense of purpose) to despair (where hope is lost) and demoralization (where meaning and purpose are lost). Psychiatry becomes involved with the more severe end of this spectrum, where meaninglessness, pointlessness, and hopelessness can lead to suicidal thinking. Klein et al. (1980) viewed the core features of demoralization as the loss of meaning and hope, causing the loss of anticipatory pleasure (although in this state consummatory pleasure is still possible, in contrast with anhedonic depression).

Empirical Studies of Demoralization

Beck first recognized that hopelessness predicted suicide independently of depression (Beck et al. 1975), and this was subsequently confirmed in psychiatric inpatients (Wetzel et al. 1980), cancer patients (Owen et al. 1994), HIV patients (Breitbart et al. 1996), suicidal adolescents (Dori and Overholser 1999), and primary care patients (Gutkovich et al. 1999). Latent trait analyses of psychopathology in patients with medical illness showed that anhedonia, anxiety, demoralization, grief, and somatization were distinct (Clarke et al. 2000).

A study group in Bologna, Italy, developed diagnostic criteria for psychosomatic disorders and looked for demoralization across a range of medical illnesses; demoralization was reported, for instance, in 31% of patients following cardiac transplantation (Grandi et al. 2001) and in 29% of patients with breast cancer (Grassi et al. 2004). In Japan, loss of meaning and hope was found in 37% of terminally ill patients (Morita et al. 2000). Clarke et al. (2005a) found significantly higher demoralization and suicidality in patients with amyotrophic lateral sclerosis and higher anhedonia among patients with advanced cancer.

Prevalence of Demoralization

Validation of the Demoralization Scale (Kissane et al. 2004) enabled estimates of the frequency of high demoralization among cancer patients at 16% (Mehnert et al. 2011). The mean score in a Dutch sample attending a methadone clinic was twice that found in a Dutch community sample (de Jong et al. 2008). Demoralization has been associated with younger age, being female, living alone, family dysfunction, high physical symptom burden, use of resignation and avoidant coping, and emotional, spiritual, and practical problems (Clarke et al. 2005a; Kissane et al. 2004; Mehnert et al. 2011). In contrast, lower levels of demoralization may be found in people reporting high spiritual meaning and a sense of coherence to their life (Boscaglia and Clarke 2007; Lethborg et al. 2006, 2007; Mullane et al. 2009).

Correlation of Anxiety, Demoralization, and Depression

Trait anxiety has been found to predict the development of both demoralization and depression (Clarke et al. 2005b), with anxiety having a higher correlation with demoralization ($r = 0.71$) than with depression ($r = 0.61$) (Mehnert et al. 2011). Feelings of subjective incompetence and a sense of existential uncertainty help to explain this association between anxiety and demoralization.

A high correlation between demoralization and clinical depression has also been shown in several studies. It is clear that patients can develop major depression with or without demoralization. Some studies have also shown cases of demoralization without depression (Kissane et al. 2004; Mehnert et al. 2011), but others have not (Mullane et al. 2009). Using one standard deviation above and below the mean to identify levels of high and low demoralization, Mehnert et al. (2011) found that 60% of participants with moderate demoralization had no clinical depression, whereas only 5% of patients with severe demoralization had no depression. The worse the patient's clinical state, the greater the likelihood of comorbid states of depression, anxiety, and demoralization.

Adjustment Disorders and Demoralization

DSM-IV criteria for adjustment disorders require a maladaptive response to a stressor event that does not meet criteria for a major mood disorder (American Psychiatric Association 1994). The subjective judgment of the clinician in determining whether an anxious or depressed affect, or behavioral change, reaches a threshold for poor coping has made this a difficult diagnostic category for clinicians from wide-ranging backgrounds to apply in medically ill patients.

In contrast, the fresh focus on the phenomenology of meaninglessness, hopelessness, and loss of purpose in life brings existential dimensions to the fore and empowers better recognition by oncologists of the lived experience of patients. Our contention is that a diagnostic category such as demoralization syndrome (see proposed criteria in Table 4–3) will have greater utility through its easier recognition, given that the criteria reflect the language that patients so commonly use when experiencing existential distress. Field trials are clearly needed to examine more comprehensively a typology of existential distress and to define diagnostic criteria for such a diagnosis.

Treatment of Depression and Demoralization

Pharmacological and psychotherapeutic treatments are combined in treating depression. Less empirical guidance is available for treating demoralization, although newer meaning-centered and dignity-conserving therapies have applicability. In the following subsections, we consider treatments of depression and demoralization in detail.

Pharmacological Treatment of Depression

The pharmacological management of depression in cancer patients is similar to that in non-cancer patients, although the frequency of symptoms of serious physical illness and the complexities of cancer treatment regimens require additional flexibility and caution. Liver function, electrolytes, and other parameters should be monitored more closely in cancer patients than is typically done in the general population, and patients undergoing active cancer treatments should be started at low dosages of medication.

Meta-analyses have demonstrated that mirtazapine, citalopram, fluoxetine, and sertraline are effective for depression in the setting of coronary artery disease, and a review of 51 studies showed that antidepressants are significantly more effective than placebos in improving symptoms of depression among patients with any physical illness (Dowlati et al. 2010; Rayner et al. 2010). Randomized controlled trials in the cancer setting have been infrequent, but reviews have found antidepressants to be effective (Lloyd-Williams 2004), and extrapolation from smaller studies and those examining patients with earlier cancers seems to confirm this finding (Price and Hotopf 2009).

Current general practice guidelines call for use of selective serotonin reuptake inhibitors (SSRIs) as first-line treatment for depression. Differences, if any, are modest in comparisons of SSRIs (Cipriani et al. 2010;

TABLE 4–3.	Proposed diagnostic criteria for demoralization syndrome

1. Loss of meaning or purpose in life

2. Loss of hope for a worthwhile future

3. Sense of being trapped or pessimistic

4. Feel like giving up

5. Unable to cope with predicament

6. Socially isolated or alienated

7. Potential suicidal thinking

8. Phenomena persist for more than 2 weeks

Source. Fava et al. 1995; Kissane et al. 2001.

Omori et al. 2010). In a few cases, particular depression treatments have been studied for their preventive benefits. For instance, paroxetine and sertraline prevent as well as treat depressive effects of interferon used for melanoma, and sertraline might have a modest direct effect against the melanoma itself (Musselman et al. 2001; Reddy et al. 2008). Case reports or small studies of depression in seriously ill patients have also documented the use of various nonstandard treatments, including ketamine (Irwin and Iglewicz 2010), scopolamine (Furey and Drevets 2006), and electroconvulsive therapy (Rasmussen and Richardson 2011). In general, however, selection of an antidepressant in the cancer population, as in the broader population, depends in large part on evaluation of possible side effects and interactions.

Monoamine oxidase inhibitors (MAOIs) should be avoided because of the risk of serotonin syndrome if MAOIs are coadministered with opiates and other medications. Tricyclic antidepressants (TCAs), mirtazapine, trazodone, and SSRIs including fluoxetine and sertraline can, in rare instances, reduce neutrophil levels, which may be serious in a patient already taking chemotherapy agents that induce neutropenia (Albertini and Penders 1978; Duggal and Singh 2005; Kasper et al. 1997). Less serious, but still an important consideration, are the anticholinergic side effects of TCAs, which can exacerbate the constipating effect of opiates, or complicate painful mucositis with dry mouth, or exacerbate delirium. Constipating effects may be particularly risky in patients with pelvic or abdominal masses.

In patients with brain lesions or other reason for risk of seizures, bupropion should be avoided and mirtazapine may also pose a risk. Although citalopram may induce seizures in overdose, therapeutic dosages have been associated, in most studies of the general population, with no increased risk of seizure or even with a decreased risk, but studies in the cancer population are lacking (Favale et al. 2003; Waring et al. 2008).

Psychostimulants are often prescribed as an adjunctive treatment of depression and to counter narcotic sedation or cancer-related fatigue. Methylphenidate is beneficial for both mood and fatigue in terminally ill patients (Hardy 2009; Minton et al. 2008). Bupropion also benefits fatigue (Cullum et al. 2004; Moss et al. 2006). Modafinil is a newer agent that may be better tolerated, but cost usually limits its use as a first-line agent (Breitbart and Alici 2010).

Patients who are having trouble sleeping may benefit from the sedating side effects of mirtazapine or the older TCAs. Serotonin-norepinephrine reuptake inhibitors (SNRIs), including venlafaxine and duloxetine, may have a coanalgesic effect when given with opiates, and TCAs similarly may treat pain. Venlafaxine and mirtazapine are effective for hot flashes in both men and women undergoing hormonal treatments (Biglia et al. 2007; Buijs et al. 2009; Loibl et al. 2007). Nausea from any nonmechanical cause can be treated with haloperidol or with olanzapine, the latter having the added advantage of treating anxiety and improving appetite (Critchley et al. 2001; Tan et al. 2009). Pruritus, a symptom associated with various malignancies, especially in the presence of renal failure or cholestasis, may respond to paroxetine or mirtazapine (Demierre and Taverna 2006; Zylicz et al. 1998).

Tamoxifen and Cytochrome P450 Interactions

Tamoxifen is a selective estrogen receptor modulator that has been shown to reduce recurrence in estrogen receptor–positive (ER+) breast cancers and is also used to treat metastatic ER+ breast cancer. Tamoxifen depends for its effect on conversion to endoxifen by the cytochrome P450 (CYP450) 2D6 enzyme. Most common antidepressants are believed to have some degree of 2D6 inhibition, and studies have shown that in patients taking tamoxifen, use of the more potent 2D6 inhibitors fluoxetine, paroxetine, and sertraline was associated with increased mortality and higher rates of cancer recurrence (Aubert et al. 2009; Kelly et al. 2010). Retrospective studies have shown that citalopram and escitalopram, which are less potent 2D6 inhibitors, do not seem to have been associated with increased cancer risk (Cronin-Fenton et al. 2010). Venlafaxine and mirtazapine are believed to be weak 2D6 inhibitors, and evidence to date suggests they are safe (Aubert et al. 2009).

Irinotecan and SSRIs

Irinotecan is a treatment for colon cancer that, like tamoxifen, is a prodrug requiring conversion to an active form by the CYP450 system. SSRIs and TCAs may increase levels of the active drug through action on the CYP450 system, but the drug combination may also rarely cause rhabdomyolysis by a mechanism that is not completely described, and antidepressants should be used cautiously in patients taking irinotecan (Richards et al. 2003).

Serotonin Syndrome

Serotonin syndrome is an autonomic dysregulation caused by excessive synaptic serotonin. Symptom onset is generally rapid, within minutes of medication administration, and symptoms may include shivering, sweating, and nausea, so that mild or early cases may be mistaken for minor infectious disease. However, patients can develop tachycardia, dilated pupils, myoclonus, and hyperreflexia, followed by psychomotor agitation, disorientation, or hypervigilance, and finally hyperthermia and hypertension so severe that shock, seizure, metabolic acidosis, renal failure, disseminated intravascular coagulation, coma, and death are possible (Kim and Fisch 2006). A number of medications in cancer care have MAOI- or SRI-like properties, and may precipitate serotonin toxicity through interaction with antidepressants; these include tramadol, opiates, and serotonin 5-HT_3 antagonist antiemetics (ondansetron, granisetron) (Lee et al. 2009; Takeshita and Litzinger 2009).The use of any antidepressant within 2 weeks of prescription of linezolid (an oxazolidinone used to treat gram-positive infections) should be avoided. Antidepressants can also precipitate a serious reaction if given with procarbazine (an alkylating hydralazine derivative used as a chemotherapy agent for lymphoma or glioblastoma), or with meperidine, which is now rarely used as an analgesic but continues to be prescribed for rigors.

Psychological Treatment of Depression

Meta-analyses of psychotherapies in cancer patients confirm clear benefits (Meyer and Mark 1995), with larger effect sizes for psychoeducation (Devine and Westlake 1995). Both individual and group psychotherapeutic interventions had "clinically powerful effects," with effectiveness increasing with the experience and skill of the therapist and the length of intervention (Sheard and Maguire 1999). In one meta-analysis, de Mello et al. (2005) reported that 8 of 13 studies showed interpersonal psychotherapy to be better than placebo in improving depression, through its focus on life transitions, grief, social isolation, and interpersonal conflicts, which are all relevant for the depressed cancer patient. Evidence for the effectiveness of psychotherapy in the cancer population seems to be growing.

Behavioral Activation Strategies

Depression is readily maintained by withdrawal and avoidance behaviors. Strategies such as scheduling, self-monitoring, rating daily levels of pleasure and accomplishment, and exploring alternative roles with rehearsal during therapy help alleviate depression (Dimidjian et al. 2006; Dobson et al. 2008).

Couple Therapy

A randomized controlled trial of active coping for couples compared with usual care in the breast cancer setting showed a reduction in women's depressive symptoms up to 6 months posttreatment in the active group (Manne et al. 2005). Couple therapy helps achieve an adaptive adjustment when body image changes (e.g., due to mastectomy, colostomy, ileal conduit, limb amputation), sexuality is affected (e.g., erectile dysfunction after prostate cancer, dyspareunia after gynecological cancers), infertility results (e.g., from chemotherapy, castration surgery), or issues of shame, guilt, doubt, despair, or depression arise, and the partner is a prime source of support.

In working with cancer patients and partners to promote effective mutual support, the clinician needs to maintain awareness of demand-withdrawal patterns that can represent a protest at the burden of illness and lead to disengagement and diminished safety. Couple therapy that identifies existential fears and supports intimacy in the face of death can do much to harness resilience and protect against demoralization and depression (Dobson et al. 2008).

Group Therapy

In cognitive-existential group therapy with early-stage cancers, the goal is to promote a supportive environment, facilitate grief work over the multiple losses, alter maladaptive cognitive patterns, enhance problem-solving and coping skills, foster a sense of mastery, and encourage review of lifestyle priorities for the future (Kissane et al. 1997). In supportive-expressive group therapy, the goals are to build bonds, express emotions, detoxify death, redefine life's priorities, fortify families and friends, enhance doctor-patient relationships, and improve coping (Classen et al. 2001). Through an emphasis on transforming existential ambivalence into creative living and promoting adherence to anticancer treatment (Kissane et al. 2004), supportive-expressive group therapy has been shown to prevent depression in treated patients compared with control subjects (Kissane et al. 2007).

Family Therapy

In a randomized controlled trial targeting palliative care patients' families at risk of poor psychosocial outcome, family focused grief therapy was shown to reduce depression and to support mourning arising from family loss due to cancer (Kissane et al. 2006). The goals of family focused grief therapy are to optimize family relational functioning through promotion of effective communication, enhanced cohesion, and adaptive resolution of conflict. The more pronounced the relational dysfunction, the greater the number of family sessions needed across the bereavement phase. In general, families with mild communication breakdown can be aided by 4–6 sessions, whereas 10–12 sessions are preferred if family dysfunction is more pronounced. Openness to discussion of death and dying and early containment of conflict prove beneficial until improved communication and closeness help family members tolerate any differences of opinion.

Therapists make use of circular questions to reveal family dynamics and offer regular summaries as a means to help families integrate understanding of their patterns of relating and coping with loss and change (Dumont and Kissane 2009). Commencing therapy while the cancer patient is still alive and present to voice his or her opinions establishes a model of family care that is preventive and cost-effective, and enables continuity of support to be carried into bereavement.

Psychological Treatment for Demoralization

Models of psychotherapy are emerging that may have greater focus in treating demoralization and other states of existential or spiritual distress. These models include dignity and meaning-centered therapies. (For further discussion of existential therapies, see Chapter 1, Appendix 1–B.)

Dignity Therapy

Dignity therapy is a brief focused intervention designed to address psychosocial and existential distress in cancer patients near the end of life (Chochinov et al. 2005). Its goals are to sustain generativity and continuity of self, maintain pride and hope, preserve one's role, alleviate concerns about being a burden to others, and, if desired, leave a legacy document that summarizes one's accomplishments and values in life. Dignity therapy seeks to celebrate life and affirm the worth of each person, making it likely to ameliorate demoralization and enrich the life lived (Dumont and Kissane 2009).

Meaning-Centered Therapy

Based on Viktor Frankl's model of logotherapy, meaning-centered psychotherapy has been delivered in group and individual formats in the setting of cancer patients receiving palliative care (Breitbart and Alici 2010). Its goals are to review concepts and sources of psychological meaning and value, as well as the impact of cancer on those meanings and values, and to acknowledge the finiteness of life and therefore highlight the value and worth of life. The therapy often focuses on the responsibility to pursue creativity and good deeds; appreciate nature, art, and humor; and take stock of the depth of meaning that sustains worthwhile living. meaning-centered psychotherapy is anticipated to be especially effective in alleviating demoralization and promoting dignity of the person.

The psychodynamic life review as a narrative approach identifies key accomplishments and personal strengths alongside any vulnerabilities, so as to frame the crisis of illness as also an opportunity for growth (Viederman 1983). The containing frame of support thus generated actively by the therapist maintains defenses and draws attention to where the value and meaning of continued life is found.

Pharmacological Treatment for Demoralization

For cancer patients with comorbid major depression and demoralization, treatment with antidepressants, as discussed previously for the treatment of depression, is indicated. When demoralization exists without comorbid depression, the mainstay of treatment is psychotherapeutic, without current research evidence to guide the use of antidepressants in more severe states of demoralization (Angelino and Treisman 2001).

Conclusion

Depression and demoralization are interrelated experiences that have a measurable effect on the lives of cancer patients and their course of illness. Treatments including both medications and psychotherapies with patients and their families have been shown to be both promising and effective in alleviating suffering and improving the quality of cancer care.

Key Clinical Points

- Depression is a very common consequence, but not a cause, of cancer.

- Demoralization develops when the meaning and purpose of life are lost, limiting coping and reducing the value anticipated in life.

- Untreated depression among cancer patients is associated with increased suicidality, decreased treatment adherence, worsened quality of life, and shorter survival.

- Identifying depression in cancer patients may be more challenging than it is in the general population owing to complex medical symptoms, confusion between grief and depression, and cultural barriers to acknowledging distress.

- Pharmacological treatment of depression in the cancer population is similar to that in the general population, but requires more attention to medical symptoms, physical vulnerabilities, and medication inter-actions.

- Individual and group psychotherapies have been shown to be effec-tive in alleviating symptoms in cancer patients with psychiatric dis-tress.

- Narrative, dignity, and meaning-centered therapies restore a sense of coherence, value, and purpose in life, helping to ameliorate demoral-ization and depression.

References

Albertini RS, Penders TM: Agranulocytosis associated with tricyclics. J Clin Psychi-atry 39:483–485, 1978

Allebeck P, Bolund C: Suicides and suicide attempts in cancer patients. Psychol Med 21:979–984, 1991

American Psychiatric Association: Diagnostic and Statistical Manual of Mental Disorders, 4th Edition. Washington, DC, American Psychiatric Association, 1994

Angelino AF, Treisman GJ: Major depression and demoralization in cancer patients: diagnostic and treatment considerations. Support Care Cancer 9:344–349, 2001

Aubert RE, Stanek EJ, Yao J, et al: Risk of breast cancer recurrence in women initiat-ing tamoxifen with CYP2D6 inhibitors. J Clin Oncol 27(suppl):18S, 2009

Azevedo RC, Leme JL, Miranda FZ, et al: Implementation of a smoke-free psychiat-ric unit in a general hospital. Rev Bras Psiquiatr 32:197–198, 2010

Beck AT, Kovacs M, Weissman A: Hopelessness and suicidal behavior. An overview. JAMA 234:1146–1149, 1975

Biglia N, Kubatzki F, Sgandurra P, et al: Mirtazapine for the treatment of hot flushes in breast cancer survivors: a prospective pilot trial. Breast J 13:490–495, 2007

Boesen EH, Boesen SH, Frederiksen K, et al: Survival after a psychoeducational intervention for patients with cutaneous malignant melanoma: a replication study. J Clin Oncol 25:5698–5703, 2007

Boscaglia N, Clarke D: Sense of coherence as a protective factor for demoralisation in women with a recent diagnosis of gynaecological cancer. Psychooncology 16:189–195, 2007

Breitbart W, Alici Y: Psychostimulants for cancer-related fatigue. J Natl Compr Canc Netw 8:933–942, 2010

Breitbart W, Rosenfeld B, Passik S: Interest in physician-assisted suicide among ambulatory HIV-infected patients. Am J Psychiatry 153:238–242, 1996

Buijs C, Mom CH, Willemse PH, et al: Venlafaxine versus clonidine for the treatment of hot flashes in breast cancer patients: a double-blind, randomized cross-over study. Breast Cancer Res Treat 115:573–580, 2009

Chochinov HM, Wilson KG, Enns M, et al: Desire for death in the terminally ill. Am J Psychiatry 152:1185–1191, 1995

Chochinov HM, Hack T, Hassard T, et al: Dignity therapy: a novel psychotherapeutic intervention for patients near the end of life. J Clin Oncol 23:5520–5525, 2005

Chwastiak LA, Rosenheck RA, Kazis LE: Association of psychiatric illness and obesity, physical inactivity, and smoking among a national sample of veterans. Psychosomatics 52:230–236, 2011

Cipriani A, La Ferla T, Furukawa TA, et al: Sertraline versus other antidepressive agents for depression. Cochrane Database of Systematic Reviews 2010, Issue 4. Art. No.: CD006117. DOI: 10.1002/14651858.CD006117.pub4.

Clarke D, Mackinnon A, Smith G, et al: Dimensions of psychopathology in the medically ill. A latent trait analysis. Psychosomatics 41:418–425, 2000

Clarke D, Kissane D, Trauer T, et al: Demoralization, anhedonia and grief in patients with severe physical illness. World Psychiatry 4:96–105, 2005a

Clarke D, McLeod J, Smith G, et al: A comparison of psychosocial and physical functioning in patients with motor neurone disease and metastatic cancer. J Palliat Care 21:173–179, 2005b

Classen C, Butler LD, Koopman C, et al: Supportive-expressive group therapy and distress in patients with metastatic breast cancer: a randomized clinical intervention trial. Arch Gen Psychiatry 58:494–501, 2001

Couper JW, Bloch S, Love A, et al: The psychosocial impact of prostate cancer on patients and their partners. Med J Aust 185:428–432, 2006

Critchley P, Plach N, Grantham M, et al: Efficacy of haloperidol in the treatment of nausea and vomiting in the palliative patient: a systematic review. J Pain Symptom Manage 22:631–634, 2001

Cronin-Fenton D, Lash TL, Sorensen HT: Selective serotonin reuptake inhibitors and adjuvant tamoxifen therapy: risk of breast cancer recurrence and mortality. Future Oncol 6:877–880, 2010

Cullum JL, Wojciechowski AE, Pelletier G, et al: Bupropion sustained release treatment reduces fatigue in cancer patients. Can J Psychiatry 49:139–144, 2004

de Figueiredo JM, Frank JD: Subjective incompetence, the clinical hallmark of demoralization. Compr Psychiatry 23:353–363, 1982

de Jong CAJ, Kissane D, Geessink R, et al: Demoralization in opioid dependent patients: a comparative study with cancer patients and community subjects. Open Addict J 1:7–9, 2008

de Mello MF, de Jesus Mari J, Bacaltchuk J, et al: A systematic review of research findings on the efficacy of interpersonal therapy for depressive disorders. Eur Arch Psychiatry Clin Neurosci 255:75–82, 2005

Demierre MF, Taverna J: Mirtazapine and gabapentin for reducing pruritus in cutaneous T-cell lymphoma. J Am Acad Dermatol 55:543–544, 2006

Derogatis LR, Morrow GR, Fetting J, et al: The prevalence of psychiatric disorders among cancer patients. JAMA 249:751–757, 1983

Devine EC, Westlake SK: The effects of psychoeducational care provided to adults with cancer: meta-analysis of 116 studies. Oncol Nurs Forum 22:1369–1381, 1995

DiMatteo MR, Hanskard-Zolnierek KB: Impact of depression on treatment adherence and survival from cancer, in Depression and Cancer. Edited by Kissane DW, Maj M, Sartorius N. Oxford, UK, Wiley-Blackwell, 2011, pp 101–124

DiMatteo MR, Lepper HS, Croghan TW: Depression is a risk factor for noncompliance with medical treatment: meta-analysis of the effects of anxiety and depression on patient adherence. Arch Intern Med 160:2101–2107, 2000

Dimidjian S, Hollon SD, Dobson KS, et al: Randomized trial of behavioral activation, cognitive therapy, and antidepressant medication in the acute treatment of adults with major depression. J Consult Clin Psychol 74:658–670, 2006

Dobson KS, Hollon SD, Dimidjian S, et al: Randomized trial of behavioral activation, cognitive therapy, and antidepressant medication in the prevention of relapse and recurrence in major depression. J Consult Clin Psychol 76:468–477, 2008

Dohrenwend B, Shrout P, Egri G, et al: Nonspecific psychological distress and other dimensions of psychopathology. Measures for use in the general population. Arch Gen Psychiatry 37:1229–1236, 1980

Dori G, Overholser J: Depression, hopelessness, and self-esteem: accounting for suicidality in adolescent psychiatric inpatients. Suicide Life Threat Behav 29:309–318, 1999

Dowlati Y, Herrmann N, Swardfager WL, et al: Efficacy and tolerability of antidepressants for treatment of depression in coronary artery disease: a meta-analysis. Can J Psychiatry 55:91–99, 2010

Duggal HS, Singh I: Psychotropic drug-induced neutropenia. Drugs Today (Barc) 41:517–526, 2005

Dumont I, Kissane D: Techniques for framing questions in conducting family meetings in palliative care. Palliat Support Care 7:163–170, 2009

Ebrahimi B, Tucker SL, Li D, et al: Cytokines in pancreatic carcinoma: correlation with phenotypic characteristics and prognosis. Cancer 101:2727–2736, 2004

Endicott J: Measurement of depression in patients with cancer. Cancer 53:2243–2249, 1984

Engel G: A psychological setting of somatic disease: the "giving up–given up" complex. Proc R Soc Med 60:553–555, 1967

Ewertz M: Bereavement and breast cancer. Br J Cancer 53:701–703, 1986

Fava G, Freyberger H, Bech P, et al: Diagnostic criteria for use in psychosomatic research. Psychother Psychosom 63:1–8, 1995

Favale E, Audenino D, Cocito L, et al: The anticonvulsant effect of citalopram as an indirect evidence of serotonergic impairment in human epileptogenesis. Seizure 12:316–318, 2003

Folkman S: Positive psychological states and coping with severe stress. Soc Sci Med 45:1207–1221, 1997

Fox BH, Stanek EJ 3rd, Boyd SC, et al: Suicide rates among cancer patients in Connecticut. J Chronic Dis 35:89–100, 1982

Frank J: Psychotherapy: the restoration of morale. Am J Psychiatry 131:271–274, 1974

Furey ML, Drevets WC: Antidepressant efficacy of the antimuscarinic drug scopolamine: a randomized, placebo-controlled clinical trial. Arch Gen Psychiatry 63:1121–1129, 2006

Ganzini L, Lee MA, Heintz RT, et al: The effect of depression treatment on elderly patients' preferences for life-sustaining medical therapy. Am J Psychiatry 151:1631–1636, 1994

Goodkin K, Antoni MH, Blaney PH: Stress and hopelessness in the promotion of cervical intraepithelial neoplasia to invasive squamous cell carcinoma of the cervix. J Psychosom Res 30:67–76, 1986

Graham NA, Frost-Pineda K, Gold MS: Tobacco and psychiatric dual disorders. J Addict Dis 26 (suppl 1):5–12, 2007

Grandi S, Fabbri S, Tossani E, et al: Psychological evaluation after cardiac transplantation: the integration of different criteria. Psychother Psychosom 70:176–183, 2001

Grassi L, Rossi E, Sabato S, et al: Diagnostic criteria for psychosomatic research and psychosocial variables in breast cancer patients. Psychosomatics 45:483–491, 2004

Grassi L, Holland JC, Johansen C, et al: Psychiatric concomitants of cancer, screening procedures, and training of health care professionals in oncology: the paradigms of psycho-oncology in the psychiatry field, in Advances in Psychiatry, Vol. 2. Edited by Christodolou GN. Athens, Greece, Beta Publishing, 2005, pp 59–66

Gruenberg E: The social breakdown syndrome—some origins. Am J Psychiatry 123:1481–1489, 1967

Gutkovich Z, Rosenthal R, Galynker I, et al: Depression and demoralization among Russian-Jewish immigrants in primary care. Psychosomatics 40:117–125, 1999

Hahn RC, Petitti DB: Minnesota Multiphasic Personality Inventory-rated depression and the incidence of breast cancer. Cancer 61:845–848, 1988

Hardy SE: Methylphenidate for the treatment of depressive symptoms, including fatigue and apathy, in medically ill older adults and terminally ill adults. Am J Geriatr Pharmacother 7:34–59, 2009

Hem E, Loge JH, Haldorsen T, et al: Suicide risk in cancer patients from 1960 to 1999. J Clin Oncol 22:4209–4216, 2004

Hooper SC, Vaughan KJ, Tennant CC, et al: Major depression and refusal of life-sustaining medical treatment in the elderly. Med J Aust 165:416–419, 1996

Ironside W: Conservation-withdrawal and action-engagement: on a theory of survivor behavior. Psychosom Med 42:163–175, 1980

Irwin SA, Iglewicz A: Oral ketamine for the rapid treatment of depression and anxiety in patients receiving hospice care. J Palliat Care 13:903–908, 2010

Kaplan GA, Reynolds P: Depression and cancer mortality and morbidity: prospective evidence from the Alameda County study. J Behav Med 11:1–13, 1988

Kasper S, Praschak-Rieder N, Tauscher J, et al: A risk-benefit assessment of mirtazapine in the treatment of depression. Drug Saf 17:251–264, 1997

Kelly CM, Juurlink DN, Gomes T, et al: Selective serotonin reuptake inhibitors and breast cancer mortality in women receiving tamoxifen: a population based cohort study. BMJ 340:c693, 2010

Kim HF, Fisch MJ: Antidepressant use in ambulatory cancer patients. Curr Oncol Rep 8:275–281, 2006

Kissane DW, Bloch S, Miach P, et al: Cognitive-existential group therapy for patients with primary breast cancer—techniques and themes. Psychooncology 6:25–33, 1997

Kissane DW, Clarke DM, Street AF: Demoralization syndrome—a relevant psychiatric diagnosis for palliative care. J Palliat Care 17:12–21, 2001

Kissane DW, Wein S, Love A, et al: The Demoralization Scale: a preliminary report of its development and validation. J Palliat Care 20:269–276, 2004

Kissane DW, McKenzie M, Bloch S, et al: Family focused grief therapy: a randomized, controlled trial in palliative care and bereavement. Am J Psychiatry 163:1208–1218, 2006

Kissane DW, Grabsch B, Clarke DM, et al: Supportive-expressive group therapy for women with metastatic breast cancer: survival and psychosocial outcome from a randomized controlled trial. Psychooncology 16:277–286, 2007

Klein D, Gittelman R, Quitkin F, et al: Diagnosis and Drug Treatment of Psychiatric Disorders: Adults and Children. Baltimore, MD, Williams & Wilkins, 1980

Kulie T, Slattengren A, Redmer J, et al: Obesity and women's health: an evidence-based review. J Am Board Fam Med 24:75–85, 2011

Lee J, Franz L, Goforth HW: Serotonin syndrome in a chronic-pain patient receiving concurrent methadone, ciprofloxacin, and venlafaxine. Psychosomatics 50:638–639, 2009

Lethborg C, Aranda S, Bloch S, et al: The role of meaning in advanced cancer-integrating the constructs of assumptive world, sense of coherence and meaning-based coping. J Psychosoc Oncol 24:27–42, 2006

Lethborg C, Aranda S, Cox S, et al: To what extent does meaning mediate adaptation to cancer? The relationship between physical suffering, meaning in life, and connection to others in adjustment to cancer. Palliat Support Care 5:377–388, 2007

Li J, Johansen C, Hansen D, et al: Cancer incidence in parents who lost a child: a nationwide study in Denmark. Cancer 95:2237–2242, 2002

Lloyd-Williams M: Are antidepressants effective in cancer patients? Prog Palliat Care 12:217–219, 2004

Loibl S, Schwedler K, von Minckwitz G, et al: Venlafaxine is superior to clonidine as treatment of hot flashes in breast cancer patients—a double-blind, randomized study. Ann Oncol 18:689–693, 2007

Louhivuori KA, Hakama M: Risk of suicide among cancer patients. Am J Epidemiol 109:59–65, 1979

Manne SL, Ostroff JS, Winkel G, et al: Couple-focused group intervention for women with early stage breast cancer. J Consult Clin Psychol 73:634–646, 2005

Massie MJ: Prevalence of depression in patients with cancer. J Natl Cancer Inst Monogr 32:57–71, 2004

McKenzie D, Clarke D, Forbes A, et al: Pessimism, worthlessness, anhedonia, and thoughts of death identify DSM-IV major depression in hospitalized, medically ill patients. Psychosomatics 51:302–311, 2010

Mehnert A, Vehling S, Höcker A, et al: Demoralization and depression in patients with advanced cancer: validation of the German version of the Demoralization Scale. J Pain Symptom Manage 42:768–776, 2011

Meyer TJ, Mark MM: Effects of psychosocial interventions with adult cancer patients: a meta-analysis of randomized experiments. Health Psychol 14:101–108, 1995

Miller KE, Adams SM, Miller MM: Antidepressant medication use in palliative care. Am J Hosp Palliat Care 23:127–133, 2006

Miller W, Seligman M, Kurlander H: Learned helplessness, depression, and anxiety. J Nerv Ment Dis 161:347–357, 1975

Minton O, Richardson A, Sharpe M, et al: A systematic review and meta-analysis of the pharmacological treatment of cancer-related fatigue. J Natl Cancer Inst 100:1155–1166, 2008

Mitchell AJ, Chan M, Bhatti H, et al: Prevalence of depression, anxiety, and adjustment disorder in oncological, haematological, and palliative-care settings: a meta-analysis of 94 interview-based studies. Lancet Oncol 12:160–174, 2011

Morita T, Tsunoda J, Inoue S, et al: An exploratory factor analysis of existential suffering in Japanese terminally ill cancer patients. Psychooncology 9:164–168, 2000

Moss EL, Simpson JS, Pelletier G, et al: An open-label study of the effects of bupropion SR on fatigue, depression and quality of life of mixed-site cancer patients and their partners. Psychooncology 15:259–267, 2006

Mullane M, Dooley B, Tiernan E, et al: Validation of the Demoralization Scale in an Irish advanced cancer sample. Palliat Support Care 7:323–330, 2009

Murphy JM, Gilman SE, Lesage A, et al: Time trends in mortality associated with depression: findings from the Stirling County study. Can J Psychiatry 55:776–783, 2010

Musselman DL, Lawson DH, Gumnick JF, et al: Paroxetine for the prevention of depression induced by high-dose interferon alfa. N Engl J Med 344:961–966, 2001

National Comprehensive Cancer Network: Distress Management Clinical Practice Guidelines, Vol. 1. Washington, DC, National Comprehensive Cancer Network, 2003

Omori IM, Watanabe N, Nakagawa A, et al: Fluvoxamine versus other anti-depressive agents for depression. Cochrane Database of Systematic Reviews 2010, Issue 3. Art. No.: CD006114. DOI: 10.1002/14651858.CD006114.pub2.

Onyike CU, Crum RM, Lee HB, et al: Is obesity associated with major depression? Results from the Third National Health and Nutrition Examination Survey. Am J Epidemiol 158:1139–1147, 2003

Owen C, Tennant C, Levi J, et al: Cancer patients' attitudes to final events in life: wish for death, attitudes to cessation of treatment, suicide and euthanasia. Psychooncology 3:1–19, 1994

Passik SD, Lowery AE: Recognition of depression and methods of depression screening in people with cancer, in Depression and Cancer. Edited by Kissane DW, Maj M, Sartorius N. Oxford, Wiley-Blackwell, 2011, pp 81–100

Persky VW, Kempthorne-Rawson J, Shekelle RB: Personality and risk of cancer: 20-year follow-up of the Western Electric Study. Psychosom Med 49:435–449, 1987

Pettingale KW, Morris T, Greer S, et al: Mental attitudes to cancer: an additional prognostic factor. Lancet 1:750, 1985

Price A, Hotopf M: The treatment of depression in patients with advanced cancer undergoing palliative care. Curr Opin Support Palliat Care 3:61–66, 2009

Rasmussen KG, Richardson JW: Electroconvulsive therapy in palliative care. Am J Hosp Palliat Care 28:375–377, 2011

Rayner L, Price A, Evans A, et al: Antidepressants for depression in physically ill people. Cochrane Database of Systematic Reviews 2010, Issue 3. Art. No.: CD007503. DOI: 10.1002/14651858.CD007503.pub2.

Reddy KK, Lefkove B, Chen LB, et al: The antidepressant sertraline downregulates Akt and has activity against melanoma cells. Pigment Cell Melanoma Res 21:451–456, 2008

Richards S, Umbreit JN, Fanucchi MP, et al: Selective serotonin reuptake inhibitor-induced rhabdomyolysis associated with irinotecan. South Med J 96:1031–1033, 2003

Roth AJ, Kornblith AB, Batel-Copel L, et al: Rapid screening for psychologic distress in men with prostate carcinoma: a pilot study. Cancer 82:1904–1908, 1998

Sheard T, Maguire P: The effect of psychological interventions on anxiety and depression in cancer patients: results of two meta-analyses. Br J Cancer 80:1770–1780, 1999

Sihvo S, Wahlbeck K, McCallum A, et al: Increase in the duration of antidepressant treatment from 1994 to 2003: a nationwide population-based study from Finland. Pharmacoepidemiol Drug Saf 19:1186–1193, 2010

Takeshita J, Litzinger MH: Serotonin syndrome associated with tramadol. Prim Care Companion J Clin Psychiatry 11:273, 2009

Tan L, Liu J, Liu X, et al: Clinical research of Olanzapine for prevention of chemotherapy-induced nausea and vomiting. J Exp Clin Cancer Res 28:131, 2009

Temoshok L, Heller BW, Sagebiel RW, et al: The relationship of psychosocial factors to prognostic indicators in cutaneous malignant melanoma. J Psychosom Res 29:139–153, 1985

van der Lee ML, van der Bom JG, Swarte NB, et al: Euthanasia and depression: a prospective cohort study among terminally ill cancer patients. J Clin Oncol 23:6607–6612, 2005

Viederman M: The psychodynamic life narrative: a psychotherapeutic intervention useful in crisis situations. Psychiatry 46:236–246, 1983

Vodermaier A, Linden W, Siu C: Screening for emotional distress in cancer patients: a systematic review of assessment instruments. J Natl Cancer Inst 101:1464–1488, 2009

Waring WS, Gray JA, Graham A: Predictive factors for generalized seizures after deliberate citalopram overdose. Br J Clin Pharmacol 66:861–865, 2008

Watson M, Haviland JS, Greer S, et al: Influence of psychological response on survival in breast cancer: a population-based cohort study. Lancet 354:1331–1336, 1999

Watson M, Homewood J, Haviland J, et al: Influence of psychological response on breast cancer survival: 10-year follow-up of a population-based cohort. Eur J Cancer 41:1710–1714, 2005

Wetzel R, Margulies T, Davis R, et al: Hopelessness, depression, and suicide intent. J Clin Psychiatry 41:159–160, 1980

Wilson KG, Chochinov HM, Skirko MG, et al: Depression and anxiety disorders in palliative cancer care. J Pain Symptom Manage 33:118–129, 2007

Zonderman AB, Costa PT Jr, McCrae RR: Depression as a risk for cancer morbidity and mortality in a nationally representative sample. JAMA 262:1191–1195, 1989

Zylicz Z, Smits C, Krajnik M: Paroxetine for pruritus in advanced cancer. J Pain Symptom Manage 16:121–124, 1998

CHAPTER 5

Counseling and Specific Psychological Treatments in Common Clinical Settings

An Overview

Carolyn Pitceathly, M.Sc.
Maggie Watson, B.Sc., Ph.D., Dip.Clin.Psych.
Anne Cawthorn, M.Sc., B.Sc., R.N.T., Dip. Hypno.

MANY CLINICIANS REFER cancer patients to psycho-oncology services for help with intractable worries or mood problems. They may see benefits in patients from psychological interventions but be unaware of how those benefits were effected. Some doctors and nurses may hold back from making a referral because they are uncertain which member of the psycho-oncology team—counselor, psychologist, psychotherapist, or psychiatrist—is likely to meet a particular patient's needs. A survey on the nature of psychosocial care delivered by oncologists indicates that only 50% of oncologists had practice-affiliated mental health professionals and less than half (47%) initiated a referral to psychosocial support services (Muriel et al. 2009).

The authors would like to acknowledge Anne Crook (M.B.A.C.P. Accred.), Counselor, Psycho-Oncology Service, Christie Hospital, Manchester, United Kingdom, for her contribution to the Counseling section of the chapter.

In this chapter, we describe some of the psychological interventions currently provided in psycho-oncology services as well as the theory that informs their delivery and evidence for efficacy. Our aim is to help clinicians feel more confident about referring patients for psychological help.

Background

Cancer diagnoses and treatments present patients with multidimensional challenges: physical, spiritual, existential, social, practical, financial, emotional, and psychological. The cancer experience may have an impact on a patient's sense of self and on relationships with family, friends, and health professionals (Akechi et al. 2004; Parle et al. 1996).

The majority of patients cope with these challenges, but a substantial minority experience significant ongoing psychological distress. Prevalence rates of psychological morbidity vary depending on the patient groups studied and the tools used to measure distress (Massie 2004), but there is general agreement that approximately 25%–30% of patients become highly distressed or develop anxiety and/or depressive disorders (Naaman et al. 2009; Osborn et al. 2006; Schneider et al. 2010; Sellick and Crooks 1999). Those problems may become chronic (Jacobsen and Jim 2008; Naaman et al. 2009), and morbidity is likely to be higher among patients with advanced disease compared with those in the early stages of illness or in remission (Massie 2004; Jacobsen and Jim 2008). The integration of psychosocial support into routine oncology practice is now widely recommended, and if psychological interventions are effective in reducing levels of psychological distress and morbidity, the benefits to patients are important.

Research Evidence

Do cancer patients benefit from psychosocial interventions? Review papers and meta-analyses of the research literature suggest that drawing clear conclusions from intervention trials is difficult because of a lack of methodological quality and standardization in reporting and variations in populations studied (Newell et al. 2002). There are differences in the psychosocial difficulties targeted and the outcomes assessed (Edwards et al. 2008). Demographic profiles, disease characteristics, treatment regimens, and distress levels in the samples also vary (Edwards et al. 2008; Jacobsen and Jim 2008). Some demographic groups or cancer sites are insufficiently or overly represented. For example, ethnic and racial minority groups and patients with advanced disease are less frequently studied (Jacobsen and Jim 2008; Newell et al. 2002; Schneider et al. 2010; Sellick and Crooks 1999; Sheard and Maguire 1999; Stanton 2005).

In spite of reservations, most reviewers conclude that psychological interventions do benefit patients. Newell et al. (2002), in a rigorous and extensive review of psychological therapies used by cancer patients, concluded that group therapy, education, counseling, and cognitive-behavioral therapy (CBT) offer the "most promise" for medium- and long-term benefits for many psychosocial outcomes. Relaxation and guided imagery appeared to provide most benefit for reducing patients' physical side effects. Findings indicate that interventions offer benefits across a range of outcomes but that no single intervention model benefits all.

Factors That Moderate the Effectiveness of Interventions

Research and clinical experience suggest that if patients are to benefit from psychological interventions, they must be struggling to cope with concerns or emotions, interventions must "fit" the problem, and patients must feel that an intervention is relevant and acceptable. Patients benefit from psychological intervention when they report measurable distress (concerns, psychological symptoms), but there is no evidence that future distress is prevented by targeting well-adjusted patients (Jacobsen and Jim 2008; Pitceathly et al. 2009; Schneider et al. 2010). Therefore, routine screening is recommended at key change points in the illness trajectory—that is, at initial diagnosis, after treatment has been completed (reentry), at recurrence, and when treatment becomes palliative (National Institute for Clinical Excellence 2004; Sellick and Crooks 1999). However, for screening programs to be effective, health professionals must be trained and be confident that a management plan is in place for patients identified with difficulties (Bidstrup et al. 2011).

The nature of a patient's psychological problem may dictate the intervention that is most effective and most durable. Osborn et al. (2006) conducted meta-analyses reviewing the impact of CBT and patient education on depression, anxiety, and quality of life. They concluded that CBT was effective for treating depression and anxiety and improving quality of life outcomes; however, although CBT had long-term benefits for quality of life, it provided only short-term benefits for depression and anxiety.

The relevance of a particular intervention in helping a distressed patient is likely to be related to the source and severity of the coping difficulties. Cancer patients with a premorbid history of depression are at greater risk of developing depressive disorders after cancer diagnosis (Parle et al. 1996; Sellick and Crooks 1999). Research with community samples has consistently shown a link between depression in response to negative life events and childhood trauma, such as bereavement, loss, neglect, and abuse (Brown and Harris 1993; Smit et al. 2004). Therefore, although patients struggling to cope with the novel challenges of cancer may respond quite quickly to a coping-based intervention, some with psychological difficulties that predate the cancer may be better served by interventions that address the contribution of early experience to current difficulties (Pitceathly et al. 2011).

The optimal intervention may be dictated by the patient's illness and treatment context. Naaman et al. (2009) reviewed psychological interventions targeting breast cancer patients. Short-term coping intervention benefited early breast cancer patients, but longer-term supportive intervention seemed more suitable for patients with advanced disease. Some evidence suggests that longer interventions confer more change (Rehse and Pukrop 2003; Schneider et al. 2010), but intensive interventions may be too demanding for patients already challenged by the effects of toxic cancer treatments (Coyne and Kagee 2001). Similarly, patients affected by traumatic experiences may have difficulty tolerating treatments that involve restraint or closed spaces. Although longer-term psychological intervention may be helpful at some stage, interventions such as hypnotherapy or relaxation to help patients tolerate essential procedures may be the most relevant in the acute situation.

Patients may have difficulty complying with interventions that demand attendance beyond routine hospital appointments, and participation rates in face-to-face psychotherapy can be variable (15%–82%, median 35%; Owen et al. 2004). Therefore, there has been a move toward use of technology. CBT for managing health problems has been successfully adapted for the Internet (Cuijpers et al. 2008). In the United Kingdom, the National Institute for Clinical Excellence (2002) appraisal of computer-delivered cognitive-behavioral therapy [CCBT] concluded that preliminary evidence supports the use of CCBT in the management of depression and some anxiety disorders in the mental health setting. Telephone outreach and computer-based CBT is likely to improve access and benefits to patients, although clinical trial evidence is at an early stage (Donnelly et al. 2000; DuHamel et al. 2010).

Patients' preferences are a key consideration in what intervention is chosen (Edwards et al. 2008; Sellick and Crooks 1999). Some patients recognize that their coping difficulties are linked to early experience but do not wish to revisit those memories. Although evidence supports the effectiveness of group interventions (Naaman et al. 2009; Schneider et al. 2010), not all patients wish to disclose their concerns to others. Some fear that hearing other patients' concerns and worries will undermine their own coping (Kissane et al. 2003). Also, some patients find the idea of computer-based therapy too impersonal, whereas others welcome the opportunity for self-management that it affords.

Often, a combined approach is more effective than a single intervention. The combination of relaxation and complementary therapies with a coping intervention may be the optimal treatment for a highly anxious patient. For depressed patients who lack the motivation and energy levels needed to engage effectively with psychological therapies (Roth and Fonagy 1996; Strong et al. 2008), antidepressant medication may be an important precursor to psychological intervention.

Regardless of the intervention chosen, evidence from cancer and community samples suggests that the effectiveness of any psychological intervention rests with the skill or competence of the therapist and the strength of the therapeutic relationship established (Bennett and Parry 2004; Davidson et al. 2004; Kissane et al. 2003; Sellick and Crooks 1999). Empathy, warmth, and the therapeutic relationship have correlated more highly with patient outcomes than have specialized treatment interventions. Meta-analyses have attributed from 50% (Horvath and Symonds 1991) to 85% (Lambert and Okiishi 1997) of the beneficial effects of therapeutic change to the quality of the alliance.

Findings relevant to psychosocial interventions for cancer patients are summarized in Table 5–1.

Tiered Approach for Provision of Psychological Support

The importance of effective, evidence-based psychological care in cancer services is recognized (National Institute for Clinical Excellence 2004), but all national health services are challenged by limited economic resources. Traditionally, psychological interventions are delivered by counselors, clinical psychologists, psychotherapists, and psychiatrists, all of whom have professional training in mental health or psychology. In an effort to make provision of psychological care more available, however, a growing number of psychological interventions have been designed to be delivered by health care staff without any professional training in psychology or mental health. Some of these interventions have shown benefits for patients in preventing the development of mood disorders among distressed cancer patients or promoting recovery for those already diagnosed with major depression (Pitceathly et al. 2009; Strong et al. 2008).

Packages for training non-psychologists in psychological methods of assessment and intervention have been welcomed in clinical practice. Given the primacy of the therapist role in determining therapeutic outcomes, the effectiveness of a non-specialist is likely to depend on the suitability of individuals selected for training and the quality of the training provided. Supervisors with relevant professional qualification and experience are essential to ensure adherence to the model of intervention and to "quality assure" programs. Specialist psychological or mental health services must also be avail-

TABLE 5–1.   Summary of findings regarding psychosocial interventions for cancer patients

Evidence supports the effectiveness of a broad range of interventions.

Illness context may determine the most helpful therapeutic approach.

The etiology of the problem and each patient's coping style inform the relevant therapeutic approach.

Patient preference is key in the choice of intervention method and context for delivery.

Combined interventions can be more effective than a single treatment approach.

The competence of the therapist or practitioner is pivotal to therapeutic outcomes.

able when patients with more complex problems are identified, to ensure optimal care for patients and appropriate staff support.

Integrating these perspectives into care, national health services have identified models of service provision that reflect a tiered approach (Hutchison et al. 2006; National Institute for Clinical Excellence 2004). All health professionals are expected to assess patients' basic psychological needs and provide psychological support, but for patients with more severe and more complex psychological difficulties, both needs assessment and provision of psychological intervention are the responsibility of health professionals with a core professional training in counseling or mental health.

In the cancer service guidance for supportive and palliative care, the National Institute for Clinical Excellence (2004) recommends a four-level model of psychological assessment and support. Broad definitions are given to the training and expertise expected of practitioners at each level. Table 5–2 summarizes these recommendations and those of the Department of Health's (2010) "Manual for Cancer Services 2008: Psychological Support Measures."

Psychological Interventions

Consistent with a model of service delivery that provides the minimum intervention necessary to achieve therapeutic change, the psychological interventions that we describe build from those that are (or should be) common practice for all social and health care professionals (Level 1) to those that are the province of health professionals with core training in clinical psychology

TABLE 5–2.	Summary of the recommendations for four-tier psychological support provision in U.K. cancer services

Level 1: All health and social care staff provide support and effective communication.

Level 2: Designated health care professionals have additional training (and supervision) in specific psychological interventions.

Level 3: Trained, accredited professionals deliver psychological interventions that adhere to specific theoretical models.

Level 4: Mental health specialists manage and treat complex psychological problems and moderate to severe mental health problems.

Source. Adapted from Department of Health 2010; National Institute for Clinical Excellence 2004.

(Level 4). We focus on psychological interventions that aim to alleviate measurable psychological distress in the form of concerns, anxiety or depressive symptoms, or mood disorders by focusing on the conditions, particularly the beliefs, thoughts, emotions, and behaviors, that maintain or increase distress.

The models of intervention and the therapeutic methods we describe are chosen to represent those currently provided in cancer care. There are commonalities between the theoretical models and modes of delivery that underpin the interventions. Effective triaging of referrals within the psycho-oncology team involves consideration of each patient's emotional or psychological difficulties, personality, and coping style, as well as practical considerations of health status and ease of access to clinic-based services. Practitioners use interventions concurrently or consecutively to meet an individual patient's needs.

Level 1: All Health and Social Care Staff

Communication Skills

The way health and social care staff communicate with patients can either support patients in adapting to the demands of the cancer and its treatment or undermine their efforts to cope.

Effective eliciting of patients' concerns and difficulties underpins the early identification and prevention of distress and mood problems. If psychological problems are found early and patients are referred for appropriate help, they will be less distressed in the longer term (Maguire and Pitceathly 2003), and if patients with high levels of concerns are recognized and helped early on, the development of mood disorders may be avoided (Pitceathly et al. 2009).

The way in which health and social care professionals deliver information is also important to patients' psychological adaptation. Patients who feel they have received too much or too little information (Fallowfield et al. 1990) or perceive that information has been delivered in an uncaring or insensitive fashion (Mager and Andrykowski 2002) experience more psychological distress.

Theory and process

The structuring of the interpersonal encounter between health professional and patient is the foundation for achieving effective communication. If clinicians need to deliver important information, patients are more likely to understand and remember it if they have had their own issues addressed first. Establishing the nature of a patient's perceptions, concerns, and needs (including psychological needs) before delivering information or advice allows for the content and form of information provided to be tailored to the patient's needs. Hearing a patient describe his or her illness perceptions and concerns can also help health professionals to deliver complex information at a pace and in a language style tailored to the individual. Information delivered in this way is likely to be better understood and remembered (Maguire and Pitceathly 2002; Silverman et al. 2005).

Assessment skills are fundamental to identifying patients who are psychologically distressed (Jacobsen and Jim 2008; Naaman et al. 2009), but does a holistic assessment of a patient's concerns and needs (i.e., medical, physical, spiritual, relationship, existential, social, practical, and emotional or psychological difficulties) constitute a psychological intervention? We think it does. Patients who have the opportunity to talk through their illness experiences, concerns, and difficulties, and who have their information needs met, feel more positive. Health professionals are able to respond to some concerns with reassurance and practical solutions. Patients may identify unhelpful coping attitudes and behaviors and start to address their own difficulties without further intervention, confirming the psychological benefits of emotional expression and "telling the story" (Pennebaker and Seagal 1999; Stanton et al. 2002).

Case Vignette

Alice, age 52 years, had been diagnosed with breast cancer. Following a mastectomy, she was on the third cycle of a six-cycle chemotherapy regimen. She was tearful at her chemotherapy appointment, and a nurse spent time talking to her. The nurse discovered that the patient lived alone but avoided going out and did not contact friends because she felt self-conscious about her appearance. She also worried about feeling so tired and what that might mean in terms of her disease. She was feeling anxious and very isolated. The nurse was able to address some of the patient's illness worries but was concerned about her social withdrawal and offered her a referral for counseling. When Alice saw the counselor, she already felt better. She had found the nurse "very understanding," and their conversation had highlighted how much she missed her friends. She had made contact again, and as a result, her embarrassment about her hair loss was considerably reduced. No further counseling appointments were planned.

Although specific psychological interventions may vary in focus and complexity, this model of assessing patients' perceptions, concerns, and psychological difficulties underpins every psychological intervention at all levels.

Target population for intervention:

- All patients at any time but particularly at key times in the illness (e.g., at diagnosis, after treatment, at recurrence, when treatment becomes palliative)

Referral pathways:

- Counseling for patients identified with persistently high levels of concerns or distress
- Mental health specialist for patients identified with symptoms of mood disorder

Level 2: Designated Health Care Professionals With Additional Training

The role of a clinical nurse specialist in U.K. cancer services includes an explicit responsibility to provide emotional support to cancer patients and their families. Therefore, these health professionals (and others with a particular interest in psychological care) are targeted for training in specific psychological interventions.

Concerns-Focused Interventions Based on Cognitive-Behavioral Methods

Psychological interventions based on cognitive-behavioral methods have been shown to prevent the development of anxiety and depressive disorders among distressed cancer patients and to promote recovery among patients who are already depressed (Greer et al. 1992; Jacobsen and Jim 2008; Osborn et al. 2006; Pitceathly et al. 2009; Sellick and Crooks 1999; Strong et al. 2008). Professionals who are not psychologists (e.g., nurses, social workers) can be trained to deliver interventions using cognitive-behavioral and problem-solving methods for the benefit of patients who are psychologically distressed (Moorey et al. 2009; Nezu et al. 2003; Pitceathly et al. 2009; Strong et al. 2008), although the evidence for impact on depressed mood is less clear (Moorey et al. 2009). If oncology nurses can use aspects of CBT to help some patients encountered in their routine practice, there is potential to destigmatize the therapeutic experience by making psychological intervention an integral part of clinical care.

Theory and process

Patients who perceive their illness to be exceptionally challenging or threatening and who feel they have limited support resources, whether actual or perceived, are less likely to persist in their efforts to cope with problems and worries. They may employ strategies that exacerbate the problem, and if coping efforts prove ineffective, they may perceive the demands of the illness as even more challenging. As concerns become more worrying and more unmanageable, patients become more distressed and eventually depressed (Parle et al. 1996).

The broad aims of coping interventions are to help patients relinquish unhelpful coping behaviors and identify more effective ways of dealing with problems, and to support patients in their efforts to employ more adaptive strategies. There is no evidence for the primacy of particular strategies; the key is to identify what will help with the identified concern and, as a result, the patient's emotional and mood difficulties. The approach is a collaborative one. Therapists work alongside patients to identify the strengths and limitations of their thinking and behavioral coping strategies. If unhelpful strategies are identified, new ways of coping are considered and tried out. Patient and therapist then review and evaluate the outcomes.

Case Vignette

Barbara, age 32 years, was diagnosed with non-Hodgkin lymphoma. She was receiving 3-weekly cycles of chemotherapy and becoming increasingly tired. Her strategy for managing her treatment was to keep life as close to normal as possible to avoid feeling that the cancer had "taken over." Her ways of achieving this included seeing her work friends regularly and taking her four dogs on daily walks of up to 4 miles.

When asked to reflect on the helpfulness of these strategies, she recognized that social visits with her friends from work were very helpful. Hearing about their lives distracted her from her illness for a while, and they kept her up to date on "work gossip" so she felt "connected" to events in the office even though she wasn't there. Her mood was always good when she got home. She also enjoyed getting outside in the fresh air with the dogs but was finding it more difficult to manage the distances she walked. She persevered because not to do so felt like a concession to the illness. However, because of the increasing tiredness, Barbara felt that the illness was "taking over" and she was becoming lower in mood.

Having acknowledged the consequence of these ways of thinking and behaving on her overall mood, Barbara decided to modify her strategy. She planned to maintain normality "within reason." Therefore, she continued to meet with friends but let her husband do the longer dog walks and accompanied him on shorter ones. As a result, she felt less tired, more in control, and better in mood. An unexpected gain from her change in strategy was that she realized she had been quite rejecting of her husband's offers of help, so the change in coping style met both their needs. She found that reflecting on her coping style and the strategies she used not only helped her to identify more effective ways of thinking and behaving but made her more aware of the impact of her coping behaviors on herself and others.

Target populations for intervention:

- Patients reporting high levels of concerns/distress
- Patients identifying coping difficulties
- Patients reporting symptoms of depression

Referral pathway:

- Psychologist or psychiatrist for patients with concerns, distress, or depressive symptoms that fail to alleviate

Relaxation

Studies have investigated the efficacy of relaxation techniques that include imagery, guided relaxation, and the more structured technique of progressive muscle relaxation. A meta-analysis of 116 studies of psychoeducational care provided to adults with cancer (Devine and Westlake 1995) found statistically significant reductions in reported levels of anxiety, depression, mood, nausea and vomiting, and pain in patients with cancer. In a study with breast cancer patients undergoing chemotherapy, Walker et al. (1999) evaluated the effectiveness of progressive muscle relaxation and guided imagery compared with standard care. Following intervention, patients who received progressive muscle relaxation and guided imagery reported less psychological distress, less emotional suppression, increased relaxation, and better quality of life than did patients receiving standard care.

Theory and process

According to Freeman (2001), progressive muscle relaxation and other muscle-based relaxation techniques are beneficial in three ways: they manipulate the autonomic responses (which are involved in the so-called flight or fight response), increase or activate the production of opiates, and promote optimal immune function. Relaxation techniques are increasingly being used by health care professionals as nonpharmacological strategies for managing a number of somatic states, including anxiety and stress, and also in health promotion.

Case Vignette

Susan, age 44 years, was becoming extremely anxious about receiving chemotherapy for her non–small cell lung cancer. To help her cope, she learned to use progressive muscle relaxation, which involved learning about the body's tension-release cycle. She was asked to make a tight fist and then release it while using her breath as a way of relieving any tension. She was then invited to get in touch with any other areas of tension in her body using the same tension-release cycle. The result was that Susan became much calmer. She was also taught to use guided imagery while undergoing chemotherapy by visualizing her treatment impacting on her malignant cells. She chose an image that suited her personally. Avoiding an aggressive image involving an attack on the cancer cells, Susan chose a gentler image in which she visualized the chemotherapy as a golden healing color that washed away the cancer cells.

Mindfulness

Theory and process

Kabat-Zinn (1996) suggests that "we practice mindfulness by remembering to be present in all our waking moments" (p. 29). Meditation using mindfulness practice is finding a place within supportive cancer care.

Often, patients focus on a predicament that cannot be changed, such as waiting for test results, treatment outcomes, and the likelihood of survival. Each of these has the potential to increase patients' anxiety and psychological distress. In addition, many patients have difficulty "being positive" because this puts them at risk of being unprepared for the shock and distress of bad news. The practice of mindfulness allows patients to be in the present moment and thus freed from negative thoughts and anxieties about the future that contribute to their psychological and emotional distress.

Case Vignette

Stan, a 68-year-old man with prostate cancer, was becoming extremely anxious about the outcome of his radiotherapy. He would have to wait a few weeks before having a scan and another 2 weeks for the results. Stan joined a mindfulness meditation group at the hospice and was taught how to "stay in the moment." He learned how to let his mind settle from its normal unsettled state by remaining focused on his breath. Gradually, his focus became more on the body, giving him a sense of being more grounded. When his mind became distracted, which it inevitably did, he used the breath as a support to keep returning to and help him gently focus on the moment. By practicing for 30 minutes a day, Stan began to teach his mind to become more focused on the present moment, thereby avoiding thoughts about the future over which he had no control.

Target populations for intervention:

- Patients who are generally anxious or stressed
- Patients who are unable to relax or who have difficulty sleeping
- Patients who become anxious about undergoing treatments or investigations, or who are having difficulty waiting for test results
- Patients who want to learn coping skills

Referral pathways:

- Psychologist or psychiatrist for patients with evidence of depression
- CBT for patients whose anxiety levels remain elevated
- Concurrent medication for patients with mood problems

Levels 3 and 4: Accredited Professionals and Mental Health Specialists

Counseling

Bower et al. (2011) conducted a review of counseling from professionally trained counselors in primary care (local community) services in the United Kingdom. The aim was to assess the effectiveness and cost-effectiveness of counseling compared with usual care from the general practitioner. Patients included in the trial had psychological and psychosocial problems considered suitable for counseling. The analysis found significantly greater clinical effectiveness in the counseling group compared with general practitioner care in the short term, but there were no additonal advantages in the long term. Levels of satisfaction with counseling were high. Overall costs of care were similar. Reviews of psychological interventions in cancer settings suggest that counseling improves quality of life (Newell et al. 2002) and benefits patients with symptoms of depression (Sellick and Crooks 1999).

Theory and process

In a review of a cancer counseling service, clients perceived that counseling helped them to come to terms with cancer and its consequences and to regain a measure of control in their lives (Boulton et al. 2001). Counseling aims to provide a therapeutic space in which the client feels safe to talk about whatever is concerning him or her and to express emotions and feelings without judgment or advice. Safety is promoted by the counselor's maintaining boundaries of confidentiality and consistency. The therapeutic qualities of empathy, unconditional positive regard, and genuineness described by Rogers (1957) facilitate the therapeutic process. Patients or clients commonly use counseling as an opportunity to talk about the impact of the illness and treatment, whether they are working through the shock of diagnosis, grieving for the losses that the illness has brought, processing the effects on their relationships, or perhaps reassessing their lives.

Counselors may work from a diverse range of models. Some of the most commonly encountered in psycho-oncology services are humanistic, psychodynamic, person-centered, existential, and systemic approaches. Flexibility is a fundamental characteristic for working in the cancer setting, and many counselors will adopt an integrative approach. Whatever the approach or core model of the counselor, the quality of the relationship with the client is the key to the therapeutic process. The case example given illustrates a psychodynamic approach.

Psychodynamic Counseling

Derived from psychoanalysis, psychodynamic psychotherapy stresses the importance of past experiences and the unconscious in shaping current behavior. The client is encouraged to talk about childhood relationships with parents and other significant people. The therapist focuses on the client-therapist relationship and in particular on the transference (when the client projects onto the therapist feelings experienced in previous significant relationships).

Case Vignette

Michael, age 35 years, was receiving intensive chemotherapy for Burkitt lymphoma. He was referred for counseling because he became increasingly distressed during an inpatient stay. He was often tearful and became very anxious when by himself in his room. He would plead with nurses to stay with him but remained inconsolable, despite their efforts to help him talk about what was worrying him. He could not identify any particular fears and was confident that treatment would be successful. He had a good network of support. The counselor was interested to know about his early history, and he told her that his mother had left him and his father when he was 3 years old. He had always thought of himself as a survivor and could not understand his dependence on the nurses. Thinking about his early experiences helped him make sense of his feelings, and he felt more able to cope with the treatment.

Target populations for intervention:

- Patients struggling to adjust to the cancer diagnosis and treatment
- Patients struggling with their emotional responses
- Patients experiencing interpersonal problems
- Patients who struggle to comply with treatments, after initial efforts from medical and nursing colleagues have not been successful
- Patients coping with end-of-life issues

Referral pathways:

- CBT or hypnotherapy if specific difficulties (e.g., social phobia or anxiety) persist
- Concurrent medication for mood problems
- Longer-term psychotherapy
- Family or couples therapy

Psychotherapies

Improved outcomes have been reported for patients who receive brief psychotherapeutic intervention in addition to routine specialist mental health treatment (Guthrie et al. 1999; Keller et al. 2000). CBT and cognitive analytic therapy (CAT) are examples of the psychotherapies offered in U.K. psychooncology services by Level 3 and 4 practitioners.

Cognitive-behavioral therapy

Research evidence. CBT research provides substantial evidence on efficacy in the treatment of depression (Clark and Fairburn 1997). The American Psychiatric Association's (2000) practice guidelines indicated that among psychotherapy methods, CBT was one of the most efficacious for treatment of major depression.

CBT was used to good effect in a large randomized controlled trial by Greer et al. (1992) in patients with locoregional cancers. Patients were initially screened for evidence of symptoms of depression and anxiety and offered an average of four sessions of CBT that had been adapted to the needs of cancer patients (referred to as adjuvant psychological therapy).

In recent years there have been concerted attempts to introduce CBT as an effective part of enhancing the psychological care of cancer patients. CBT is not appropriate for patients with organic mental syndromes such as psychosis, schizoaffective disorders, or delirium; patients with these syndromes should be referred for psychiatric assessment and care.

Theory and process. CBT represents a pragmatic, brief, structured approach to managing psychological problems that cancer patients experience throughout the disease trajectory. CBT is a collaborative problem-focused therapy in which patient and therapist agree on positive changes that might be integrated into the patient's daily life to help lift mood (Horne and Watson 2011). Therapy focuses on interactions between thoughts, feelings, and behaviors, and provides patients with a rational formulation of the problems they are experiencing. In cancer services, CBT is often adapted to focus on problem solving; issues to be resolved are targeted and worked on using techniques that have an impact on thinking and the degree or intensity of negative ruminations. Behavioral techniques are usually straightforward to grasp and seem to apply generally across the patient spectrum.

Case Vignette

Ann felt unable to join close friends at social events because she was afraid she would become anxious and tearful. This was based on her thought that "if my friends ask how I am, I will break down in front of them and be an embarrassment to everyone." This attitude contributed to her refusing to attend important social events, including her best friend's twenty-fifth wedding anniversary. She had developed a social phobia.

Ann was encouraged to try two strategies that might help her to cope by using behavioral experiments. This involved her testing the idea that when friends talked to her about her health, her only response was to become tearful. To achieve this she needed to plan ahead for how she would put herself into social situations where she might test out the idea.

To increase the likelihood that she would engage with this behavioral experiment, aimed at challenging her negative thoughts, Ann was asked to construct a plan in advance whereby she might remove herself from the situation if she became overwhelmed. The aim was not to encourage her to further avoid the situation but to get her to think, "How would I deal with the situation if my fears are confirmed and I do start to cry? What options do I have?" She was invited to play out this scenario within the therapy session so that she could rehearse her response. During her therapy session, she practiced replies she might make to everyday social situations (e.g., a response to the simple question "How are you?"). During therapy she was encouraged further to talk about her concerns regarding cancer to try to discover what aspects were upsetting to her and consider how she might accommodate to her fears.

Target populations for intervention:

- Patients reporting high unremitting levels of concerns/distress
- Patients reporting symptoms of depression
- Patients reporting complex relational/social problems

Referral pathway:

- Psychologist or psychiatrist for patients with concerns, distress, or depressive symptoms that fail to be alleviated

Cognitive analytic therapy

Recent reporting of the use of CAT in cancer services suggests that benefits are seen in clinical practice (Pitceathly et al. 2011). Although no research evidence yet supports this clinical experience, trials of CAT have been conducted in a range of clinical populations, including patients with medical co-morbidities. In an early study of patients with poorly controlled type 1 diabetes (Fosbury et al. 1997), patients benefited more from CAT than from education in the form of information, advice, and support from a clinical nurse specialist. A valid and reliable measure of CAT competency has been developed (Bennett and Parry 2004) that will further contribute to the methodological robustness of trials.

Theory and process.   CAT was developed in the United Kingdom by Anthony Ryle in response to the needs of the National Health Service for brief psychotherapeutic treatments. CAT is an integrative model of psychotherapy. Initially informed by other models, including cognitive-behavioral approaches and psychoanalytic object relations theory, the theoretical base for CAT has continued to be developed, incorporating ideas from Vygotsky's activity theory and Bakhtin's concept of a dialogical self (Ryle 1990; Ryle and Kerr 2002).

In CAT the major focus is on the social and relational origins of the self. Early relational experiences (in CAT, termed *reciprocal roles*) may range from very positive to very negative. The following are two examples:

- caring and valuing (parent) ↔ cared for and valued (child)
- attacking, abusing (parent) ↔ attacked, vulnerable, sullied (child)

Early relational experiences are internalized and then determine the way people manage themselves, their relationships with others, and their response to life events such as a cancer diagnosis. Patterns of coping responses and behaviors aimed at managing or avoiding unbearable feelings associated with negative role positions (e.g., having been abused or abandoned) and achieving more desirable positions are termed *reciprocal role procedures*. These procedures may have unplanned consequences that maintain the problems that bring a patient to therapy.

The activity of therapy is collaborative. In the first few sessions of therapy, patient and therapist develop an understanding together of how current problems originated in early relational experience (RRs) and how they are maintained (RRPs). A summary of those understandings (termed the reformulation) is shared with the patient in the form of a letter. Together, patient and therapist map the reformulation on a diagram that makes the RRs and RRPs explicit. The diagram is used throughout the therapy to explore reenactments of problem RRPs and to recognize positive outcomes from revised responses. Monitoring of the patterns in daily life and in relationships is the vehicle for revision. The therapist-patient relationship is a key context for experiencing more positive reciprocal roles. Patient and therapist write a

letter to each other at the end of therapy (the goodbye letter). The letter
recalls the patient's goals for therapy, identifies what has been achieved, and
notes what challenges remain. The letters and the diagram can become tools
to support patients as they continue working to achieve their goals after
therapy has ended.

The relational focus of CAT is particularly relevant in the cancer setting.
Cancer is often perceived as a powerful, controlling, and intrusive "other."
Patients respond in ways that aim to regain some control, such as by seeking
to be well informed. Some responses are less adaptive. The applications of
CAT in a psycho-oncology service range from a single-session reformula-
tion to full therapy (16–24 sessions).

Case Vignette: One-Session Reformulation

Carl, age 35 years, became irritable and uncooperative with the demands of
ward routines and with delays in tests or treatment times. Staff realized that
these uncertainties compounded the "loss of control" he experienced in
relation to the illness and his hospital admission. Acknowledging the impact
of the diagnosis in relational terms helped him to identify tools for addressing the difficulties he experienced. He worked out strategies with the nursing
staff to keep him more updated regarding plans for tests and procedures and
thereby reduced his sense of helplessness in relation to his treatment. No
further intervention was necessary.

Case Vignette: Sixteen-Session CAT

Emily, age 58 years, "ignored" early signs of her breast cancer and, when
eventually diagnosed, failed to attend appointments for important procedures. She had agreed to surgery but was reluctant to accept chemotherapy
treatment because it meant regular visits to the cancer center. She was terri-
fied that her cancer would return because she had failed to comply with
treatment, and she became depressed.

In her first therapy session, Emily described her childhood. Her parents
worked hard and went out drinking at night, leaving her alone at home
(reciprocal role: overlooking/distracted↔unseen/vulnerable). She tried
hard to gain positive attention from them by behaving well and helping in the
house. At age 10, she was sexually abused for some months by a man lodging
with them (reciprocal role: abusing↔violated/powerless). She felt she could
not tell anyone or "make a fuss" and had tried to "block out" both the memories and the unbearable feelings associated with them.

Emily experienced the cancer as intrusive, powerful, and overwhelming
(in CAT terms, she experienced it as a "reenactment" of her childhood
trauma). As in childhood, she coped by not thinking about it and tried to "just
get on with life," so the prospect of a 6-month chemotherapy regimen challenged her efforts to maintain normality. She experienced the well-
intentioned efforts of medical staff to explain the benefits of further treatment as pressuring. She recognized that, although her inclination was to

"resist" and "avoid" treatments, she was afraid of losing the support of her medical team and reducing her chance of cure. She felt confused and anxious.

In therapy, Emily reflected on the origins of her ways of managing difficult emotions. These understandings left her feeling more in control, and she then became more respectful of herself and her difficulties. The medical team helped her to feel supported and less overwhelmed by providing information in amounts that she could manage, and she decided to pursue treatment.

The team anticipated that the end of therapy would mean the loss of a supportive, respectful relationship for Emily. Perhaps understandably, considering her early relationships, she became "too busy" to attend the later sessions.

Target populations for intervention:

- Patients whose emotional responses to illness or treatments seem out of proportion and overwhelming to themselves and those caring for them
- Patients who have received other psychological or psychiatric interventions, but benefits have been partial or absent
- Patients who describe current psychological or interpersonal problems but recognize that their difficulties predated the cancer diagnosis
- Patients who find that their memories of past abuse or bereavement seem to be suddenly "in the present" in a way that is alarming and distressing

Hypnotherapy

Evidence supports the medical utility of hypnotherapy. In a review of the literature, Patterson and Jenson (2003) concluded that hypnotherapy was an effective treatment for both acute and chronic pain. Hypnotherapy can effect psychological as well as physical benefits. Lang et al. (2000) investigated the effectiveness of self-hypnotic relaxation as a means of reducing discomfort and adverse effects during medical procedures. The hypnotherapy groups had fewer intraoperative adverse events, flattened pain levels, and decreased anxiety levels. Lang et al. (2008) continued this investigation with a second trial of patients undergoing tumor treatments. Patients in the hypnosis group, compared with controls, experienced lower levels of pain and anxiety and needed less analgesia.

Theory and process

Derbyshire et al. (2009) and Mohr et al. (2005) used positron emission tomography to investigate whether hypnotherapy works and if so how it works. Both studies found that hypnosis moderated brain function during the reduction in perceived pain. The investigators agreed that certain areas in the limbic system appear to be involved in the analgesic effect.

Hypnotherapy is increasingly being used as a stand-alone therapy or as a useful adjunct to other conventional and integrated therapeutic modalities (Cawthorn and Mackereth 2010). Hypnotherapy has been defined as a psychological intervention that helps the individual to achieve a natural trance state (Zahourek 2001). The aim is to effect changes in both conscious and unconscious states of mind. The therapist acts as a facilitator of the therapeutic process. Therapists work in a variety of ways informed by an individual assessment of each patient's difficulties.

One way is through the use of diagnostic imagery where ideas or information become available from the unconscious. This information is not always accessible in the rational mind, so the images can prove illuminating to both patient and therapist. Images might include how patients see their cancer, how they view chemotherapy, or whether they see themselves as whole following surgery. This information may be valuable of itself, or may form the basis for the therapist's work using hypnotherapy techniques.

Case Vignette

Michelle, age 24 years, was recovering from treatment for oral cancer. She experienced severe anxiety when having blood tests at the follow-up clinic. During trance she was asked to scan her body to access any images she wanted to change. To her surprise the skin on her right arm looked extremely fragile and that explained why she was reluctant to have blood taken and why she pulled her arm away. Using imagery, Michelle was able to use her breath in order to bring healing colored light into the area. This resulted in her seeing her right arm as normal again and she was able to have venipuncture.

Referral pathways:

- CBT or hypnotherapy if specific difficulties (e.g., social phobia or anxiety) persist
- Concurrent medication for mood problems

Therapeutic imagery

Some patients continue to have negative images of events that occurred prior to their diagnosis. These could include a history of physical and sexual abuse or a variety of traumatic events. For some, the trauma can be attributed to their cancer treatments or investigations. Whatever the cause, these add to the difficulties that patients experience. Through hypnotherapy techniques, negative images can be changed to help a patient regain a sense of control.

Case Vignette

Claire, age 46 years, had difficulty accepting her newly reconstructed breast. On hearing her narrative, the therapist realized that Claire linked her breast cancer with her abusive ex-partner. While deeply relaxed, she was invited to put the partner's face in a television screen. Then she changed the color to black and white, turned the volume down, and shrunk the image to a size that was small and insignificant. Following the intervention, Claire felt much more in control, and the link between her ex-partner and the new breast was severed.

Working With Anxiety, Panic, and Phobia

Coming to terms with the diagnosis of a life-threatening illness such as cancer, or managing challenging investigations and treatments can cause acute distress, anxiety, phobia, or development of a panic state. The capacity to become anxious serves an important role in people's lives, serving to make individuals cautious. Understanding anxiety and learning how to manage it can help patients tolerate the challenges they face.

Phobia is "characterized by an excessive, irrational fear of a specific object or situation, which is avoided at all costs or endured with great distress" (Choy et al. 2007, p. 267). Phobias are extremely challenging when linked with cancer treatments or investigations. For example, a patient experiencing a phobic response to chemotherapy may be hyperventilating, distressed, and/or angry when attending for treatment. Effective techniques that can be employed to reprogram the person's view of the object or situation include desensitization or phobia cures that are based on neurolinguistic programming techniques (Rushworth 1999).

Panic is an extreme form of anxiety with marked autonomic nervous system arousal, and it has a number of uncomfortable signs and symptoms, leading the patient to have a fight, flight, or freeze reaction.

Case Vignette

Jane, age 46 years, remained very anxious on completion of her treatment for breast cancer. She went to the emergency department with chest pains on two separate occasions, but all the tests were normal. Working with Jane, the therapist found that she was frightened of dying and was holding herself in the brace position (hence the chest pains). In trance she was taught how to find a safe place that she could use when she felt anxious. She was also invited to look for an anxiety dial and see if she wanted to turn it down. She saw it as 9 out of 10 and chose to turn it down to 4. These techniques helped Jane feel much more in control of her anxiety, with her level remaining at 4 out of 10.

Target populations for intervention:

- Patients willing to access information in their unconscious to help them cope with their cancer or subsequent treatments
- Patients who are anxious or depressed or who exhibit existential anxiety
- Patients for whom the cancer or treatments have raised issues relating to abuse or trauma

- Patients with unresolved symptoms such as pain, nausea, and vomiting
- Patients with body image issues or sexual problems

Referral pathways:

- Psychologist or psychiatrist if depression or anxiety persists
- Concurrent medication if required
- Relationship or family therapy

Conclusion

The psychological and counseling interventions described in this chapter can be found in psycho-oncology services worldwide, but the provision of psychological support and intervention in cancer care is not consistent. There is wide variation regionally, nationally, and internationally in the size of psycho-oncology services, their structure, the professional makeup of the therapeutic team, and the range and nature of interventions provided. There are also differences in the training and supervision offered for health professionals to learn to provide "nonspecialist" psychological support and intervention. The result of these inconsistencies is that not every patient who might benefit from the interventions described in this chapter will be able to access them. More positively, some patients will benefit from interesting and innovative approaches to the emotional and psychological care of cancer patients that we have not been able to address.

Key Clinical Points

- Research and clinical evidence supports the benefits of psychological interventions.

- Patients need access to a range of interventions in terms of type of therapy and the context for delivery (i.e., individual, couples, family, group).

- Patients should be routinely assessed as part of oncology practice to establish the type and extent of any psychological problems.

- Routinely assessing for psychological and emotional problems helps clinicians develop their skills and destigmatizes coping difficulties and emotional problems for patients.

- Patients will wait for doctors and nurses to show interest in emotional problems. Responsibility lies with clinicians to ask.

- Simpler emotional problems can be managed using effective communication behaviors that all clinicians can adopt.

- More complex and enduring problems need to be triaged to clarify what level of intervention is needed.

- All cancer clinicians should have access to mental health professionals who will work alongside the oncology teams in managing patients.

- Patients with well-managed psychological problems do better in terms of improved quality of life, better adherence to treatment, and reduced use of clinical consultations and community (general practitioner) services.

References

Akechi T, Okuyama T, Sugawara Y, et al: Major depression, adjustment disorders, and post-traumatic stress disorder in terminally ill cancer patients: associated and predictive factors. J Clin Oncol 22:1957–1965, 2004

American Psychiatric Association: Diagnostic and Statistical Manual of Mental Disorders, 4th Edition, Text Revision. Washington, DC, American Psychiatric Association, 2000

Bennett D, Parry G: A measure of psychotherapeutic competence derived from cognitive analytic therapy. Psychother Res 14:176–192, 2004

Bidstrup PE, Johansen C, Mitchell AS: Screening for cancer-related distress: summary of evidence from tools to programmes. Acta Oncol 50:194–204, 2011

Boulton M, Boudioni M, Mossman J, et al: "Dividing the desolation": clients views on the benefits of a cancer counselling service. Psychooncology 10:124–136, 2001

Bower P, Knowles S, Coventry PA, et al: Counselling for mental health and psychosocial problems in primary care. Cochrane Database of Systematic Reviews 2011, Issue 9. Art. No.: CD001025. DOI: 10.1002/14651858.CD001025.pub3.

Brown GW, Harris T: Aetiology of anxiety and depressive disorders in an inner-city population. 1. Early adversity. Psychol Med 23:143–154, 1993

Cawthorn A, Mackereth PA: Integrative Hypnotherapy Complementary Approaches in Clinical Care. Edinburgh, Scotland, Churchill Livingstone, 2010

Choy Y, Fryer AJ, Lipsitz JD: Treatment of specific phobias in adults. Clin Psychol Rev 27:226–286, 2007

Clark DM, Fairburn CG (eds): The Science and Practice of Cognitive Behaviour Therapy. Oxford, UK, Oxford University Press, 1997

Coyne J, Kagee A: More may not be better in psychosocial interventions for cancer patients. Health Psychol 20:458–459, 2001

Cuijpers P, van Straten A, Andersson G: Internet-administered cognitive behavior therapy for health problems: a systematic review. J Behav Med 31:169–177, 2008

Davidson K, Scott J, Schmidt U, et al: Therapist competence and clinical outcome in the Prevention of Parasuicide by Manual Assisted Cognitive Behaviour Therapy Trial: the POPMACT study. Psychol Med 34:855–863, 2004

Department of Health: Manual for cancer services 2008: psychological support measures. August 2010. Available at: www.dh.gov.uk/en/Publicationsandstatistics/Publications/PublicationsPolicyAndGuidance/DH_118818. Accessed July 26, 2012.

Derbyshire SW, Whalley MG, Oakley DA: Fibromyalgia and its modulation by hypnotic and non-hypnotic suggestion: an fMRI analysis. Eur J Pain 13:542–550, 2009

Devine EC, Westlake S: The effects of psycho-educational care provided to adults with cancer: meta-analysis of 116 studies. Oncol Nurs Forum 22:1369–1381, 1995

Donnelly JM, Kornblith AR, Fleishman S, et al: A pilot study of interpersonal psychotherapy by telephone with cancer patients and their partners. Psychooncology 9:44–56, 2000

DuHamel KN, Mosher CE, Winkel G, et al: Randomized clinical trial of telephone-administered cognitive-behavioral therapy to reduce post-traumatic stress disorder and distress symptoms after hematopoietic stem-cell transplantation. J Clin Oncol 28:3754–3761, 2010

Edwards AGK, Hulbert-Williams N, Neal RD: Psychological interventions for women with metastatic breast cancer. Cochrane Database of Systematic Reviews 2008, Issue 3. Art. No.: CD004253. DOI: 10.1002/14651858.CD004253.pub3.

Fallowfield L, Hall A, Maguire GP, et al: Psychological outcomes of different treatment policies in women with early breast cancer outside a clinical trial. BMJ 301:575–580, 1990

Fosbury JA, Bosley CM, Ryle A, et al: A trial of cognitive analytic therapy in poorly controlled type 1 diabetes patients. Diabetes Care 20:959–964, 1997

Freeman LW: Research on mind-body effects, in Complementary and Alternative Medicine: A Research Based Approach. Edited by Freeman LW, Lawlin GF. London, Mosby, 2001, pp 34–65

Greer S, Moorey S Baruch JD, et al: Adjuvant psychotherapy for patients with cancer: a prospective randomised trial. BMJ 304:675–680, 1992

Guthrie E, Moorey J, Margison F, et al: Cost-effectiveness of brief psychodynamic-interpersonal therapy in high utilizers of psychiatric services. Arch Gen Psychiatry 56:519–526, 1999

Horne D, Watson M: Cognitive-behavioural therapies in cancer care, in Handbook of Psychotherapy in Cancer Care. Edited by Watson M, Kissane D. London, Wiley-Blackwell, 2011, pp 15–26

Hovarth AO, Symonds BD: Relationship between working alliance and outcome in psychotherapy: a meta-analysis. J Couns Psychol 38:139–149, 1991

Hutchison SD, Steginga SK, Dunn J: The tiered model of psychosocial intervention in cancer: a community based approach. Psychooncology 15:541–546, 2006

Jacobsen PB, Jim HS: Psychosocial interventions for anxiety and depression in adult cancer patients: achievements and challenges. CA Cancer J Clin 58:214–230, 2008

Kabat-Zinn J: Full Catastrophe Living. London, Piatkus Books, 1996

Keller MB, McCullough JP, Klein DN, et al: A comparison of nefazodone, the cognitive behavioral-analysis system of psychotherapy, and their combination for the treatment of chronic depression. N Engl J Med 342:1462–1470, 2000

Kissane DW, Bloch S, Smith GC, et al: Cognitive-existential group psychotherapy for women with primary breast cancer: a randomised controlled trial. Psychooncology 12:532–546, 2003

Lambert MJ, Okiishi JC: The effects of the individual psychotherapist and implications for future research. Clinical Psychology: Science and Practice 4:66–75, 1997

Lang EV, Benotsch EG, Fick LJ, et al: Adjuvant non-pharmacological analgesia for invasive medical procedures: a randomised trial. Lancet 355:1486–1490, 2000

Lang EV, Berbaum KS, Pauker SG, et al: Beneficial effects of hypnosis and adverse effects of empathic attention during percutaneous tumor treatment: when being nice does not suffice. J Vasc Interv Radiol 19:897–905, 2008

Mager WM, Andrykowski MA: Communication in the cancer "bad news" consultation: patient perceptions and psychological adjustment. Psychooncology 11:35–46, 2002

Maguire P, Pitceathly C: Key communication skills and how to acquire them. BMJ 325:697–700, 2002

Maguire P, Pitceathly C: Improving the psychological care of cancer patients and their relatives. The role of specialist nurses. J Psychosom Med 55:469–474, 2003

Massie JM: Prevalence of depression in patients with cancer. J Natl Cancer Inst Monogr 32:57–71, 2004

Mohr C, Binkofski S, Erdmann C, et al: The anterior cingulate cortex contains distinct areas dissociating external from self-administered painful stimulation: a parametric fMRI study. Pain 114:347–357, 2005

Moorey S, Cort E, Kapari M, et al: A cluster randomized controlled trial of cognitive behaviour therapy for common mental disorders in patients with advanced cancer. Psychol Med 39:713–823, 2009

Muriel AC, Hwang VS, Kornblith A, et al: Management of psychosocial distress by oncologists. Psychiatr Serv 60:1132–1134, 2009

Naaman S, Radwan K, Fergusson D, et al: Status of psychological trials in breast cancer patients: a report of three meta-analyses. Psychiatry 72:50–69, 2009

National Institute for Health and Clinical Excellence: Guidance on the use of computerised cognitive behavioural therapy for anxiety and depression. Technology Appraisal Guidance No. 51. October 2002. Available at: www.nice.org.uk/nicemedia/pdf/51_ccbt_full_guidance.pdf. Accessed July 26, 2012.

National Institute for Clinical Excellence: Improving supportive and palliative care for adults with cancer. March 2004. Available at: www.nice.org.uk/CSGSP. Accessed July 26, 2012.

Newell SA, Sanson-Fisher RW, Savolainen NJ: Systematic review of psychological therapies for cancer patients: overview and recommendations for future research. J Natl Cancer Inst 94:558–584, 2002

Nezu A, Nezu C, Felgoise S, et al: Project Genesis: assessing the efficacy of problem-solving therapy for distressed adult cancer patients. J Consult Clin Psychol 71:1036–1048, 2003

Osborn R, Demoncada A, Feuerstein M: Psychosocial interventions for depression, anxiety, and quality of life in cancer survivors: meta-analyses. Intl J Psychiatry Med 36:13–34, 2006

Owen JE, Klapow JC, Roth DL, et al: Improving the effectiveness of adjuvant psychological treatment for women with breast cancer: the feasibility of providing online support. Psychooncology 13:281–292, 2004

Parle M, Maguire P: Exploring relationships between cancer, coping, and mental health. Psychosocial Oncol 13:27–50, 1995

Parle M, Jones B, Maguire P: Maladaptive coping and affective disorders in cancer patients. Psychol Med 26:735–744, 1996

Patterson DR, Jenson MP: Hypnosis and clinical pain. Psychol Bull 129:495–521, 2003

Pennebaker J, Seagsl J: Forming a story: the health benefits of narrative. J Clin Psychol 55:1243–1254, 1999

Pitceathly C, Maguire P, Fletcher I, et al: Can a brief psychological intervention prevent anxiety or depressive disorders in cancer patients? A randomised controlled trial. Ann Oncol 20:928–934, 2009

Pitceathly C, Tolosa I, Kerr I, et al: Cognitive analytic therapy in psycho-oncology, in Handbook of Psychotherapy in Cancer Care. Edited by Watson M, Kissane D. London, Wiley-Blackwell, 2011, pp 27–35

Rehse B, Pukrop R: Effects of psychosocial interventions on quality of life in adult cancer patients: meta-analysis of 37 published controlled outcome studies. Patient Educ Couns 50:179–186, 2003

Rogers C: The necessary and sufficient conditions of therapeutic personality change. J Consult Psychol 21:95–103, 1957

Roth A, Fonagy P: What Works for Whom? A Critical Review of Psychotherapy Research. New York, Guilford, 1996

Rushworth C: Making a Difference in Cancer Care: Practical Techniques in Palliative and Curative Treatment, 2nd Edition. London, Souvenir Press, 1999

Ryle A: Cognitive-Analytic Therapy: Active Participation in Change. A New Integration in Brief Psychotherapy. London, Wiley, 1990

Ryle A, Kerr I: Introducing Cognitive Analytic Therapy: Principles and Practice. London, Wiley, 2002

Schneider S, Moyer A, Knapp-Oliver S, et al: Pre-intervention distress moderates the efficacy of psychosocial treatment for cancer patients: a meta-analysis. J Behav Med 33:1–14, 2010

Sellick S, Crooks D: Depression and cancer: an appraisal of the literature for prevalence, detection, and practice guideline development for psychological interventions. Psychooncology 8:315–333, 1999

Sheard T, Maguire P: The effect of psychological interventions on anxiety and depression in cancer patients: results of two meta-analyses. Br J Cancer 80:1770–1780, 1999

Silverman J, Kurtz S, Draper J: Skills for Communicating With Patients. Oxford, UK, Radcliffe, 2005

Smit F, Beekman A, Cuijpers P, et al: Selecting key variables for depression prevention: results from a population-based prospective epidemiological study. J Affect Disord 81:241–249, 2004

Stanton A: How and for whom? Asking questions about the utility of psychosocial interventions for individuals diagnosed with cancer. J Clin Oncol 23:4818–4820, 2005

Stanton AL, Danoff-Burg S, Sworowoski LA, et al: Randomized, controlled trial of written emotional expression and benefit finding in breast cancer patients. J Clin Oncol 20:4160–4168, 2002

Strong V, Waters R, Hibberd C, et al: Management of depression for people with cancer (SMaRT oncology 1): a randomised trial. Lancet 372:40–48, 2008

Walker LG, Walker MB, Ogston K, et al: Psychological, clinical and pathological effects of relaxation training and guided imagery during primary chemotherapy. Br J Cancer 80:262–268, 1999

Zahourek RP: Trance and suggestion: timeless interventions and implications for nurses in the new millennium. Holist Nurs Pract 15:73–82, 2001

CHAPTER 6

Genetic Counseling and Testing for Hereditary Cancers

Psychosocial Considerations

Allison M. Burton-Chase, Ph.D.
Ellen R. Gritz, Ph.D.
Susan K. Peterson, Ph.D., M.P.H.

ADVANCES IN genetics and genomics have broadened understanding of the basis of many common, chronic diseases, including cancer, and have brought about changes in the delivery of health care in oncology and other specialties. Genetic counseling and testing for inherited predisposition to cancer are an integral part of cancer prevention and oncology care, and the results of genetic testing for inherited cancers are increasingly used to define cancer risk and identify treatment or prevention strategies for high-risk individuals.

Since genetic testing for hereditary cancers became clinically available over a decade ago, psychosocial research has investigated motivations and decisions regarding genetic testing. The focus of much of the research to date has been on the psychological impact of genetic risk notification, effects on family and interpersonal relationships, and factors that influence the uptake (i.e., the decision to utilize or adopt the recommendation) of risk reduction options (e.g., screening, risk-reducing surgery, or chemoprevention).

In this chapter, we discuss the relevant literature on these topics for hereditary cancer syndromes and the implications for clinical practice. Although we discuss a variety of hereditary cancers, we focus mainly on hereditary breast and ovarian cancer syndrome and Lynch syndrome because they are the two most widely studied. Clinicians can use the findings from these studies to aid in their understanding of what motivates people to seek genetic counseling and testing, what they hope to gain from it, and how they cope with the results of testing. Ultimately, this information can be integrated into cancer prevention and treatment decisions.

Overview of Genetic Counseling and Testing for Hereditary Cancer Syndromes

Analysis of DNA from blood or saliva is used to identify specific gene mutations associated with known inherited cancer syndromes. Persons with such mutations have lifetime cancer risks that are substantially higher than in the general population. For example, men with a mutation in a mismatch repair gene (e.g., *MLH1, MSH2, MLH6, PMS1)* associated with Lynch syndrome have a 74%–82% lifetime risk of developing colorectal cancer, and women with such a mutation have a 30%–54% and a 40%–60% lifetime risk of developing colorectal and endometrial cancers, respectively (Lindor et al. 2006). Table 6–1 shows examples of germline gene mutations associated with common cancers in several hereditary cancer syndromes. These mutations are highly penetrant yet rare, and are estimated to account for a small percentage of the associated cancers. As an example, mutations related to Lynch syndrome are estimated to account for 2%–4% of all colorectal cancers (Lynch et al. 2008). Table 6–2 shows examples of germline gene mutations associated with rare cancer syndromes. Although rare, these cancer syndromes can be very devastating due to the early onset of illness and the predisposition to multiple types of primary cancers.

Identification of a cancer-predisposing gene mutation has implications for clinical and preventive care. Individuals with these known gene mutations are often advised to consider undergoing increased cancer screening or surveillance, preventive surgery, or chemoprevention (Lindor et al. 2006). The results of genetic testing have implications not only for the person who undergoes testing but also for his or her family members. Many cancer-predisposing gene mutations are inherited in an autosomal dominant pattern; thus, children are at 50% risk of inheriting such mutations from their parents. When an individual learns about his or her own risk for an inher-

TABLE 6–1. Hereditary cancer syndromes

Syndrome	Predominant tumor types	Gene(s) causing syndrome
Basal cell nevus syndrome; Gorlin syndrome	Basal-cell cancer	*PTCH*
Cowden syndrome	Breast cancer, thyroid cancer, endometrial cancer	*PTEN*
Familial adenomatous polyposis	Adenomatous polyps of the colon/rectum, gastrointestinal cancers, papillary thyroid cancer	*APC*
Familial atypical mole malignant melanoma syndrome/hereditary dysplastic nevus syndrome	Cutaneous malignant melanoma, pancreatic cancers	*CDKN2A* (p16/p14), *CDK4*
Hereditary breast and ovarian cancer syndrome	Breast cancer, ovarian cancer	*BRCA1, BRCA2*, probably other gene(s)
Hereditary prostate cancer	Prostate cancer	*HPC1/RNASEL, HPC2/ELAC2, MSR1*, other gene(s)
Juvenile polyposis syndrome	Multiple juvenile polyps in the gastrointestinal tract, colorectal and gastrointestinal malignancies	*SMAD4, BMPR1A*
Lynch syndrome/hereditary nonpolyposis colorectal cancer	Colorectal and endometrial cancer	*MLH1, MSH2, MSH6, PMS1, PMS2*

Source. Adapted from Lerman C, Shields AE: "Genetic Testing for Cancer Susceptibility: The Promise and the Pitfalls," *Nature Reviews Cancer* 4(3): 235–241, 2004; and Michigan Cancer Genetics Alliance: "Testing for Hereditary Cancer Predisposition Syndromes and Genetic Counseling, November 2009.

TABLE 6–2. Examples of rare hereditary cancer syndromes

Syndrome	Predominant tumor types	Gene(s) causing syndrome
Hereditary retinoblastoma	Pediatric retinal tumors	*RB1*
Li-Fraumeni syndrome	Breast cancers, soft-tissue sarcomas, tumors, adrenocortical tumors, leukemia	*TP53, CHEK2*
Multiple endocrine neoplasia type I	Primary hyperparathyroidism, pancreatic islet cell tumors, anterior pituitary tumors	*MEN1*
Multiple endocrine neoplasia type II	Medullary thyroid cancer, pheochromocytomas, mucosal neuromas	*RET*
Peutz-Jeghers syndrome	Gastrointestinal-tract cancer, breast cancer, testicular cancers, gynecological malignancies	*STK11/LKB1*
von Hippel-Lindau syndrome	Renal-cell cancer, retinal and central nervous system hemangioblastomas, pheochromocytomas	*VHL*
Wilms tumor	Nephroblastoma	*WT1*

Source. Adapted from Lerman C, Shields AE: "Genetic Testing for Cancer Susceptibility: The Promise and the Pitfalls," *Nature Reviews Cancer* 4(3): 235–241, 2004; and Michigan Cancer Genetics Alliance: "Testing for Hereditary Cancer Predisposition Syndromes and Genetic Counseling, November 2009.

ited predisposition toward cancer, he or she is also gaining valuable information about family members' genetic risk status, particularly for first-degree
relatives such as children, siblings, and parents.

Leading professional organizations in oncology and genetics describe
genetic testing for hereditary cancers as part of a process of care that
includes comprehensive cancer risk assessment, pretest and posttest genetic
counseling, and informed consent (Robson et al. 2010). A referral for hereditary cancer risk assessment, and possibly genetic testing, may be warranted
for persons who have a personal and/or family health history with features
that are suggestive of a pattern of inherited cancers. These features include
1) early onset of cancer; 2) more than one primary cancer in an individual;
3) cancers occurring in multiple generations on the same side of the family;
4) a constellation of cancers consistent with specific cancer syndromes (e.g.,
breast and ovarian, or colon and endometrial); 5) rare cancers, with or without additional cancers in the family (e.g., retinoblastoma, adrenocortical
carcinoma); 6) unusual presentation of cancer; 7) uncommon tumor histol-
ogy; and 8) geographic or ethnic populations known to be at risk for hereditary cancer due to a founder effect (e.g., Ashkenazi Jewish heritage and
BRCA1/BRCA2 mutations) (Weitzel et al. 2011). Genetic testing may be
considered if an individual's personal and/or family health history is suspicious for a genetic predisposition to cancer, if there is a clinically valid test
available, and if the results of testing will impact recommendations for cancer risk management or will help clarify family members' cancer risks (Weitzel et al. 2011).

Several clinical guidelines now include genetic testing and risk management recommendations for certain hereditary cancer syndromes (Weitzel
et al. 2011). For example, the National Society for Genetic Counselors recommends the following for developing and implementing a comprehensive
genetic counseling program: 1) information collected at intake should
include a thorough personal medical history and a three- to four-generation
family medical history; 2) the risk assessment process should include using
personal and family medical history to determine average, moderate, or increased cancer risk; 3) genetic testing should be offered when individuals
meet the appropriate criteria (see previous paragraph); 4) an informed consent process should be followed prior to genetic testing; 5) disclosure of genetic test results should include personalized interpretation of results,
cancer risk reassessment, and identification of at-risk relatives; and 6) psychosocial assessment is critical and should be conducted as part of the pretest and posttest genetic counseling program (Riley et al. 2012).

A study comparing international guidelines for genetic counseling and testing reported that referral patterns, costs of services, and who provides the genetic counseling vary by country (Meiser et al. 2006). A recent article compared

the national guidelines and recommendations for referral to genetic testing for hereditary breast and ovarian cancer (HBOC) syndrome from the United Kingdom, France, the Netherlands, and Germany (Gadzicki et al. 2011). Although each of these countries is relying on the same knowledge base to inform their guidelines, some differences exist in referral patterns. For example, a small number of families would be referred for genetic testing in one country but not another; this group includes small families, families in which a mutation is transmitted through the paternal line, and families in which all of the cancer-affected family members are deceased (Gadzicki et al. 2011). These countries also had some very important similarities, including providing genetic testing within the framework of genetic counseling and first offering testing to the cancer-affected individual in a family, which suggest that once a family is identified as being at risk for the gene mutation, the care they receive is very similar across countries (Gadzicki et al. 2011).

Genetic education and counseling by health care providers with adequate knowledge and/or training in cancer genetics are essential to the genetic testing process, and should be initiated as part of cancer risk assessment. When genetic testing is an option, genetic counseling can facilitate informed decision making regarding the option to test or not to test, allowing persons to consider the risks, benefits, and potential medical and psychosocial consequences (Schneider 2002). Test results should be disclosed in the context of genetic counseling to ensure that the implications of the results for the individual tested, as well as his or her family, are understood and to facilitate consideration of the psychological, social, medical, and genetic ramifications. Follow-up counseling and consultation with medical and genetics specialists can be beneficial, because they provide further opportunities for updating cancer risk status, considering options for risk management (e.g., cancer screening, preventive surgery), and discussing implications for family members.

Attending to psychosocial concerns is an essential component of the genetic counseling and testing process. During cancer risk assessment and prior to genetic testing, it is important to identify and explore potential psychological issues and concerns that may affect decisions to undergo testing, responses to test results, and adoption of risk management recommendations. This process includes exploring motivations for seeking cancer risk information; beliefs regarding the causes of cancer; personal and family experiences with cancer and the emotions, concerns, or fears related to those experiences; perceptions about personal risk for developing cancer; and general psychological issues, such as depression or anxiety. Persons considering testing also are encouraged to anticipate potential responses to the various testing outcomes, as well as their resources for coping with those outcomes. In addition, consideration of the family context and available support systems is important throughout the counseling and testing process. Health care providers offering genetic counseling and testing should attempt to assess when a referral to a mental health professional may be beneficial, particularly when there are factors suggesting risk of adverse psychological outcomes after assessment of cancer risk status or disclosure of results (discussed in later section "Psychological Impact of Undergoing Genetic Counseling and Testing").

Uptake of Genetic Counseling for Hereditary Cancers

The complex process of genetic testing for inherited cancer susceptibility requires decisions regarding whether to seek counseling, undergo mutation testing, and receive test results. Upon receipt of genetic test results, individuals face additional decisions, including whether to share the information with others (e.g., family members and health care providers) and how best to manage their cancer risk (e.g., screening and prophylactic surgery). Two common hereditary cancer syndromes for which people undergo genetic counseling and testing are HBOC syndrome and Lynch syndrome. Demographic, clinical, and psychosocial factors associated with genetic testing participation have been identified in these populations; however, comparisons of uptake rates across studies may be challenging. The primary reason for this difficulty is that study procedures and methodology vary; for example, it is common practice for studies to recruit participants from familial cancer registries or clinical settings, and for free genetic counseling and testing to be offered as part of research protocols. Also, accurate assessment of uptake rates is complicated by the fact that the genetic counseling and testing process is a multistep process that includes multiple points at which an individual may decline or discontinue participation, as well as the lack of standard methodology for defining and reporting uptake rates (Bowen et al. 1999).

Genetic Testing for HBOC Syndrome– Related Mutations

Individuals who may be at risk for HBOC syndrome, based on personal and family health history, undergo testing for *BRCA1* and *BRCA2* mutations, and reported testing uptake rates have varied widely. In a systematic review, genetic testing uptake rates averaged 59% across all studies and ranged from 20% to 96% (Ropka et al. 2006). Having a personal or family history of breast or ovarian cancer was associated with testing uptake, as were methodological features of the studies, such as the use of convenience sampling strategies and offering of free counseling for study participation, (Ropka et al. 2006).

Other factors that also have been associated with greater uptake rates across studies include psychosocial factors, such as the presence of cancer-specific distress and the perceived risk of developing breast or ovarian cancer, and family factors, such as having children or having a greater number of cancer-affected relatives (Lerman et al. 1997; Meiser 2005; Ropka et al. 2006). In a comparison of international studies regarding attitudes toward genetic counseling and testing for HBOC syndrome, the three most consistently endorsed perceived benefits of testing included learning about children's risk, enabling an improved basis for decision making about screening and/or prophylactic surgery, and relieving uncertainty (Meiser et al. 2006). To date, many demographic factors, such as age, education level, and marital status, show no consistent pattern of affecting genetic testing uptake rates (Lerman et al. 1997; Meiser 2005; Ropka et al. 2006).

Very little information is available regarding the characteristics of genetic testing decliners. The limited data on decliners of *BRCA1/BRCA2* mutation testing suggest that compared with individuals who accepted genetic testing, decliners are more likely to be male, unmarried, childless, and younger; to have fewer cancer-affected relatives; and to have lower levels of cancer worry (Foster et al. 2004; Lerman et al. 1998). The data also suggest that individuals may decline genetic testing due to the perceived potential negative impacts, including concerns about the effects of a positive test result on employment status or eligibility for life insurance and worries about one's own health or children's health (Foster et al. 2004). Similar patterns were seen in international studies; the most frequently cited barriers toward genetic testing include concerns about insurance, concerns about the effects of testing on the family, and lack of trust in the results (Meiser et al. 2006). Scant data are available regarding longer-term psychological effects of declining *BRCA1/BRCA2* genetic testing. One study reported a significant increase in depression rates in decliners from *BRCA1-* and *BRCA2*-linked families (from 26% at the baseline [pretest] assessment to 47% at 1- and 6-month follow-up assessments), whereas rates among known carriers and noncarriers remained unchanged or decreased, respectively (Lerman et al. 1998).

When comparing testing uptake rates across countries, the data indicate significant variability both within and between countries (Meiser et al. 2006). Uptake rates vary from 29% to 89% in the United Kingdom, from 26% to 82% in the United States, and from 44% to 84% in Australia, Canada, France, Germany, and the Netherlands (Meiser et al. 2006). These international differences in uptake rates may be attributable to factors such as the variation in cost and infrastructure for genetic counseling and testing, the real or imagined potential for discrimination based on the test results, and cultural differences (Meiser et al. 2006).

Genetic Testing for Lynch Syndrome– Related Mutations

Individuals who are identified as being at risk for Lynch syndrome undergo genetic testing for mutation in a mismatch repair gene (*hMLH1, hMSH2, hMLH6, PMS1*). Across studies, uptake rates for Lynch syndrome–related mutations have ranged from 14% to 59% (Aktan-Collan et al. 2000; Hadley et al. 2003; Lerman et al. 1999; Lynch et al. 1997). Factors such as cost, test characteristics, and the context in which counseling and testing were offered may account for the variability in uptake rates.

Having a personal history of cancer, a greater number of affected relatives, a greater perceived risk of developing colorectal cancer, more frequent thoughts about colorectal cancer, and greater perceived social support are factors that have been associated with uptake of Lynch syndrome genetic testing (Aktan-Collan et al. 2000; Codori et al. 1999; Gritz et al. 1999; Hadley et al. 2003; Lerman et al. 1999). Additionally, an individual's desire to learn about his or her mutation status may be motivated by the belief that testing will help family members (Vernon et al. 1999). Those who decline testing may be more likely to report depressive symptoms, be less likely to have received prior colorectal cancer screening, and have a lower perceived ability to cope with mutation-positive test results (Codori et al. 1999; Lerman et al. 1999). Concerns about potential insurance discrimination, the effects of genetic testing on one's family, and emotional reactions to genetic test results have also been cited as reasons for declining genetic testing for Lynch syndrome (Hadley et al. 2003).

Taken together, the research results to date indicate that both clinical and psychological factors have been positively associated with the decision to undergo genetic testing for Lynch syndrome. Clinical factors include having a personal history of cancer and having a greater number of cancer-affected relatives, whereas psychological factors include a greater perceived risk of developing cancer and greater distress or worries related to cancer. An individual's decisions about undergoing genetic counseling and testing appear to be influenced by a strong motivation to gain knowledge about why he or she was diagnosed with cancer and/or about his or her family members' cancer risk (Meiser 2005). Individuals may choose to undergo genetic testing to reduce cancer-related distress and to feel reassured. Although little is known about test decliners, concerns about the impact of the testing on practical matters, such as employment and insurance, may influence testing decisions; however, due to the lack of available data, little is known about the long-term consequences of such decisions.

Psychological Impact of Undergoing Genetic Counseling and Testing

Psychological consequences associated with undergoing genetic counseling and testing have been a primary concern of both researchers and clinicians since the testing first became available. Longitudinally designed studies have assessed individuals before genetic counseling, after counseling, and for various lengths of time after disclosure of mutation status and have examined psychological distress outcomes—most commonly, depression, anxiety, and cancer-specific worries or distress. Individuals receiving mutation-positive, mutation-negative, and inconclusive/uninformative results have all been included in these studies, and most of the research to date has focused on the psychological impact of genetic testing in cancer-unaffected persons. A small number of studies have examined the effects on persons diagnosed with cancer.

HBOC Syndrome

A review of studies that evaluated psychological outcomes among cancer-unaffected women who had received genetic testing for HBOC syndrome found that mutation carriers, in general, experienced few, if any, serious effects up to 1 year after disclosure of results and that noncarriers may gain psychological benefits from testing (Meiser 2005). The psychological outcomes that have been examined in this population include anxiety, depression, general distress, and cancer-specific distress (Meiser 2005). For cancer-unaffected noncarriers, research to date has demonstrated that mean scores on psychological outcome measures either improved or did not change (Meiser 2005; Schwartz et al. 2002). For unaffected carriers, studies have found that distress following disclosure of mutation status did not change relative to baseline or increased over the short term (Meiser 2005; Schwartz et al. 2002; van Roosmalen et al. 2004). It is important to note that levels generally remained in the normal ranges and often did not indicate the presence of clinically significant distress. In regard to long-term psychological impact of genetic testing for HBOC syndrome, one study examined anxiety and distress up to 5 years after the disclosure of results in both mutation carriers and noncarriers (van Oostrom et al. 2003). Distress levels did not differ between the two groups up to 1 year following disclosure; however, mean scores on anxiety and depression measures increased from the 1-year to the 5-year follow-up points (van Oostrom et al. 2003). Factors associated with long-term distress in this study included the presence of cancer-specific distress at the time of testing, having young children, and having lost a family member to breast or ovarian cancer (van Oostrom et al. 2003). Notably, the majority of mutation carriers had undergone risk-reducing surgery during the 5-year follow-up time period, which could possibly confound the distress outcomes (Meiser 2005). In general, the research findings that are available to date suggest that notification of positive mutation carrier status does not appear to result in serious psychological distress. However, additional research is needed to further explore the long-term psychological impact of genetic testing.

Although the majority of studies have focused on psychological outcomes of cancer-unaffected women who underwent *BRCA1/BRCA2* genetic testing, data focusing on the experience of women who have been diagnosed with cancer are more limited. The focus on unaffected women in earlier studies may have been attributable to an early assumption that the impact of genetic risk notification for cancer-affected women is attenuated by their prior cancer diagnosis; however, findings from some studies of affected carriers dispute that assumption. Although strong declines in well-being were reported by affected *BRCA1/BRCA2* carriers in one study, particularly among those who had been diagnosed with cancer within the previous year, cancer-affected carriers more often experienced no change in distress levels over time after disclosure of results (Meiser 2005; Schwartz et al. 2002; van Roosmalen et al. 2004). It is possible that affected women may underestimate their own emotional response to receiving a mutation-positive test result, which in turn may exacerbate distress. Evidence for this was reported in one study, which showed that affected *BRCA1* carriers experienced higher levels of anger and worry after disclosure than they had anticipated (Dorval et al. 2000). In addition, the underestimation of postdisclosure distress by these women was associated with higher levels of general distress at the 6-month follow-up point (Dorval et al. 2000). Mutation testing is typically initiated in a cancer-affected individual, and being the first person identified as a mutation carrier in one's family may pose an additional psychological burden (Bonadona et al. 2002).

The limited data that are available regarding individuals who receive uninformative genetic test results suggest that these individuals may not experience the same decrease in distress as those who receive a true negative result (Schwartz et al. 2002). Understanding the meaning of inconclusive results may be difficult, and accurately communicating their meaning to family members may be challenging (Hallowell et al. 2002).

There appear to be no systematic differences across international studies that have examined the psychological impact of genetic counseling and testing; however, most research has been undertaken in Western countries and there has been relatively low diversity in the study samples (Meiser et al. 2006).

Additional research involving non-Western populations and higher numbers of minorities has been called for to address this issue (Meiser et al. 2006).

Lynch Syndrome

Longitudinal studies of psychological outcomes after genetic testing for Lynch syndrome–related mutations with relatively short follow-up periods (2 weeks to 1 month) indicated that carriers may experience increased general distress (Aktan-Collan et al. 2001; Gritz et al. 2005), cancer-specific distress (Meiser et al. 2004), or cancer worries (Gritz et al. 2005), relative to their pretest assessments. Although the carriers' distress often was significantly higher immediately postdisclosure (when compared with noncarriers), the effects were short term, subsided during the course of the first year postdisclosure, and returned to pretest distress levels by the 1-year postdisclosure time point (Aktan-Collan et al. 2001; Gritz et al. 2005; Meiser et al. 2004). Noncarriers experienced a reduction or no change in distress up to 1 year following results disclosure, indicating that they may derive psychological benefit from testing (Aktan-Collan et al. 2001; Collins et al. 2007; Gritz et al. 2005; Meiser et al. 2004). As for HBOC syndrome, fewer data are available on the long-term (more than 1 year) psychological impact of Lynch syndrome genetic counseling and testing. In a study that evaluated psychological outcomes up to 3 years postdisclosure, carriers' and noncarriers' mean scores on measures of depression, anxiety, and cancer-specific distress were similar to baseline scores (pregenetic testing) (Collins et al. 2007). The only exception was that noncarriers showed a decrease in cancer-specific distress scores that was significantly lower than that of carriers and that dropped below pretest levels through the 1- and 3-year study follow-up periods (Collins et al. 2007).

Individuals who present with relatively higher scores on measures of general or cancer-specific distress prior to undergoing genetic testing may be at higher risk of psychological distress following disclosure of test results (Esplen et al. 2003; Gritz et al. 2005; van Oostrom et al. 2006; Vernon et al. 1997, 1999). In a sample of colorectal cancer patients undergoing genetic testing, higher levels of depressive symptoms and/or anxiety were found among women, younger persons, nonwhites, individuals with less formal education, and individuals with fewer and less satisfactory sources of social support (Vernon et al. 1997). From this study population, a subgroup of individuals who showed higher levels of psychological distress, lower quality of life, and lower social support was identified (Gritz et al. 1999). These individuals were more likely to worry about finding out that they tested positive for a Lynch syndrome mutation and being able to cope with learning their test results (Gritz et al. 1999). In a longitudinal follow-up study after the disclosure of test results, a subgroup with the same psychosocial characteristics (higher levels of psychosocial distress, lower quality of life, and lower social support) experienced higher levels of general distress and distress specific to the experience of having genetic testing within the year after disclosure, regardless of mutation status (Gritz et al. 2005). At all study time points, higher levels of depression and anxiety were reported by nonwhites and those with lower education compared with whites and those with higher education, respectively (Gritz et al. 2005). Other factors that have been identified to predict higher levels of distress postdisclosure include having a history of major or minor depression, higher pretest levels of cancer-specific distress, having a greater number of cancer-affected first-degree relatives, greater grief reactions, and greater emotional illness–related representations (Murakami et al. 2004; van Oostrom et al. 2006). Further research in this area is warranted; however, evidence from these limited studies suggests that it is important to identify individuals who may be at risk for experiencing psychiatric distress and to offer them additional psychological support throughout the genetic counseling and genetic testing process.

Family Communication About Genetic Testing and Inherited Cancer Risk

Individuals who undergo genetic testing for cancer receive results that provide information not only for themselves, but also for their biological relatives. The index case, or the first person in the family to be tested, often becomes the gatekeeper for this important family health information (Peterson 2005). In most cases, it is largely the responsibility of family members, rather than health care providers, to communicate genetic risk information within families. Educating individuals on the importance of communicating test results to family members is considered an integral part of the genetic counseling and testing process (American Society of Clinical Oncology 2003). Studies have shown that individuals generally are willing to share their genetic test results with at least some of their relatives and that they are willing to do so within a few weeks after disclosure (Gaff et al. 2005; Mesters et al. 2005; Peterson et al. 2003; Stoffel et al. 2008). Communication of this information most commonly occurs with first-degree relatives, such as siblings, parents, or children, rather than with more distant relatives (Gaff et al. 2005; Mesters et al. 2005; Peterson et al. 2003; Stoffel et al. 2008).

Individuals are motivated to share genetic risk information for various reasons, including 1) having a desire to increase family awareness about health care options and predictive genetic testing, 2) increasing their emotional support, and 3) having a perceived moral obligation and responsibility to help their family members (Gaff et al. 2005; Mesters et al. 2005; Peterson et al. 2003; Stoffel et al. 2008). Although communicating about genetic risk information is typically seen as an open process, individuals have reported some barriers; specifically, lack of a close relationship, not wanting family members to worry, concerns about family members not understanding the results, and lack of contact with certain family members have all been cited as reasons for non-disclosure (Stoffel et al. 2008). The following factors were associated with being less likely to disclose results: 1) at-risk individuals were considered too young to receive the information (i.e., children), 2) information about the hereditary cancer risk had previously created conflict in the family, and 3) relatives were assumed to be uninterested in information about testing (Mesters et al. 2005; Stoffel et al. 2008). Discussions about hereditary cancer risk appear to be inhibited by the prior existence of conflict, and this relationship seems to be even stronger if the discussions involve disclosure of bad news (Mesters et al. 2005).

Studies have indicated that some probands (the first person in the family to test positive for a gene mutation) reported feeling particularly obliged to inform family members about a hereditary cancer risk (Mesters et al. 2005). Additionally, probands often became advocates in their families and strongly encouraged their family members to undergo genetic counseling and testing for the known mutation (Peterson et al. 2003). The dissemination of hereditary cancer information may be affected by some gender and family role differences. Specifically, one study found that female probands were more comfortable than male probands discussing genetic information; additionally, male probands showed a greater need for professional support during the family communication process (Gaff et al. 2005). Mothers and older family members may be particularly influential members of the family network in regard to communicating health risk information, and studies indicate that they are more likely to be involved in communication about *BRCA1/BRCA2* or Lynch syndrome mutation results (Ashida et al. 2011; Koehly et al. 2003). When compared with probands and other at-risk individuals who have undergone genetic testing, mutation-negative individuals, persons who chose not to be tested, and spouses of at-risk persons have reported not feeling as personally involved with the risk communication process (Peterson et al. 2003). Families who are more comfortable and open with cancer-related discussions may be more receptive to and accepting of news about genetic risk (Mesters et al. 2005).

Family members use a variety of modes of communication to disclose genetic risk information, including in-person discussions, telephone calls, and written contact (Gaff et al. 2005; Mesters et al. 2005; Peterson et al.

2003). Although not considered central or necessary to the successful risk communication in families, communication aids, such as a genetic counseling summary letter or Lynch syndrome booklet, were viewed in one study as helpful adjuncts to the communication process (Gaff et al. 2005). Health care providers may play an important role in facilitating family communication. Specifically, studies have suggested that recommendations by health care providers to inform relatives about hereditary cancer risk may encourage communication about Lynch syndrome (Mesters et al. 2005). In addition, evidence suggests that support by health care professionals may be helpful in overcoming barriers to communicating genetic risk information to family members (Koehly et al. 2003).

Decision Making and Psychological Consequences Associated With Risk Management Recommendations

Carriers of *BRCA1/BRCA2* or Lynch syndrome–associated mutations are advised to follow medical management recommendations for reducing their cancer risk. These recommendations include options for screening and risk-reducing surgery. The reduction of cancer morbidity and mortality in families with HBOC syndrome and Lynch syndrome is one of the primary goals of genetic testing. For clinicians to effectively manage patients with hereditary cancer syndromes, it is imperative that they develop an understanding of factors that influence patients' decisions regarding risk reduction options, barriers to adoption of the recommendations, and the effects on quality of life and psychological adjustment.

HBOC Syndrome

Breast Cancer Risk Management Strategies

Several strategies, including screening, surgery, and chemoprevention, are recommended as options to mitigate breast cancer risk in individuals with *BRCA1/BRCA2* mutations. Screening recommendations for *BRCA1/ BRCA2* mutation carriers include monthly breast self-examination starting in adulthood, semi-annual clinical breast examination beginning at age 25, and annual mammography and breast magnetic resonance imaging (MRI) beginning at age 25–35 years, with recommendations being tailored based on earliest age of cancer onset in the family (Howard et al. 2009; Petrucelli et al. 2011). Recent research indicates that MRI screening may be able to detect cancers in women with *BRCA1/BRCA2* mutations that would have been missed with standard mammography; however, some cancers (e.g., ductal carcinoma in situ) are not identified by MRI (Petrucelli et al. 2011). As a result, the screening recommendations for *BRCA1/BRCA2* mutation carriers now include a breast MRI in addition to the standard mammogram (Howard et al. 2009; Petrucelli et al. 2011).

Prophylactic surgical options for carriers of the *BRCA1/BRCA2* mutation include risk-reducing mastectomy (RRM) and risk-reducing salpingo-oophorectomy (RRSO). Evidence indicates that RRM reduces breast cancer risk by approximately 90%, but uptake rates vary widely across studies (Howard et al. 2009; Petrucelli et al. 2011). One study comparing uptake rates of RRM in nine countries found that women from the United States had the highest uptake rates (36.3%) (Metcalfe et al. 2008). In a review of international studies, RRM uptake rates varied significantly within and between countries, with rates ranging from 2% in Australia to 54% in the Netherlands (Meiser et al. 2006). Factors found to be associated with RRM uptake include 1) personal factors, such as younger age or having a family history of breast cancer; 2) psychosocial factors, such as a desire for reduction of cancer-related stress; 3) recommendations of the health care provider; and 4) cultural or health care system factors (Howard et al. 2009).

Tamoxifen has been approved as a chemopreventive agent for women at high risk for developing breast cancer; however, few studies exist on women with *BRCA1/BRCA2* mutations. In the general population, tamoxifen decreases breast cancer risk by an estimated 50% and is most beneficial in women with an elevated risk for breast cancer who are younger than age 50 (Petrucelli et al. 2011). Tamoxifen may be more effective in women with *BRCA2* mutations due to the differential effects on estrogen receptor (ER)–positive and ER-negative cancers (Petrucelli et al. 2011). Studies have demonstrated that tamoxifen is effective in reducing rates of ER-positive cancer, but not ER-negative cancer, which is what is predominantly found in women with *BRCA1* mutations (Petrucelli et al. 2011). A study that compared uptake rates of tamoxifen in cancer-unaffected mutation carriers across nine countries found that no participants in France, Italy, Holland, and Norway reported using this chemopreventive medication, whereas only small percentages reported using the drug in other countries (12.4% for the United States, 11% for Israel, 9.8% for Canada, 6.4% for Poland, and 5.0% for Austria) (Metcalfe et al. 2008). In women without breast cancer, having had a prior oophorectomy was related to having taken tamoxifen; 15.6% of women who had undergone this procedure had used tamoxifen, whereas only 1.7% who had not undergone the procedure had used this medication (Metcalfe et al. 2008). As with all treatment options, tamoxifen has potential side effects; therefore, the decision to recommend this chemopreventive agent should be based on individual physician-patient consultations.

Research indicates that a substantial percentage (45.8%) of *BRCA1/ BRCA2* mutation carriers who are at risk for a first primary breast cancer do not choose to undergo prophylactic surgery or to take chemopreventive medications (Metcalfe et al. 2008). In this international sample, 19.5% of these women had had at least one MRI and 75.0% had had a mammogram (Metcalfe et al. 2008). Differences in health care systems, cost and availability of services, and variations in cancer risk management recommendations (e.g., the use of MRI) may account for some of the differences (Metcalfe et al. 2008).

Gynecological Cancer Risk Management Strategies

Although efficacy data for these risk reduction options are lacking, transvaginal ultrasound (TVU) and serum CA-125 testing every 6 months to screen for ovarian cancer are included as potential risk management recommendations for *BRCA1/BRCA2* mutation carriers (Daly et al. 2006; Lu 2008). Not surprisingly, positive *BRCA1/BRCA2* mutation status was the most consistent predictor of ovarian cancer screening use after testing; however, greater perceived risk of developing ovarian cancer, having a greater number of ovarian cancer–affected relatives, and physician recommendation also were positively associated with adherence to ovarian cancer screening following mutation testing (Howard et al. 2009).

High-risk women who choose to have an RRSO have a reduction in both breast and ovarian cancer risk, including an 85%–90% reduction in lifetime ovarian cancer risk for *BRCA1/BRCA2* carriers (Rebbeck et al. 2002). It is also important to note that RRSO results in infertility and surgically induced menopause, which in turn may increase risk for other health conditions such as osteoporosis and heart disease (Howard et al. 2009). Given the complexity of this decision for women, it is not surprising that the uptake rates for RRSO among *BRCA1/BRCA2* carriers following genetic testing vary widely (ranging from 5% to 78% across studies) (Howard et al. 2009). One study compared RRSO uptake rates in nine countries and found that in every country other than Poland (34.9%), at least half of the women surveyed had had oophorectomies, ranging from 52.1% in Austria to 73.5% in Norway (Metcalfe et al. 2008). Approximately half of the women reported having the procedure prior to genetic counseling and testing and the other half after receiving their positive genetic test results; however, this study was unable to differentiate between oophorectomies that were conducted solely for the purpose of cancer prevention and those done for other reasons (Metcalfe et al. 2008). A review article comparing international uptake rates of RRSO found that Germany reported the lowest rates (8%), Australia and the United Kingdom were in the middle (23%–29%), and Canada and the Netherlands had the highest rates (50%–64%) (Meiser et al. 2006).

Research indicates that the factors influencing the decision to have an RRSO are complex. Specifically, clinical factors associated with uptake of RRSO include the following: 1) positive *BRCA1/BRCA2* mutation status, 2) prior breast cancer diagnosis or RRM, and 3) a family history of ovarian cancer (Howard et al. 2009). There are also psychosocial and other factors associated with uptake, including greater perceived benefits of surgery, higher perceived cancer risk, older age, already having children, and the limitations of current ovarian screening options (Howard et al. 2009). The research to date suggests that there is a psychological benefit to undergoing RRSO. Specifically, individuals who undergo RRSO report reductions in cancer worry and in perceived risk of developing cancer, although the long-term effects of this procedure merit further attention in the literature (Howard et al. 2009). The currently available evidence indicates that some women continue to experience cancer-specific distress as well as dissatisfaction with their body image and reduced quality of sexual functioning following RRSO (Howard et al. 2009).

For premenopausal women, the decision to undergo RRSO carries additional consequences. As previously stated, infertility and surgically induced menopause are end results of this procedure (Howard et al. 2009). Women have indicated a variety of reasons for not undergoing or for delaying the decision to have RRSO, including the desire for childbearing, worries about feeling a loss of femininity, and concerns about long-term use of hormone replacement therapy (Howard et al. 2009). To facilitate decision making about RRSO, it is vital that women receive appropriate information and counseling on the possible physical and emotional postsurgery effects, including premature menopause, and on the benefits and risks of hormone replacement therapy.

Lynch Syndrome

Colorectal Cancer Risk

The current screening recommendation for individuals at risk for Lynch syndrome–associated colorectal cancer is to undergo a colonoscopy every 1–2 years beginning at age 20–25 years or starting 10 years younger than the first known case in the family, whichever is younger (Lindor et al. 2006). Cancer-unaffected individuals have been assessed to compare colonoscopy use prior to and up to 1 year following genetic counseling and testing in several studies. Mutation carriers were more likely to have had a colonoscopy following genetic testing than were noncarriers and those who declined testing (73% vs. 16% vs. 22%), and their colonoscopy use increased from 36% to 73% in the year following disclosure of test results (Claes et al. 2005). Among noncarriers, colonoscopy rates decreased in the year following notification of genetic test results (Collins et al. 2005; Hadley et al. 2004). Factors associated with an increased likelihood of having a colonoscopy within 1 year after the disclosure of results included testing positive for a DNA mismatch repair MMR gene mutation, being older, and expressing greater perceived control over colorectal cancer (Collins et al. 2005; Hadley et al. 2004; Halbert et al. 2004). The findings from studies examining longer-term colorectal screening behaviors suggest that improvements in colorectal screening behaviors among MMR gene mutation carriers may be maintained over time. Adherence to colorectal screening ranged from 73% to 100% among persons with a genetic or clinical diagnosis of Lynch syndrome in studies with follow-up periods ranging from 1 to 18 years after genetic testing and/or risk counseling (Bleiker et al. 2005; Collins et al. 2007; Wagner et al. 2005). Factors associated with nonadherence to screening recommendations have included greater perceived barriers to screening and greater embarrassment regarding colorectal screening procedures (Wagner et al. 2005). *MMR* mutation carriers have expressed positive attitudes toward future colorectal cancer screening. In one study, 94% of carriers stated an intention to have annual or biannual colonoscopy in the future, suggesting a favorable outcome for long-term screening adherence (Claes et al. 2005). Among noncarriers in the same study, 64% indicated that they did not intend to have colonoscopy in the future or were unsure, which suggests that noncarriers also need to be given up-to-date information about appropriate screening recommendations for the general population (Claes et al. 2005). Taken together, these studies indicate that genetic testing for Lynch syndrome may motivate individuals to maintain or improve recommended colorectal screening. However, screening rates reported in these studies are often less than optimal, and further research is needed to identify barriers to screening as well as to develop and evaluate interventions that encourage colonoscopy use among individuals who are not adherent.

Individuals who undergo colonoscopy more frequently than recommended by guidelines also merit further attention by researchers and clinicians. In one study, hypervigilant colorectal cancer screening behavior was reported within the year following disclosure of genetic test results by both carriers and noncarriers of the Lynch syndrome mutation (Hadley et al. 2004). Specifically, approximately half of the 35% of mutation carriers and 13% of noncarriers actually underwent colorectal cancer screening more often than was recommended (Hadley et al. 2004). A number of factors could be contributing to this hypervigilant screening behavior, including inappropriate advice by health care providers and persistent worry about colorectal cancer risk. The overutilization of screening results in higher health care costs and unnecessary patient risks; therefore, it is important for researchers and clinicians to better understand why people may adopt hypervigilant screening practices.

Gynecological Cancer Risk

Gynecological cancer screening is included as a risk management recommendation for women with Lynch syndrome, although this strategy has no proven efficacy in the early detection of endometrial cancer. The current guidelines include the option of annual endometrial biopsy with TVU for women with a suspected or documented mismatch repair mutation beginning at age 30–35 years (Lindor et al. 2006). Data on adherence to endometrial cancer screening in Lynch syndrome are sparse, and the studies that do exist have included very small sample sizes. Generally, existing data suggest that mutation carriers do not universally adopt gynecological cancer screening, although there appears to be an increase in screening uptake following genetic counseling and testing. Of women enrolled in a Lynch syndrome registry who had received genetic counseling and risk assessment with or without genetic testing, 69% reported having undergone at least one endometrial biopsy (Yang et al. 2006). Similar studies have reported that approximately 53% of carriers underwent endometrial biopsy and 47%–86% underwent TVU within 1–3 years after disclosure of test results (Claes et al. 2005; Collins et al. 2007). One recent study assessed the feasibility of concurrently performing endometrial biopsies and colonoscopies for women with Lynch syndrome and found that this approach is clinically feasible and that patients rated the combined procedure higher in regard to satisfaction and convenience (Huang et al. 2011). Patients in that study also reported lower levels of pain with this procedure when compared with previous biopsies performed in the office setting and reported that they would be more likely to adhere to current screening recommendations if they were presented with the option to undergo colonoscopy and endometrial biopsies as combined procedures (Huang et al. 2011).

Data regarding the use of risk-reducing hysterectomy (RRH) or RRSO among women with Lynch syndrome are limited. One study of individuals who had undergone genetic testing for Lynch syndrome suggested that consideration of risk-reducing surgery may have motivated interest in testing (Lynch et al. 1997). Of women in this study, 69% reported considering RRH and RRSO prior to receiving their genetic test results; however, the study did not assess whether these women ultimately followed through with risk-reducing surgery after they received their test results (Lynch et al. 1997). In a longitudinal study of cancer-unaffected women who underwent genetic testing for Lynch syndrome, 5% indicated that if they tested positive for a mutation, they would have an RRH and an RRSO (Collins et al. 2007). Two of the women in this study (out of 13 women who tested positive for a gene mutation) who had undergone an RRH before genetic testing underwent RRSO within 1 year after testing; by 3 years following disclosure of results, risk-reducing surgery was not elected by any other female mutation carriers (Collins et al. 2007). As for individuals with HBOC syndrome, the decision to undergo risk-reducing surgery is complex, and individual preferences, such as delaying surgery until childbearing has been completed, may contribute to the relatively low uptake of RRH and RRSO among women with Lynch syndrome. There is evidence showing the efficacy of hysterectomy and oophorectomy in reducing the occurrence of endometrial and ovarian cancers for Lynch syndrome, and the continued dissemination of these efficacy data over time may increase provider recommendations about risk-reducing surgery and influence patients to choose this option more frequently (Schmeler et al. 2006).

Clinical genetic testing for hereditary cancer syndromes has significantly impacted the care of patients and families who are affected by these deleterious mutations. The impact of the genetic counseling and testing process includes clinical ramifications, such as the need for appropriate medical management; psychological ramifications, such as the potential for distress responses; and social ramifications, such as the communication of risk among family members. The ability to properly diagnose and provide appropriate medical management for these individuals and their family members can lead to improvements in cancer survivorship as well as quality of life. Individuals affected by these gene mutations are presented with a variety of options for risk management, and many of the individuals have adopted the recommended strategies to reduce or manage their cancer risk. By partnering with their health care providers, individuals are able to resolve uncertainty about their personal and familial risk and to obtain information to guide future health care decisions. There is a growing body of literature in this area; however, many questions remain unanswered. Additional research is needed to assess the long-term psychosocial impact of genetic testing, genetic risk notification, and adoption of risk reduction recommendations at both the individual and family levels. As science and health care continue to progress, it is imperative that professionals address current gaps in knowledge to inform the delivery of optimal clinical services for high-risk hereditary cancer populations.

Key Clinical Points

- There is increasing identification of inherited cancer-predisposing gene mutations that make genetic counseling an important option.

- For individuals at risk for hereditary cancer syndromes, considerations addressed during genetic counseling include deciding whether to undergo genetic testing, concerns about disclosed results, whether to communicate results to family members, and other psychosocial issues.

- Hereditary risk assessment is particularly important for ovarian, breast, and colorectal malignancies. Decision aids such as booklets and interactive computer technology can facilitate greater use of genetic counseling and testing.

- Positive test results may foster subclinical anxiety and distress that warrant clinical attention, but such results also may resolve uncertainty about risk and allow positive action toward reducing risks.

- For individuals found to be at genetic risk, increased screening, riskreducing surgery, and chemotherapy are important options.

References

Aktan-Collan K, Mecklin JP, Järvinen H, et al: Predictive genetic testing for hereditary non-polyposis colorectal cancer: uptake and long-term satisfaction. Int J Cancer 89:44–50, 2000

Aktan-Collan K, Haukkala A, Mecklin JP, et al: Psychological consequences of predictive genetic testing for hereditary non-polyposis colorectal cancer (HNPCC): a prospective follow-up study. Int J Cancer 93:608–611, 2001

American Society of Clinical Oncology: American Society of Clinical Oncology policy statement update: genetic testing for cancer susceptibility. J Clin Oncol 21:2397–2406, 2003

Ashida S, Hadley DW, Goergen AF, et al: The importance of older family members in providing social resources and promoting cancer screening in families with hereditary cancer syndromes. Gerontologist 51:833–842, 2011

Bleiker EM, Menko FH, Taal BG, et al: Screening behavior of individuals at high risk for colorectal cancer. Gastroenterology 128:280–287, 2005

Bonadona V, Saltel P, Desseigne F, et al: Cancer patients who experienced diagnostic genetic testing for cancer susceptibility: reactions and behavior after the disclosure of a positive test result. Cancer Epidemiol Biomarkers Prev 11:97–104, 2002

Bowen DJ, Patenaude AF, Vernon SW: Psychosocial issues in cancer genetics: from the laboratory to the public. Cancer Epidemiol Biomarkers Prev 8:326–328, 1999

Claes E, Denayer L, Evers-Kiebooms G, et al: Predictive testing for hereditary nonpolyposis colorectal cancer: subjective perception regarding colorectal and endometrial cancer, distress, and health-related behavior at one year post-test. Genet Test 9:54–65, 2005

Codori AM, Petersen GM, Miglioretti DL, et al: Attitudes toward colon cancer gene testing: factors predicting test uptake. Cancer Epidemiol Biomarkers Prev 8:345–351, 1999

Collins V, Meiser B, Gaff C, et al: Screening and preventive behaviors one year after predictive genetic testing for hereditary nonpolyposis colorectal carcinoma. Cancer 104:273–281, 2005

Collins VR, Meiser B, Ukoumunne OC, et al: The impact of predictive genetic testing for hereditary nonpolyposis colorectal cancer: three years after testing. Genet Med 9:290–297, 2007

Daly MB, Axilbund JE, Bryant E, et al: Genetic/familial high-risk assessment: breast and ovarian. J Natl Compr Canc Netw 4:156–176, 2006

Dorval M, Patenaude AF, Schneider KA, et al: Anticipated versus actual emotional reactions to disclosure of results of genetic tests for cancer susceptibility: findings from p53 and BRCA1 testing programs. J Clin Oncol 18:2135–2142, 2000

Esplen MJ, Urquhart C, Butler K, et al: The experience of loss and anticipation of distress in colorectal cancer patients undergoing genetic testing. J Psychosom Res 55:427–435, 2003

Foster C, Evans DG, Eeles R, et al: Non-uptake of predictive genetic testing for BRCA1/2 among relatives of known carriers: attributes, cancer worry, and barriers to testing in a multicenter clinical cohort. Genet Test 8:23–29, 2004

Gadzicki D, Evans DG, Harris H, et al: Genetic testing for familial/hereditary breast cancer-comparison of guidelines and recommendations from the UK, France, the Netherlands and Germany. J Community Genet 2:53–69, 2011

Gaff CL, Collins V, Symes T, et al: Facilitating family communication about predictive genetic testing: probands' perceptions. J Genet Couns 14:133–140, 2005

Gritz ER, Vernon SW, Peterson SK, et al: Distress in the cancer patient and its association with genetic testing and counseling for hereditary non-polyposis colon cancer. Cancer Research, Therapy, and Control 8:35–49, 1999

Gritz ER, Peterson SK, Vernon SW, et al: Psychological impact of genetic testing for hereditary nonpolyposis colorectal cancer. J Clin Oncol 23:1902–1910, 2005

Hadley DW, Jenkins J, Dimond E, et al: Genetic counseling and testing in families with hereditary nonpolyposis colorectal cancer. Arch Intern Med 163:573–582, 2003

Hadley DW, Jenkins JF, Dimond E, et al: Colon cancer screening practices after genetic counseling and testing for hereditary nonpolyposis colorectal cancer. J Clin Oncol 22:39–44, 2004

Halbert CH, Lynch H, Lynch J, et al: Colon cancer screening practices following genetic testing for hereditary nonpolyposis colon cancer (HNPCC) mutations. Arch Intern Med 164:1881–1887, 2004

Hallowell N, Foster C, Ardern-Jones A, et al: Genetic testing for women previously diagnosed with breast/ovarian cancer: examining the impact of BRCA1 and BRCA2 mutation searching. Genet Test 6:79–87, 2002

Howard AF, Balneaves LG, Bottorff JL: Women's decision making about risk-reducing strategies in the context of hereditary breast and ovarian cancer: a systematic review. J Genet Couns 18:578–597, 2009

Huang M, Sun C, Boyd-Rogers S, et al: Propsective study of combined colon and endometrial cancer screening in women with Lynch syndrome: a patient-centered approach. J Oncol Practice 7:43–47, 2011

Koehly LM, Peterson SK, Watts BG, et al: A social network analysis of communication about hereditary nonpolyposis colorectal cancer genetic testing and family functioning. Cancer Epidemiol Biomarkers Prev 12:304–313, 2003

Lerman C, Schwartz MD, Lin TH, et al: The influence of psychological distress on use of genetic testing for cancer risk. J Consult Clin Psychol 65:414–420, 1997

Lerman C, Hughes C, Lemon SJ, et al: What you don't know can hurt you: adverse psychologic effects in members of BRCA1-linked and BRCA2-linked families who decline genetic testing. J Clin Oncol 16:1650–1654, 1998

Lerman C, Hughes C, Trock BJ, et al: Genetic testing in families with hereditary nonpolyposis colon cancer. JAMA 281:1618–1622, 1999

Lindor NM, Peterson GM, Hadley DW, et al: Recommendations for the care of individuals with an inherited predisposition to Lynch syndrome: a systematic review. JAMA 296:1507–1517, 2006

Lu KH: Hereditary gynecologic cancers: differential diagnosis, surveillance, management and surgical prophylaxis. Fam Cancer 7:53–58, 2008

Lynch HT, Lemon SJ, Karr B, et al: Etiology, natural history, management, and molecular genetics of hereditary nonpolyposis colorectal cancer (Lynch syndromes): genetic counseling implications. Cancer Epidemiol Biomarkers Prev 6:987–991, 1997

Lynch HT, Lynch JF, Lynch PM, et al: Hereditary colorectal cancer syndromes: molecular genetics, genetic counseling, diagnosis and management. Fam Cancer 7:27–39, 2008

Meiser B: Psychological impact of genetic testing for cancer susceptibility: an update of the literature. Psychooncology 14:1060–1074, 2005

Meiser B, Collins V, Warren R, et al: Psychological impact of genetic testing for hereditary non-polyposis colorectal cancer. Clin Genetics 66:502–511, 2004

Meiser B, Gaff C, Julian-Reynier C, et al: International perspectives on genetic counseling and testing for breast cancer risk. Breast Dis 27:109–125, 2006

Mesters I, Ausems M, Eichhorn S, et al: Informing one's family about genetic testing for hereditary non-polyposis colorectal cancer (HNPCC): a retrospective exploratory study. Fam Cancer 4:163–167, 2005

Metcalfe KA, Birenbaum-Carmeli D, Lubinski J, et al: International variation in rates of uptake of preventive options for BRCA1 and BRCA2 mutation carriers. Int J Cancer 122:2017–2022, 2008

Murakami Y, Okamura H, Sugano K, et al: Psychologic distress after disclosure of genetic test results regarding hereditary nonpolyposis colorectal carcinoma. Cancer 101:395–403, 2004

Peterson SK: The role of the family in genetic testing: theoretical perspectives, current knowledge, and future directions. Health Educ Behav 32:627–639, 2005

Peterson SK, Watts BG, Koehly LM, et al: How families communicate about HNPCC genetic testing: findings from a qualitative study. Am J Med Genet C Semin Med Genet 119C:78–86, 2003

Petrucelli N, Daly MB, Feldman GL: BRCA1 and BRCA2 hereditary breast and ovarian cancer, in GeneReviews (Internet). Edited by Pagon RA, Bird TD, Dolan CT, et al. Seattle, WA, University of Washington, Seattle, 2011

Rebbeck TR, Lynch HT, Neuhausen SL, et al: Prophylactic oophorectomy in carriers of BRCA1 or BRCA2 mutations. N Engl J Med 346:1616–1622, 2002

Riley BD, Culver JO, Skrzynia C, et al: Essential elements of genetic cancer risk assessment, counseling, and testing: updated recommendations of the National Society of Genetic Counselors. J Genet Couns 21:151–161, 2012

Robson ME, Storm CD, Weitzel J, et al: American Society of Clinical Oncology policy statement update: genetic and genomic testing for cancer susceptibility. J Clin Oncol 28:893–901, 2010

Ropka ME, Wenzel J, Phillips EK, et al: Uptake rates for breast cancer genetic testing: a systematic review. Cancer Epidemiol Biomarkers Prev 15:840–855, 2006

Schmeler KM, Lynch HT, Chen LM, et al: Prophylactic surgery to reduce the risk of gynecologic cancers in the Lynch syndrome. N Engl J Med 354:261–269, 2006

Schneider K: Counseling About Cancer: Strategies for Genetic Counseling. New York, Wiley-Liss, 2002

Schwartz MD, Peshkin BN, Hughes C, et al: Impact of BRCA1/BRCA2 mutation testing on psychologic distress in a clinic-based sample. J Clin Oncol 20:514–520, 2002

Stoffel EM, Ford B, Mercado RC, et al: Sharing genetic test results in Lynch syndrome: communication with close and distant relatives. Clin Gastroenterol Hepatol 6:333–338, 2008

van Oostrom I, Meijers-Heijboer H, Lodder LN, et al: Long-term psychological impact of carrying a BRCA1/2 mutation and prophylactic surgery: a 5-year follow-up study. J Clin Oncol 21:3867–3874, 2003

van Oostrom I, Meijers-Heijboer H, Duivenvoorden HJ, et al: Experience of parental cancer in childhood is a risk factor for psychological distress during genetic cancer susceptibility testing. Ann Oncol 17:1090–1095, 2006

van Roosmalen MS, Stalmeier PF, Verhoef LC, et al: Impact of BRCA1/2 testing and disclosure of a positive test result on women affected and unaffected with breast or ovarian cancer. Am J Med Genet A 124A:346–355, 2004

Vernon SW, Gritz ER, Peterson SK, et al: Correlates of psychologic distress in colorectal cancer patients undergoing genetic testing for hereditary colon cancer. Health Psychol 16:73–86, 1997

Vernon SW, Gritz ER, Peterson SK, et al: Intention to learn results of genetic testing for hereditary colon cancer. Cancer Epidemiol Biomarkers Prev 8:353–360, 1999

Wagner A, van Kessel I, Kriege MG, et al: Long term follow-up of HNPCC gene mutation carriers: compliance with screening and satisfaction with counseling and screening procedures. Fam Cancer 4:295–300, 2005

Weitzel JN, Blazer KR, Macdonald DJ, et al: Genetics, genomics, and cancer risk assessment: state of the art and future directions in the era of personalized medicine. CA Cancer J Clin August 19, 2011 [Epub ahead of print]

Yang K, Allen B, Contad P, et al: Awareness of gynecologic surveillance in women from hereditary non-polyposis colorectal cancer families. Fam Cancer 5:405–409, 2006

CHAPTER 7

Dimensional Psychopharmacology of the Cancer Patient

Massimo Biondi, M.D.
Massimo Pasquini, M.D.

> Disease is somatic; the suffering from it, psychic.
>
> Martin H. Fischer

Over the last twenty years, the detection and treatment of depression in cancer patients have been constantly improving, as has the recognition of anxiety, activation, and insomnia; health preoccupation; phobias and obsessional thoughts about the disease; and, in some instances, almost full-blown posttraumatic stress disorder after major surgery or near-end-of-life experiences. As a result of these developments, clinicians in many countries no longer hold the view that depression could be "the rule" for patients who have lost their health, who are undergoing multiple invasive diagnostic procedures, who may face unavoidable mutilation due to surgical interventions, and who may suffer side effects of chemotherapies. Nor is the belief now common that anxiety might be "normal" for those living with a new uncertain future or under the threat of a possibly fatal recurrence. Symptoms of demoralization, depression, fear, and anxiety are now well recognized as some of the main psychological needs to address in the clinical care of cancer patients. Also, the impact that suffering has on quality of life and adherence to or compliance with treatments is better recognized. Over these past two decades, psychopharmacological interventions have become prominent therapeutic resources in the care of distress and psychopathological suffering.

In this chapter, we propose that the traditional *categorical* approach to psychiatric diagnosis presented in DSM-IV (American Psychiatric Association 1994) could be better integrated with a *dimensional* approach for assessing and treating the complex and multifaceted psychopathological suffering of cancer patients. Although this is a preliminary view, this combined approach could be of interest in many clinical settings and may better address individual needs of distressed cancer patients. The traditional categorical diagnostic approach is based on the fulfillment of standardized criteria for disorders. These categories guide the protocols for treatments—for example, counseling or psychotherapy is used for mild major depression; antidepressants for moderate-to-severe major depression; anxiolytics or psychotherapy for demoralization or adjustment reactions; antipsychotics for delirium; and so on. In our clinical experience, this approach has some limitations. Treatments might be improved by adding a dimensional approach—that is, by recognizing prominent components of presenting psychopathology in a given patient and addressing them with drugs according to their different mechanisms impinging on circuits and neurotransmitters. We recognize that the application of such a dimensional model in psychiatry is at a very early phase and that in psycho-oncology it is even more tentative. However, our preliminary experience with this new approach is promising, and we believe the model might enrich patient care.

Another issue we address is the importance of communication skills for introducing patients to psychotropic drug treatment, with a focus on presenting drug information and, according to a biopsychosocial perspective, conveying to the patient the usefulness of taking medication. We discuss that cancer itself is for any person a severe, major life stress event, putting the individual at risk for exhaustion of physical and mental coping resources, and we suggest that drug and psychological treatments can be used together—rather than being mutually exclusive or conflicting—to help in overcoming distress, anxiety, demoralization, or depression. Psychotherapeutic and psychopharmacological treatments can be viewed as allies and may be tailored according to each patient's specific needs and psychopathological dimensions, rather than only according to standardized treatment protocols.

We do not provide in this chapter a systematic review of the evidence on psychotropic drug treatment in cancer patients, which the reader can find elsewhere in several updated reviews (Chong et al. 2011; Rodin et al. 2007). In discussion of psychotropic drugs, we intentionally do not include classifications, mechanisms of action, pharmacokinetics, and dosages. We do not describe treatment options for psychotic, bipolar, substance abuse, and other psychiatric disorders because of their wide prevalence and limited direct association with malignant diseases. We do, however, recommend taking advantage of the side effects of drugs (e.g., prescribing antidepressants to treat other symptoms) and include a section focusing on referral to a psychiatrist for psychopathological assessment and psychotropic drug treatment.

Shift From Categorical to Dimensional Diagnosis and Treatment Approaches in Psychiatry and Psychosomatic Medicine

DSM-IV (American Psychiatric Association 1994) discussed the issue of diagnosis according to a categorical approach (viewing mental illness as a category or a discrete entity) rather than a dimensional approach (describing a clinical picture according to its main psychopathological components, along a continuum from normalcy to pathology). The dimensional approach to psychiatric diagnosis was considered to be at too early a stage of development for systematic application in clinical practice and was not regarded as well suited for epidemiological, research, or legal purposes. The dimensional approach was nonetheless interesting and intriguing to many clinicians, particularly in relation to difficulties with and criticisms of DSM-IV in some clinical areas (see Pancheri 1995 for a review). Psychopathology is the discipline that systematically organizes the descriptive pictures of personal experiences. As formulated by Jaspers (1913/1964), psychopathology denotes real, conscious psychic events that have consequences and relationships. According to the categorical model, diagnostic criteria are summed only until a specified number is deemed to be present; at this point, the diagnosis is said to be valid.

The dimensional representation of psychopathology has a different structure from the categorical model. The model is cumulative in that the number of diagnostic features observed is an index of the degree to which the diagnostic entity is present (Blashfield and Livesley 1999). The concept of psychopathological dimension is derived from psychometrics and is defined as an altered psychic function phenomenologically expressing itself through a set of symptoms or signs indicating and specifying an altered function on a continuum ranging from extreme pathology to normality (Pancheri 1995). This approach is especially useful in psycho-oncology, given that DSM-IV does not provide for adequate depiction of depressive disorders associated with cancer. Furthermore, the lack of a clear border between pathology and normality helps in the comprehension of depressive states in the oncology setting, allowing the identification of points along the continuum from sadness through demoralization to depression in the same patient. Given its atheoretical assumption, this approach should be able to identify psychopathological dimensions that are not categorically expected.

Studies conducted on patients with primary unipolar depression revealed the presence of anger or an activation dimension (Biondi et al. 2005; Pasquini et al. 2004) not included in the DSM-IV criteria for depressive disorder but already described by ancient Greek physicians. An anger dimension was also detected in depressed cancer patients using a simple dimensional rating scale (Pasquini et al. 2006). A dimensional diagnosis of depression implies that clinicians have to listen more accurately to the principal complaints of the patient. Many elements are at work, such as the doctor-patient relationship, patient's expectations and needs, patient's personality and psychological status, and the severity of discomfort. With cancer patients, psychiatrists have to accurately describe the stress-related nature of depression and its relation to the immune system. Problems linked to this type of approach include the identification and definition of significant dimensions and the validation of the diagnostic system.

The categorical and the dimensional approaches are complementary and represent two successive phases of the process aiming at therapy optimization. We suggest that a categorical diagnosis be determined first, to broadly frame the patient's clinical condition; this can be followed by a dimensional diagnosis, which serves to establish the best possible therapy. In fact, dimensional diagnosis entailing a reclassification of psychotropic drugs provides the opportunity for using drugs according to a pathophysiological rationale so far not followed. According to Pancheri's (1995) view, the pathophysiology of a given psychopathological dimension (sadness, fear, anger, activation, impulsivity, obsessivity, apathy, reality distortion, etc.) could be better matched with a specific drug acting on a neurotransmitter circuit than to a diagnostic DSM-IV category—that is, a more specific psychotropic drug treatment can be planned following a dimensional approach to psychopathology. From this perspective, we do not consider anxiety or adjustment disorders as separate entities from depression. Consequently, treatment strategies discussed in this chapter not only refer to DSM-IV diagnoses but also integrate dimensional principles. Although evidence to this point has been anecdotal and limited as concerns clinical trials, we suggest considering a "dimensionally oriented" drug treatment, which in our experience well integrates the traditional DSM-IV categorical approach.

Treating Psychopathological Syndromes: The Usefulness of a Dimensional Instrument in Clinical Practice

Many clinical instruments allow for a dimensional approach in psychiatry and psychosomatic medicine. These include the Symptom Checklist–90—Revised (SCL-90-R; Derogatis 1994) and the Brief Psychiatric Rating Scale (Overall and Gorham 1962). Due to the clinical realities of time pressures, Pancheri et al. (1999) developed a specific psychopathological tool, La Scala di Valutazione Rapida Dimensionale (Rapid Dimensional Assessment Scale [SVARAD]). The SVARAD was adapted to use in psycho-oncology as a rapid, efficient means of determining the individual's placement on a continuum between pathology and normality. It is a reliable and valid "dimensional" tool for use in both research and clinical settings.

The SVARAD is a 10-item instrument specifically developed for the rapid assessment of some major psychopathological dimensions. A validation study showed that the SVARAD has satisfactory interrater reliability, content validity, and criterion validity (Pancheri et al. 1999). The items are rated on a 5-point scale ranging from 0 to 4, with higher scores indicating greater severity. Scores of 1 indicate the presence of a condition intermediate between normality and psychopathology, whereas scores of 2 or more indicate the presence of symptoms of definite clinical relevance.

The items explore the following dimensions: apprehension/fear, sadness/demoralization, anger/irritability, obsessionality, apathy, impulsiveness, reality distortion, thought disorganization, somatic preoccupation/somatization, and activation. Every dimension has been defined based on both psychopathological and functioning criteria. The following are examples of criteria in several of the dimensions:

- Sadness/demoralization: self-dislike, pessimism, reduced creativity, anhedonia
- Anger/irritability: irritation, anger, resentment; irritability, quarrelsomeness, hostility; verbal or physical violence
- Impulsiveness: the tendency to suddenly behave in an inadequate or potentially harmful way, without sufficient reflection on the causes or the consequences of one's own actions
- Activation: increased motor activity, acceleration of ideas, disinhibition, increased energy and self-confidence, euphoria, irritability

Obviously, in the clinical setting of oncology, in which demoralization and depression are quite distinct phenomena, the sadness/demoralization definition reflects limitations, and if a clear-cut distinction between these phenomena is needed, we suggest other instruments (see Chapter 4, "Demoralization and Depression in Cancer"). Similarly, if a rapid assessment is necessary, other instruments are recommended (see Chapter 9, "Rapid Psychometric Assessment of Distress and Depression for the Clinician"). However, the SVARAD has proven to be useful in assessing psychological conditions associated with serious physical illness.

Several factors may be used to guide treatment. For example, different dimensions may prevail in the clinical presentation of a categorical diagnosis of depressive disorder. As shown in Figure 7–1, three patients who received a diagnosis of depression differed greatly in their suffering. If the apathy dimension prevails, the patient should take an antidepressant with a dopaminergic or noradrenergic profile. The presence of insomnia (on the activation dimension) and anxiety might suggest the employment of an antagonist at the postsynaptic serotonin 5-HT_2 and 5-HT_3 receptors and a histamine H_1 antagonist, such as mirtazapine or trazodone. When anger/irritability is the predominant dimension, a combination of a selective serotonin reuptake inhibitor (SSRI) and an anticonvulsant, most often valproate, may produce benefit (Pasquini et al. 2007) (see Figure 7–2).

Psychological Suffering of Cancer Patients as a Response to the Stress of Illness: The Role for a Dimensional Assessment and Treatment

The psychological and psychopathological suffering of cancer patients could be viewed as the response to the stress of illness, at both a physical and an emotional level, as a severe, long-lasting stressful event that engages resources and might exhaust mind and body. The resulting distress and suffering are composite and multidimensional, resulting from event characteristics, temperament, personality, coping resources, and resilience, with varying degrees and components of psychopathology. Anxiety, depression, anger, and other psychological and psychopathological dimensions can be better conceptualized as responses, resulting from the distressing power of the cancer event. The uncertainty of illness, the bad news about diagnosis, the loss of a previously healthy status and hope for the future, the stress of

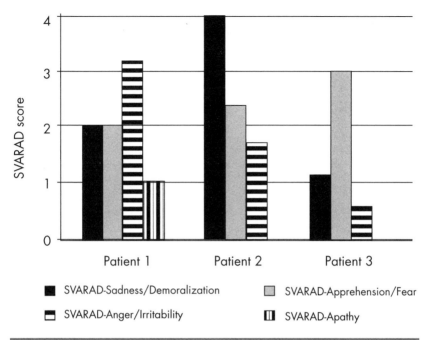

FIGURE 7–1. Three different clinical presentations of depression according to a dimensional approach.
Note. SVARAD=Scala di Valutazione Rapida Dimensionale (Rapid Dimensional Assessment Scale) (Pancheri et al. 1999).

undergoing chemotherapy or surgery, and living under the threat of recurrence all contribute to a multifaceted psychopathology.

Individuals with these same stressors might receive the same categorical diagnosis of moderate major depression, *but each individual's dimensions might strongly differ, leading to quite distinct treatment needs,* not the same as an identical diagnosis would appear to suggest. The dimensional diagnosis approach could overcome the distinctions among subthreshold major depression, a mild or moderate episode of major depression or adjustment disorder, generalized anxiety disorder comorbid with mood disorder, and mixed depressive-anxiety disorder. The best fitting criteria are less interesting than the exploration of several dimensions, their severity, their duration, and the shape of the profile of suffering.

Moreover, this approach underscores the impact of stress on the brain, specifically on brain neurotransmitters such as norepinephrine, serotonin, and dopamine. Their related circuitries are involved in the stress response to the protracted stress exposure, and their activity is linked to the patho-

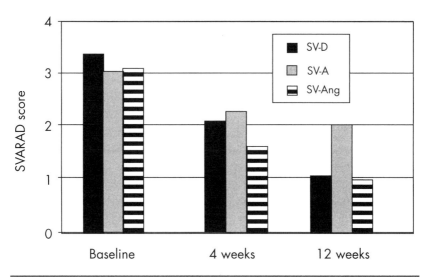

FIGURE 7–2. Effectiveness of the combination of a selective serotonin reuptake inhibitor (SSRI) with an anticonvulsant in hostile depression.
Note. Significant decrease on Scala di Valutazione Rapida Dimensionale (SVARAD; Pancheri et al. 1999) scores from baseline to 4 and 12 weeks.* SV-D = SVARAD Depressive factor; SV-A = SVARAD Anxiety factor; SV-Ang=SVARAD Anger/Irritability factor.
*All values were significant at $P<0.001$.

physiology of the psychopathological dimensions. Loss-induced depression is an interesting model of how psychological events translate into steady brain circuitry modification of serotonergic and noradrenergic transmission (Biondi and Picardi 1996). In other words, the dimensional diagnosis view minimizes the relevance of discussing the differences among categories while suggesting that psychopharmacological and psychotherapeutic interventions or counseling both act on a common ground at a brain level through different pathways (Biondi 1995), best fitting the needs of a biopsychosocial model of disease (Engel 1977).

This approach could be useful in psycho-oncology, where psychological interventions and psychotropic drug treatment can be integrated to support the individual during very difficult phases of his or her life (Biondi et al. 1995; Grassi et al. 2003). According to this view, we better conceptualize antidepressants as antistress agents rather than psychotropic drugs—that is, turning the word *antidepressant* into another term, an "antistress pill." This will give a different model of intervention in depression—as well as distress and its related psychopathological dimensions—in cancer. It will help caring personnel and patients to better understand depression/demoralization and to accept an antidepressant as a specific therapy. Destigmatization will eventually ensue.

In summary, distinguishing major depression from demoralization or adjustment disorder is difficult, and the ability to make this differential diagnosis is an essential skill of consultant-liaison psychiatrists (O'Keeffe and Ranjith 2007; see Chapter 4, "Demoralization and Depression in Cancer"). According to a dimensional view of cancer-induced distress and suffering, clinicians must also assess fear, apprehension, feelings of anger and irritability, apathy and passivity, somatic preoccupation and obsessional thoughts, activation and restlessness, and possible reality distortion and disorganization. A profile of psychopathological dimensions—better than a diagnostic category—can be better seen as strongly related to an underlying pathophysiology of brain circuits subjected to chronic stress. They—and not a diagnostic category—should be addressed as targets of drug treatment. The term *antistress pills,* rather than *psychotropic drugs,* as related to the enduring stress of facing illness, could thus lead to destigmatization of psychotropic drug treatment and a greater acceptance of the proposition by the patients.

Dimensional Psychopharmacology in Oncology Settings

In this section, we review the scanty literature to suggest some perspectives of a dimensional psychopharmacological approach to specific dimensions of psychopathology in cancer, adding discussion of our clinical samples and experience.

Sadness/Demoralization Dimension

Anxiety, sleep disturbances, and depression/demoralization are the more common complaints among cancer patients. Although aiding sleep with drugs or treating anxiety is well accepted in clinical practice, depression is a subject of controversy. Several difficulties and barriers are already present for recognizing and treating depression (Greenberg 2004), especially in older patients (Weinberger et al. 2011). If a dimensional approach is applied to diagnosis, the following question may arise: Why should an antidepressant be prescribed to a cancer patient if he or she is not suffering from a depressive disorder, but rather has an adaptation disorder or is displaying a natural emotional reaction? The benefits of antidepressants in cancer patients are debated. Some clinicians wonder why cancer patients should take antidepressants, and many patients question their antidepressant prescriptions because they deny having psychological problems.

We would answer that antidepressants can benefit cancer patients in several ways. First, they can be used to treat depression, which can otherwise cause cancer patients to have greater emotional suffering and limitation of psychosocial functioning and freedom, impaired quality of life, a negative impact on family relationships and attitudes toward work and activities, and difficulty with compliance to medical treatments. Second, antidepressant treatment can counteract the stress of coping with cancer by improving brain serotonergic and noradrenergic neurotransmissions, which are under long-term pressure during the long, exhausting phases of cancer diagnosis and treatment. Antidepressant treatment could be better viewed as an antistress intervention, rather than as only a mood-sustaining intervention or a drug for treating mental disorders. Third, treating depression in patients with metastatic breast cancer may result in longer survival (Giese-Davis et al. 2010). This effect is attributable to many factors, not only to strengthening of emotional and psychological well-being and improving quality of patients' lives, but also to improved neuroimmune modulation (Musselman et al. 2001; Reiche et al. 2004). Indeed, it is well known that treating depression may reduce chronic inflammatory reactions of cancer.

Finally, antidepressants are not simply symptomatic drugs, although they are used to treat several symptoms, such as pain or hot flashes. When prescribed to a cancer patient who has depression, they have to be considered as a disease-modifying or, more accurately, a syndrome-modifying treatment. Although SSRIs are the most widely prescribed antidepressants in many countries, they are not necessarily a first-line treatment strategy for depressive cancer patients. Medications that are often useful include tricyclic antidepressants (TCAs); dual-acting antidepressants such as venlafaxine, duloxetine, mirtazapine, and mianserin; and noradrenergic agents such as maprotiline or reboxetine. Drugs such as agomelatine and *S*-adenosyl-methionine, which act through alternative mechanisms, have still to be assessed for their possible use in mild or moderate depression in cancer patients. Recent reviews of controlled trials of high-dose omega-3 supplementation in low to moderate depression in psychiatric patients support a possible indication; to our knowledge, no similar controlled trial has been done in cancer patients.

In our view, antidepressant treatment can address several needs of cancer patients. Psychotropic drugs, along with psychological interventions, may help patients cope with the long-term distress of confronting cancer.

A thorough discussion of the limitations of the trials in psycho-oncology is beyond the scope of this chapter. We emphasize, however, that although Kim and Fisch (2006) stated that antidepressants are often prescribed for cancer patients, clinical psycho-oncologists cannot currently rely on the same strong and systematic evidence of effectiveness drawn from meta-analyses, multicenter controlled trials of antidepressants, and long-term efficacy studies as do psychiatrists. The reasons for the lack of adequate antidepressant trials in patients with cancer has been previously discussed by Fisch (2004), who stressed the relevance of the patients' perceived stigma of a psychiatric disorder in minimizing a depressive condition. Nevertheless, clinicians in psycho-oncology often cannot follow uncritically the suggestions from treatment guidelines for major depression in psychiatry but must adopt different principles, drug choices, dosages, titration schedules, and side-effect risks according to cancer type, stage, and metabolic condition. Table 7–1 shows available data on the effectiveness of antidepressants for depressive disorders in cancer patients.

Methodological shortcomings, small sample sizes, different specific types of cancer, different antidepressants, and different primary outcomes are the main problems that render the trials difficult to compare. Based on the sparse existing data, the evidence remains inconclusive.

Apprehension/Fear Dimension

Feelings of anxiety, preoccupation, excessive worry, and apprehension, as well as psychic (i.e., cognitive) symptoms and especially somatic symptoms of anxiety (e.g., muscular tension, sweating, tachycardia, palpitations, shortness of breath, gastrointestinal symptoms) are very common complaints early in the diagnostic phases of cancer and later during treatment. Diagnoses of panic disorder or generalized anxiety disorder are uncommon, whereas subsyndromal clinical pictures may be common and well recognized through a dimensional approach. Episodic treatments with benzodiazepines—preferably those without active metabolites and a conjugated hepatic excretion, such as lorazepam or oxazepam—may be helpful; in the majority of cases, they should be prescribed at low dosages and for a limited period of time. The prescription might be circumscribed to some specific days or linked in a timely fashion to invasive procedures, to attenuate the stress of waiting for critical clinical responses and preparation for invasive procedures, and to reduce conditioned nausea and vomiting in some patients undergoing chemotherapy. The dependence potential of benzodiazepines should be assessed for every patient and balanced according to a risk/benefit ratio. In our 30 years of experience, development of benzodiazepine dependence in oncological patients under common conditions is very rare. Persistent apprehension and fear are common among patients with posttraumatic stress syndromes. Pharmacological intervention for posttraumatic stress disorder in patients affected by malignant diseases could be of some usefulness, although the paucity of scientific literature hampers any therapeutic suggestion. Very little is known about medication choices for

TABLE 7–1.   Antidepressant trials

Study	Treatment groups	Study population	Instruments	Symptomatic improvement at the end of the treatment
Costa et al. 1985	Mianserin; placebo	73 Women with breast or gynecological cancer affected by MDD	HAM-D ZSRDS CGI	Mean HAM-D score at 4 weeks = 8.19 for mianserin group vs.13.2 for placebo; significantly more responders in mianserin group
Razavi et al. 1996	Fluoxetine; placebo	115 Patients with mixed cancer diagnosis and MDD or adjustment disorder	HADS MADRS	HADS<8 in 11% of fluoxetine group vs. 7% of placebo group
Fisch et al. 2003	Fluoxetine; placebo	163 Patients with advanced cancer and depression	BZSDS	Greater improvement in BZSDS scores in fluoxetine group (24.44–21.14) than placebo group (23.09–22.54)
Holland et al. 1998	Fluoxetine; desipramine	40 Women with cancer on active treatment and with MDD, or HAM-D>14	HAM-D CGI	HAM-D and CGI scores significantly decreased for both medications; improvement in pain and mood in fluoxetine group
Razavi et al. 1999	Trazodone; clorazepate	18 Women with breast cancer and adjustment disorder, or HADS≥14	HADS SCL-90 CGI	Improvement on CGI scale in 90.9% of trazodone group vs. 57.1% of clorazepate group
Pezzella et al. 2001	Paroxetine; amitriptyline	179 Women with breast cancer and MDD, or MADRS≥16	MADRS CGI	In both groups, CGI severity scores decreased similarly; ≥50% reduction in MADRS in 43.7% of paroxetine group vs. 37.9% of amitriptyline group

TABLE 7–1. Antidepressant trials *(continued)*

Study	Treatment groups	Study population	Instruments	Symptomatic improvement at the end of the treatment
Morrow et al. 2003	Paroxetine; placebo	549 Cancer patients undergoing chemotherapy assessed for fatigue	CES-D	Significant reduction in CES-D scores in paroxetine group (14.8–12.0) vs. placebo group (15.8–14.8); no difference in fatigue
Musselman et al. 2006	Paroxetine; desipramine; placebo	35 Women with breast cancer affected by MDD	HAM-D	No difference between groups; mean HAM-D change: 11.27 for placebo group, 10.09 for desipramine group, 7.62 for paroxetine group
Roscoe et al. 2005	Paroxetine; placebo	94 Women with breast cancer receiving at least 4 cycles of chemotherapy	CES-D	More significant drop in CES-D in paroxetine group (14.7–8.8) vs. placebo group (14.7–12.6)
Lydiatt et al. 2008	Citalopram; placebo	23 Patients with head and neck cancer	HAM-D UW-QOL CGI	On CGI Severity scale, 15% of citalopram group vs. 60% in placebo group rated as at least mildly ill; quality of life deteriorated in both groups but less so in citalopram group

Note. BZSDS=Brief Zung Self-Reporting Depression Scale; CES-D=Center for Epidemiologic Studies Depression Scale; CGI=Clinical Global Impression Scale; HADS=Hospital Anxiety and Depression Scale; HAM-D=Hamilton Depression Rating Scale; MADRS=Montgomery-Åsberg Depression Rating Scale; MDD=major depressive disorder; SCL–90=Symptom Checklist–90; UW-QOL=University of Washington Quality of Life Questionnaire; ZSRDS=Zung Self-Rating Depression Scale.

psychological posttraumatic symptoms in cancer patients. However, following the same principles as above, clinicians may protect the sleep-wake cycle and reduce the activation of the fear circuitry.

Anger/Irritability Dimension

Anger and aggression are complex social behaviors involving several brain circuits and mediators, including neurotransmitters, androgens, cytokines, and enzymes (Nelson and Chiavegatto 2001). Among them, 5-HT has a prominent role. Impulsivity, anger behavior, and high aggressiveness are correlated with low cerebrospinal fluid 5-hydroxyindoleacetic acid concentrations and with decreased central 5-HT activity and turnover. Potentiation of 5-HT levels by several drugs decrease aggression, anger, and impulsive behavior (Lesch and Merschdorf 2000). Fluoxetine significantly reduced anger attacks in several studies (Fava et al. 1993). In our experience, very low dosages of TCAs (e.g., 25–50 mg/day clomipramine or amitriptyline) or low dosages of citalopram or escitalopram could be considered if the sadness dimension is prominent.

Together with possible psychological interventions dealing with the meaning of anger reactions, anger attacks, irritability with family members, self-deprecation, and guilt, mood stabilizers are very useful for patients in whom depressive rumination and anger prevail over the other dimensions. Being angry is common among cancer patients, mostly during early phases of the disease. However, in the context of a normality-pathology continuum of mood, anger may turn into self-directed irritability and dysphoria, which are frequently undetected among depressed patients. In such cases, adding valproate or oxcarbazepine to an antidepressant could be successful.

Activation Dimension

Difficulties in falling asleep are common symptoms of anxiety and may benefit from short-acting sleep inducers, such as triazolam, zolpidem, zaleplon, or ramelteon. In contrast, middle-of-the-night and late-night insomnia are common symptoms underlying depression. These symptoms slowly remit under a specific antidepressant treatment as depression subsides after 2–3 weeks. Benzodiazepines (lorazepam, temazepam) may be useful during the first weeks. Trazodone or low-dose dopamine D_2 antagonists may be useful. Mirtazapine is effective as both an adjuvant analgesic and an antiemetic, and it has sedative and appetite-stimulant properties (Pasquini et al. 2006; Theobald et al. 2002; Thompson 2000). The sedative properties, which are particularly useful in depression with insomnia, are best perceived at low dosages. As an alternative, when insomnia is the predominant and more distressing dimension of a depressive episode, a first-line choice might be trazodone, considering its rapid efficacy and safety, or mianserin (a mixed noradrenergic-serotonergic antidepressant with sedative properties).

Benzodiazepines are very useful as an augmentation option for depressive states with a pronounced dimension of somatic or psychic anxiety. However, we recommend withdrawing the benzodiazepines as soon as the antidepressant shows efficacy.

Insomnia without a clear anxiety component is often a manifestation of an activation dimension. In these cases, adding quetiapine or olanzapine at low dosages is indicated.

Persistent diurnal activation, with restlessness, increased psychomotor activity, preoccupation, tension, and angst, often suggests a dysphoric condition, whereas agitated depression suggests a mixed mood state. Agitated depression requires mood-stabilizing agents or low-dose D_2 antagonists such as haloperidol, trifluoperazine, quetiapine, or olanzapine, or other atypical antipsychotics; antidepressants should be avoided until activation subsides, at which time they could be introduced at a low dosage to treat the sadness-demoralization dimension, if present.

Apathy Dimension

Apathy is a psychopathological dimension involved in several conditions with an intact cognitive system and often found with anhedonia, avolition, blunted affect, reduced motivation and activity, lack of drive, and anergia to constitute a significant component of disorders such as depression, schizophrenia, and substance dependence, as well as neuropsychiatric diseases such as Parkinson's disease and dementia. Several studies point to a dysfunction of the prefrontal-subcortical dopaminergic circuits in apathy (Guimarães et al. 2008), with a hypoactive dopaminergic system as one of the main neural correlates; noradrenergic circuits are also involved. Methylphenidate, amphetamine-related compounds, pemoline, bupropion, amantadine, pramipexole, ropinirole, and bromocriptine are drugs with prevalent dopaminergic activity. These agents, as well as compounds acting on noradrenergic transmission (among them desipramine, nortriptyline, mianserin, mirtazapine, and reboxetine), low-dose amisulpride and sulpiride (which stimulate dopaminergic activity, especially in the prefrontal cortex, due to their preferential inhibition of D_2 autoreceptors), and monoamine oxidase inhibitors (MAOIs) are useful to treat the apathy dimension in several psychiatric disorders.

Although only very limited evidence is currently available in psycho-oncology, some of these drugs could be considered for treating apathy in cancer patients. Grassi et al. (2004) and Torta et al. (2007) reported successful outcomes from using reboxetine and amisulpride, respectively, in depressed cancer patients. These agents are not the most favored first-line antidepressants (Eyding et al. 2010); however, the noradrenergic properties of reboxetine and the prodopaminergic action of amisulpride are indicated in depression associated with apathy, fatigue, and cognitive disturbances. In our outpatient clinic, we often efficaciously prescribe low dosages of preferential norepinephrine reuptake inhibitors (e.g., desipramine or trimipramine).

Obsessionality and Somatic Preoccupation/ Somatization Dimensions

Serotonergic agents such as SSRIs and clomipramine are well-recognized treatments for obsessive-compulsive disorder (Abramowitz et al. 2008) and the spectrum of related disorders, including hypochondriasis (Abramowitz et al. 2008). Obsessive personality traits predict a better response to antidepressant serotonergic drugs in depressed patients. According to our experience, low-dose SSRIs can benefit unmotivated, repetitive hypochondriacal thoughts in cancer patients. Similarly, low dosages of clomipramine (50–75 mg) may be effective, but caution is needed because of the side-effect profile (dry mouth, dizziness, orthostatic hypotension).

Reality Distortion and Thought Disorganization Dimensions: Delusion and Confusional States (Delirium)

Reality distortion and thought disorganization are to different extents common as psychopathological aspects of the psychotic disorders. Psychotic disorders, manic episodes, and other major psychiatric disorders, however, are uncommon among cancer patients. To be more precise, these conditions in cancer patients most typically represent a preexisting condition not associated with cancer. A psychotic disorder due to medical conditions (e.g., brain tumors, metastases, metabolic imbalance) or their treatment may also occur. In these cases, clinicians should plan treatment strategies according to pharmacodynamic interactions and clinical presentations. Corticosteroids may induce manic states; in such situations, we recommend stopping chemotherapy until the manic state is resolved. More difficult to manage is chemotherapy in patients with schizophrenia who are undergoing clozapine treatment. Because clozapine can induce neutropenia, the decision to continue chemotherapy is debatable (Liu et al. 2010). Thus, the role of the consultation-liaison psychiatrist is vital when a comorbid severe mental disorder could represent a barrier to cancer treatment (Howard et al. 2010). D_2 antagonists, such as haloperidol, and $5\text{-HT}_2/D_2$ blockers are well recognized drugs of choice.

Delusions are a rare primary or secondary condition in oncology patients, whereas reality distortion and disorganization are more frequently related to acute or subacute confusional states (delirium), a serious and common complication in cancer patients (Caraceni and Grassi 2003). Although the causes of delirium often are not directly linked to cancer, several medical conditions, such as polypharmacotherapy, might be implicated. This is one of the reasons for the lack of specificity and clinical significance of pharmacological trials in oncology settings. Delirium, however, can be treated successfully if the diagnosis is made early. The first-line approach to treating delirium is to identify the underlying causes and, where possible, correct them. An imbalance between cholinergic and dopaminergic activity underlies the pathophysiology of delirium (Trzepacz 2000); therefore, typical antipsychotics are considered to be first-line agents for treating it. In a double-blind, randomized trial, haloperidol and chlorpromazine were found to be equally effective (Breitbart et al. 1996). According to a Cochrane review, risperidone and olanzapine were also effective (Lonergan et al. 2007). Subcutaneous administration of olanzapine seems to be well tolerated in patients with advanced cancer (Elsayem et al. 2010). In a recent randomized controlled trial carried out in patients with delirium, but not cancer, the group treated with quetiapine improved more rapidly than the group given placebo (Tahir et al. 2010). In a comparative study, aripiprazole was as effective as haloperidol but with fewer side effects in patients with delirium (Boettger et al. 2011).

Summary

The examples of dimensional approaches to psychopharmacology provided throughout this section demonstrate the remarkable similarity between the dimensional approach and the tailored-therapy approach (Table 7–2). A clinician's choice of antidepressants typically is based on a patient's clinical depressive disorder presentation rather than on the categorical diagnoses. Indeed, a gold-standard therapy requires a focus on the more distressing patient dimensions. In other words, the serotonergic dysfunction related to the pathophysiology of depression does not imply that clinicians have to treat depression by employing serotonin-enhancing agents only. Furthermore, the aforementioned lack of evidence-based data for the psychopharmacological treatment of cancer-related depression may turn things in favor of the employment of other antidepressants.

Case Vignette

Ellen is a 50-year-old woman affected by breast cancer. She underwent radical mastectomy followed by breast reconstruction and adjuvant hormonal therapy. She developed a depressive state with a prominent anergic component

1 year after cancer diagnosis. The clinical psychologist who first assessed her psychological status suggested psychiatric assessment. Several factors made Ellen more vulnerable, such as discomfort with body image and intimate relationships. Furthermore, she was working as a fitness trainer in a high school. When the consultation-liaison psychiatrist met her, she reported low mood, emptiness, loss of interests and pleasure in doing things, poor concentration, and thinking slowness that had gradually developed over an 8-month period. Dissociative symptoms were excluded after a careful interview. Ellen's main concern involved her work; she felt that she could no longer move in the correct way or wear sportswear. She was taking tamoxifen with minimal side effects. Due to the ongoing tamoxifen treatment, the clinician chose the D_2 blocker amisulpride to avoid interference with cytochrome P450 2D6 (CYP2D6) inhibition. The clinician also prescribed oral trimipramine beginning at 25 mg/day and up-titrated in 10 days to 100 mg/day. After 1 month of this treatment, Ellen's symptoms decreased and she experienced improvement in her overall energy. However, her self-confidence was not modified as expected. Regular monitoring of prolactin was planned. The improvement was stable for 1 year, when, in agreement with Ellen and her psychologist, the clinician gradually discontinued trimipramine.

Common Drug Interactions

Applying dimensional psychopharmacology in oncology is difficult due to the many drug interactions. The consultation-liaison psychiatrist should not prescribe drugs that interfere with primary medications. For example, tamoxifen is an antagonist of estrogen receptors that is currently used for the treatment of both early and advanced estrogen receptor–positive breast cancer. Nowadays, it is well recognized that potent CYP2D6 inhibitors, such as paroxetine, reduce endoxifen, a tamoxifen metabolite, to a concentration that increases the risk of death from breast cancer (Kelly et al. 2010), whereas other antidepressants that do not inhibit CYP2D6, such as citalopram, escitalopram, and venlafaxine, will be tolerable. In these cases, consultation-liaison psychiatrists might support oncologists and primary care practitioners when treating patients. In addition, interactions between opioids and serotonergic antidepressants may lead to the development of serotonin syndrome. In these cases, slow titration and careful follow-up are needed.

Caution also is recommended in combining the chemotherapeutic agent irinotecan and SSRIs because of possible rhabdomyolysis (Richards et al. 2003). A prodopaminergic antidepressant that may increase levels of prolactin is not recommended in women with breast cancer. Although SSRIs might increase prolactin, results from a recent study show no increased risk of breast cancer with long-term use (Ashbury et al. 2010). Anticholinergic side effects of TCAs have to be taken into account for patients affected by colorectal, bladder, and prostate cancers.

TABLE 7–2. Dimensionally oriented drug treatments

Psychopathological dimension	Suggested psychotropic drugs
Sadness/demoralization	Serotonergic and noradrenergic drugs Dual-acting drugs (serotonergic and noradrenergic) MAOIs High-dose omega-3 supplements
Apprehension/fear	BDZs Serotonergic and noradrenergic compounds (SSRIs, TCAs) Dual-acting drugs (serotonergic and noradrenergic)
Anger/irritability	Mood stabilizers (anticonvulsants) Low-dose serotonergic drugs or TCAs or low-dose SSRIs
Activation and impulsiveness	Mood stabilizers (anticonvulsants) D_2 or $D_2/5\text{-HT}_2$ antagonists (low-dose typical and atypical antipsychotics) BDZ or non-BDZ hypnoinducers Antihistaminics and antidepressants with high antihistaminic sedative properties
Apathy	Dopaminergic drugs Noradrenergic drugs Dual-acting agents Low-dose sulpiride or amisulpride MAOIs
Obsessionality and somatic preoccupation/somatization	Serotonergic drugs (SSRIs; clomipramine)
Thought disorganization and reality distortion	D_1 and D_2 antagonists; $D_2/5\text{-HT}_2$ antagonists

Note. BDZ=benzodiazepine; D_1=dopamine 1 receptor; D_2=dopamine 2 receptor; 5-HT=serotonin; MAOI=monoamine oxidase inhibitor; SSRI=selective serotonin reuptake inhibitor; TCA=tricyclic antidepressant.

Hence, the psychopharmacological treatment of cancer patients requires specific knowledge, experience, and caution. It also is important for clinicians to remember that the most important international guidelines for the treatment of depressive disorders are not applicable in patients with cancer.

Psychotropic Drugs
to Target Somatic Symptoms

Knowledge of chemical neurotransmissions underlying psychological symptoms is helpful in treating other cancer-related problems. Notably, many side effects that are induced by oncological medications can benefit from psychotropic drugs. Nausea, reduced appetite, hot flashes, sleep disturbances, cognitive impairment, fatigue, and pain are often treated with antidepressant or antianxiety agents and dosage increases.

The principal mechanism of the analgesic effect is related to the inhibition of norepinephrine or serotonin reuptake or both. Nociceptors, ascending and descending pain pathways, are connected through a complex neurocircuitry. Norepinephrine, serotonin, γ-aminobutyric acid (GABA), and glutamate are fully integrated at central and peripheral levels. Monoamines also regulate neurokinins, which are involved in neurogenic inflammation and pain, and may also have psychological effects (they have been hypothesized to have a role in developmental anxiety, depression, and psychosis). Pain perception consists of sensory, cognitive, and affective components. The latter are the target of antidepressants by modulating the peripheral pain fibers, which are rich in serotonin and norepinephrine fibers. However, the cognitive component of pain also involves many central areas, such as the anterior insula, somatosensory cortex, hypothalamus, periaqueductal gray, and anterior cingulate cortex. Opioids modulate both spinal and higher ascending pain perception pathways.

Across a series of studies, several antidepressants were found to be effective analgesics, the prototypical drug being amitriptyline (Saarto and Wiffen 2007). Other studies reported the effectiveness of SSRIs and serotonin-norepinephrine reuptake inhibitors (SNRIs) in the treatment of pain (Eardley and Toth 2010; Lee and Chen 2010).

The National Institute for Health and Clinical Excellence (U.K.) has indicated the SNRI duloxetine as a first-line treatment for the management of neuropathic pain (Tan et al. 2010). Interestingly, about six times as many antidepressant trials have been reported for cancer-related pain as for cancer-related depression. We believe that this difference represents a cultural bias or stigma.

The differential diagnosis of depression and cancer-related fatigue is not simple. Fatigue is a unique symptom in some cases but a feature of a depressive state in others. Fatigue in many cases represents the direct side effect of chemotherapy or radiotherapy and is not linked to depression. Despite a sound rationale, no evidence currently supports the use of antidepressants for the treatment of cancer-related fatigue (Minton et al. 2010).

Nausea and decreased appetite are often burdensome symptoms that have a strong impact on the distress component of cancer. These symptoms may worsen in patients taking SSRIs, due to interference with $5\text{-}HT_3$ receptor function. The rather weak antiserotonergic activity of SSRI antidepressants may lead to pharmacodynamic competition with ondansetron, an antiemetic widely used in cancer patients, which is a strong $5\text{-}HT_3$ inhibitor. Mirtazapine, an antagonist at the postsynaptic serotonin receptors ($5\text{-}HT_2$ and $5\text{-}HT_3$), is effective as both an adjuvant analgesic and an antiemetic, and it also has sedative and appetite-stimulating properties. Some open studies provide preliminary data regarding its efficacy (Kim et al. 2008; Theobald et al. 2002).

Hot flashes are experienced by two-thirds of women with a history of breast cancer (Carpenter et al. 1998). SSRIs and venlafaxine are effective in the management of hot flash symptoms, but venlafaxine has been studied more extensively than other antidepressants (Bordeleau et al. 2010; Carpenter et al. 2007; Loprinzi et al. 2009) and, more importantly, it is safe to use in combination with tamoxifen. The exact mechanism of action by which these medications alleviate hot flashes is still unknown, although hot flashes have been linked to serotonin-norepinephrine imbalance. These neurotransmitter systems are involved in hypothalamic thermoregulatory processes.

Aromatase inhibitors and tamoxifen are widely used as adjuvant therapy in women with early-stage endocrine-responsive breast cancer. These agents, however, may induce cognitive impairment and insomnia. The latter is usually treated with benzodiazepines by oncologists. Once a depressive state is excluded, several drugs, such as the antidepressant trazodone or the atypical antipsychotic quetiapine, may be used to restore sleep architecture (Davis 2007; Pasquini et al. 2009). Benzodiazepines are sedative, but they tend to disrupt the physiological sleep structure.

Chemotherapy-induced paresthesias are very common. They are due to acute neurosensory toxicity. Paresthesias are usually treated with venlafaxine, pregabalin, and gabapentin, for which efficacy is generally reported. Unfortunately, recovery from paresthesias is generally incomplete, and a long time is needed for neurons to regenerate. Paresthesias, which may be neglected if dealt with superficially, may mask other underlying subthreshold conditions. In fact, in clinical practice we see many apparently nondepressed patients, referred for a second opinion for treatment of paresthesias, who perceive the existence of their underlying disorder indirectly, through the decreased ability to carry on normal daily activities or the loss of pleasure in previously pleasurable activities.

Psychiatric Referral for Psychopharmacological Treatment

Referral of an oncology patient to a psychiatrist and prescription of psycho-pharmacological treatment require that specific communication skills are possessed by oncologists, general practitioners, and psychologists for referring, and by psychiatrists for suggesting a drug treatment. We believe that in most cases drug treatment should be delivered by a trained psychiatrist, if possible. Psychotropic drug treatment requires specific knowledge, skills, and practice. For example, prescribing an SSRI might appear to be an easy task for every medical professional, but it requires specific skills regarding careful psychopathological and risk assessment, because agitation, increased suicide risk and thoughts, insomnia, anger and dyscontrol, increased anxiety, hypomania, and dysphoria are well-known effects of antidepressant treatment in certain patients, and only a well-trained psychiatrist will effectively handle these issues.

Prescribing psychotropic drugs is not only a matter of determining which drug and which dosage or titration should be used. It also involves effective communication and a good patient-doctor relationship, together with a wider view of treatment, based on both pharmacological and non-pharmacological interventions, including psychotherapy, involvement of family members, and support. Information to the patient, consensus, and empowerment are decisive ingredients for psychopharmacological treatment and to ensure motivation and compliance. For patients who never previously suffered from psychological disorders, the oncologist's suggestion to refer to a psychiatrist can induce resistance, criticism, and disbelief. Patients with a previous history of psychopathology (minor or major diagnoses) are more able to recognize the need for a referral.

Referral to a psychiatrist and the recommendation of a psychopharmacological treatment should be better viewed within the framework of a larger psychosocial intervention, which is a matter of communication. Because providing information is important, in our practice we inform patients that clinical research worldwide has demonstrated that about one-half of patients with cancer have some form of severe demoralization or depression, sometimes despair, and that many cancer patients suffer from acute or chronic anxiety, as well as sleep disorders. We add that confronting cancer threat and facing the disease process, diagnostic procedures, and different kinds of interventions are potential severe stressors, requiring all the physical and mental resources of an individual for a long time, potentially months or years. Such chronic stressors also have a biological cost and require the recruitment of every available physical and mental resource. Antidepressants and antianxiety agents may support the organism in facing the psychophysical costs of neoplastic disease, and they may preserve sleep architecture integrity and favor natural resource restoration. They can support psychological and biological adaptation of the body. We wait for questions and give answers, according to our knowledge, balancing the benefits and disadvantages of treatment. The discussion often concerns fears about side effects, interactions with the disease, tolerability, dependence potential, and care alternatives. Erroneous beliefs are investigated and worked through during such discussion. We present the pros and cons of psychotropic drug prescription and ask the patient to decide whether to accept or refuse such prescription. In some cases, patients can delay decisions for some weeks. After information has been provided and consensus has been reached, we present treatment choices and their rationales. After further discussion and clarification, we prescribe and schedule future visits. We contact the referring oncologist or practitioner for any clarification that may be needed. If possible, a family member participates in this process of information sharing and decision making.

Psychopharmacology and Humanization of Care: Integration Into a Global Therapeutic Project for Health

Psychotropic drug treatment can address a great deal of distress and suffering, but several needs of a cancer patient require an integrated approach shared among different sources. Comprehensive treatment should address both the behavioral and the psychosocial aspects of suffering; protect the sleep-wake cycle; restore energy, psychopathology, and other distress-related dimensions; and treat somatic aspects such as pain. However, many challenges cannot be addressed by psychotropic drugs, including sadness for the loss of previous health conditions and life planning, preoccupation with the progress of disease, threat for life, feelings of guilt or shame, anger with fate ("Why me?"), a sense of loneliness and sometimes despair, issues concerning dignity, dealing with side effects of treatments, facing recurrences and difficult phases of illness, difficulties in communication with family and children about illness, and emerging existential and meaning-of-life issues. Although drugs may help provide the energy needed to deal with these challenges, to control anxiety, and to maintain or restore sleep quality, those other challenges require a parallel specific intervention on behalf of a psycho-oncologist. Providing the best available psychotropic drug treatment, therefore, should be carried out not as a stand-alone intervention, but within a care network, allowing the patient to keep in touch with other caring figures (oncologist, surgeon, psychiatrist, psychologist, etc.) according to the phase of illness. To achieve humanization of care, we need patients to perceive themselves at the center of this frame and in their caring professionals' minds, and caring teams need to keep patients "in their mind."

Conclusion

In this chapter, we have stressed the usefulness of the psychopharmacological approach for cancer patients, addressing some psychological and psychopathological issues. We suggest that—along with considering the evidence of efficacy of drug treatments and related available guidelines—we might better design tailor-cut treatments if we integrate a new psychopathological dimensional approach with the categorical diagnostic one, which is strictly based on DSM-IV criteria. Although it is at an initial stage, the dimensional perspective may allow clinicians to tailor-cut psychotropic drug treatment according to different major psychopathological dimensions, such as sadness, anxiety, activation, anger, obsessiveness, reality distortion, and so on, thus differentiating treatments in patients with the same categorical diagnosis. According to our clinical experience, the international guidelines for the pharmacological treatment of psychiatric disorders do not fit the needs of cancer patients having the same disorders or symptoms. In other words, flexibility in this context is essential. The dimensional perspective allows more accurate individualization of psychotropic drug management than categorical diagnosis. Considering discrete dimensions of sadness, anxiety, activation, anger, obsessions, reality distortion, and other elements, the clinician can tailor management for each patient. The SVARAD can help make this assessment in a more efficient and reliable manner. Psycho-oncologists have to consider and balance both the tailored therapy approach and the dimensional approach in their decisional algorithms. Obviously, an ongoing psychosocial intervention is the prerequisite of any psychotropic prescription. Even more important, the psychiatrist's contribution in alleviating psychological distress is strongly associated to his or her ties with the oncologists. Psychiatrists should participate in meetings with the entire oncology staff so as to suggest patient types that could obtain benefit from referral and psychiatric consultation, as well as to promote the oncologists' communication skills in communicating the need for psychiatric referral and, possibly, psychotropic drug treatment. Clear and constant communication between psychiatrists and oncologists will allow any treatment to work better.

Key Clinical Points

- Research evidence from clinical trials of psychotropic agents in oncology is limited.

- Dimensional psychopharmacology involves prescribing based on psychopathological issues rather than diagnostic category. As a result, not all patients with a diagnosis of, say, major depression, will receive the same drug or a similar antidepressant treatment. They will receive instead a drug treatment tailored according to their main psychopathology and their specific depressive syndrome profile.

- Side effects of antidepressants (e.g., sedation) and antipsychotics can be exploited to benefit the patient.

- Psychotropic drugs are often used for other symptoms, such as pain, paresthesias, hot flashes, and nausea, without a primary psychiatric indication.

- Psychotropic drug treatment should be used as part of a larger psychosocial intervention, including counseling, psychotherapy, or other resources, according to needs of different patients and available programs.

- Bidirectional communication between the consultation-liaison psychiatrist and oncologists is strongly recommended. The process of referral requires specific communication skills.

- Providing information to the patient about the pros and cons of psychotropic drug treatment, about psychotropic drug choice and expected effects, about drug safety and side-effect risks, about obtaining consent, and about "empowerment" is crucial for motivation, future participation in care, and maximization of the treatment risk-benefit ratio.

References

American Psychiatric Association: Diagnostic and Statistical Manual of Mental Disorders, 4th Edition. Washington, DC, American Psychiatric Association, 1994

Ashbury JE, Lévesque LE, Beck PA, et al: A population-based case-control study of Selective Serotonin Reuptake Inhibitors (SSRIs) and breast cancer: the impact of duration of use, cumulative dose and latency. BMC Med 8:90, 2010

Biondi M: Beyond the brain-mind dichotomy and toward a common organizing principle of pharmacological and psychological treatments. Psychother Psychosom 64:1–8, 1995

Biondi M, Picardi A: Clinical and biological aspects of bereavement and loss-induced depression: a reappraisal. Psychother Psychosom 65:229–245, 1996

Biondi M, Costantini A, Grassi L: La Mente e il Cancro. Rome, Italy, Il Pensiero Scientifico, 1995

Biondi M, Picardi A, Pasquini M, et al: Dimensional psychopathology of depression: detection of an "activation" dimension in unipolar depressed outpatients. J Affect Disord 84:33–39, 2005

Blashfield RK, Livesley WJ: Classification, in Oxford Textbook of Psychopathology. Edited by Millon T, Blaney PH, Davis RD. New York, Oxford University Press, 1999, pp 3–28

Boettger S, Friedlander M, Breitbart W, et al: Aripiprazole and haloperidol in the treatment of delirium. Aust NZ J Psychiatry 45:477–482, 2011

Bordeleau L, Pritchard KI, Loprinzi CL, et al: Multicenter, randomized, cross-over clinical trial of venlafaxine versus gabapentin for the management of hot flashes in breast cancer survivors. J Clin Oncol 28:5147–5152, 2010

Breitbart W, Marotta R, Platt MM, et al: A double-blind trial of haloperidol, chlorpromazine, and lorazepam in the treatment of delirium in hospitalized AIDS patients. Am J Psychiatry 153:231–237, 1996

Caraceni A, Grassi L: Delirium: Acute Confusional States in Palliative Medicine. New York, Oxford University Press, 2003

Carpenter JS, Andrykowski MA, Cordova M, et al: Hot flashes in post-menopausal women treated for breast carcinoma: prevalence, severity, correlates, management and relation to quality of life. Cancer 82:1682–1691, 1998

Carpenter JS, Storniolo AM, Johns S, et al: Randomized, double-blind, placebo-controlled crossover trials of venlafaxine for hot flashes after breast cancer. Oncologist 12:124–135, 2007

Chong Guan NG, Boks MPM, Zainal NZ, et al: The prevalence and pharmacotherapy of depression in cancer patients. J Affect Disord 131:1–7, 2011

Costa D, Mogos I, Toma T: Efficacy and safety of mianserin in the treatment of depression of women with cancer. Acta Psychiatr Scand 320:85–92, 1985

Davis MP: Does trazodone have a role in palliating symptoms? Support Care Cancer 15:221–224, 2007

Derogatis LR: The SCL-90-R: Administration, Scoring, and Procedures Manual, 3rd Edition. Minneapolis, MN, National Computer Systems, 1994

Eardley W, Toth C: An open-label, non-randomized comparison of venlafaxine and gabapentin as monotherapy or adjuvant therapy in the management of neuropathic pain in patients with peripheral neuropathy. J Pain Res 3:33–49, 2010

Elsayem A, Bush SH, Munsell MF: Subcutaneous olanzapine for hyperactive or mixed delirium in patients with advanced cancer: a preliminary study. J Pain Symptom Manage 40:774–782, 2010

Engel G: The need for a new medical model: a challenge for biomedicine. Science 196:129–136, 1977

Eyding D, Lelgemann M, Grouven U, et al: Reboxetine for acute treatment of major depression: systematic review and meta-analysis of published and unpublished placebo and selective serotonin reuptake inhibitor controlled trials. BMJ 341:C4737, 2010

Fava M, Rosenbaum JF, Pava JA, et al: Anger attacks in unipolar depression, Part 1: clinical correlates and response to fluoxetine treatment. Am J Psychiatry 150:1158–1163, 1993

Fisch M: Treatment of depression in cancer. J Natl Cancer Inst Monogr 32:105–111, 2004

Fisch MJ, Loehrer PJ, Kristeller J, et al: Fluoxetine versus placebo in advanced cancer outpatients: a double-blinded trial of the Hoosier Oncology Group. J Clin Oncol 21:1937–1943, 2003

Giese-Davis J, Collie K, Rancourt KM, et al: Decrease in depression symptoms is associated with longer survival in patients with metastatic breast cancer: a secondary analysis. J Clin Oncol 29:413–420, 2011

Grassi, L, Biondi M, Costantini A: Manuale Pratico di Psicooncologia. Rome, Italy, Il Pensiero Scientifico, 2003

Grassi L, Biancosino B, Marmai L, et al: Effect of reboxetine on major depressive disorder in breast cancer patients: an open-label study. J Clin Psychiatry 65:515–520, 2004

Greenberg DB: Barriers to the treatment of depression in cancer patients. J Natl Cancer Inst Monogr 32:127–135, 2004

Guimarães HC, Levy R, Teixeira AL, et al: Neurobiology of apathy in Alzheimer's disease. Arq Neuropsiqiatr 66:436–443, 2008

Holland JC, Romano SJ, Heiligenstein JH, et al: A controlled trial of fluoxetine and desipramine in depressed women with advanced cancer. Psychooncology 7:291–300, 1998

Howard LM, Barley EA, Davies E, et al: Cancer diagnosis in people with severe mental illness: practical and ethical issues. Lancet Oncol 11:797–804, 2010

Jaspers K: Psicopatologia Generale (1913). Rome, Italy, Il Pensiero Scientifico Editore, 1964

Kelly CM, Juurlink DN, Gomes T, et al: Selective serotonin reuptake inhibitors and breast cancer mortality in women receiving tamoxifen: a population based cohort study. BMJ 340:1–8, 2010

Kim HF, Fisch MJ: Antidepressant use in ambulatory cancer patients. Curr Oncol Rep 8:275–281, 2006

Kim SW, Shin IS, Kim JM, et al: Effectiveness of mirtazapine for nausea and insomnia in cancer patients with depression. Psychiatry Clin Neurosci 62:75–83, 2008

Lee YC, Chen PP: A review of SSRIs and SNRIs in neuropathic pain. Expert Opin Pharmacother 11:2813–2825, 2010

Lesch KP, Merschdorf U: Impulsivity, aggression and serotonin: a molecular psychobiological perspective. Behav Sci Law 18:581–604, 2000

Liu F, Mahgoub NA, Kotbi N: Continue or stop clozapine when patient needs chemotherapy? J Neuropsychiatry Clin Neurosci 22:451–455, 2010

Lonergan E, Britton AM, Luxenberg J: Antipsychotics for delirium. Cochrane Database of Systematic Reviews 2007, Issue 2. Art. No.: CD005594. DOI: 10.1002/14651858.CD005594.pub2.

Loprinzi CL, Barton DL, Sloan JA, et al: Newer antidepressants for hot flashes—should their efficacy still be up for debate? Menopause 16:184–187, 2009

Lydiatt WM, Denman D, McNeilly DP, et al: A randomized, placebo-controlled trial of citalopram for the prevention of major depression during treatment for head and neck cancer. Arch Otolaryngol Head Neck Surg 134:528–535, 2008

Minton O, Richardson A, Sharpe M, et al: Drug therapy for the management of cancer-related fatigue. Cochrane Database of Systematic Reviews 2010, Issue 7. Art. No.: CD006704. DOI: 10.1002/14651858.CD006704.pub3.

Morrow GR, Hickok JT, Roscoe JA, et al: Differential effects of paroxetine on fatigue and depression: a randomized, double-blind trial from the University of Rochester Cancer Center Community Clinical Oncology Program. J Clin Oncol 21:4635–4641, 2003

Musselman DL, Miller AH, Porter MR, et al: Higher than normal plasma interleukin-6 concentrations in cancer patients with depression: preliminary findings. Am J Psychiatry 158:1252–1257, 2001

Musselman DL, Somerset WI, Guo Y, et al: A double-blind, multicenter, parallel-group study of paroxetine, desipramine, or placebo in breast cancer patients (stages I, II, III, and IV) with major depression. J Clin Psychiatry 67:288–296, 2006

Nelson RJ, Chiavegatto S: Molecular basis of aggression. Trends Neurosci 24:713–720, 2001

O'Keeffe N, Ranjith G: Depression, demoralisation or adjustment disorder? Understanding emotional distress in the severely medically ill. Clin Med 7:478–481, 2007

Overall JE, Gorham DR: The brief psychiatric rating scale. Psychol Rep 10:799–812, 1962

Pancheri P: Approccio dimensionale e approccio categoriale alla diagnosi psichiatrica. Giornale Italiano di Psicopatologia 1:8–23, 1995

Pancheri P, Picardi A, Gaetano P, et al: Validazione della scala per la valutazione rapida dimensionale "SVARAD." Rivista di Psichiatria 34:84–93, 1999

Pasquini M, Picardi A, Biondi M, et al: Relevance of anger and irritability in outpatients with major depressive disorder. Psychopathology 37:155–160, 2004

Pasquini M, Biondi M, Costantini A, et al: Detection and treatment of depressive and anxiety disorders among cancer patients: feasibility and preliminary findings from a liaison service in an oncology division. Depress Anxiety 23:441–448, 2006

Pasquini M, Picardi A, Speca A, et al: Combining an SSRI with an anticonvulsant in depressed patients with dysphoric mood: an open study. Clin Pract Epidemiol Ment Health 3:3, 2007

Pasquini M, Speca A, Biondi M: Quetiapine for tamoxifen-induced insomnia in women with breast cancer. Psychosomatics 50:159–161, 2009

Pezzella G, Moslinger-Gehmayr R, Contu A, et al: Treatment of depression in patients with breast cancer: a comparison between paroxetine and amitriptyline. Breast Cancer Res Treat 70:1–10, 2001

Razavi D, Allilaire JF, Smith M, et al: The effect of fluoxetine on anxiety and depression symptoms in cancer patients. Acta Psychiatr Scand 94:205–210, 1996

Razavi D, Kormoss N, Collard A, et al: Comparative study of the efficacy and safety of trazodone versus clorazepate in the treatment of adjustment disorders in cancer patients: a pilot study. J Int Med Res 27:264–272, 1999

Reiche EM, Nunes SO, Morimoto HK: Stress, depression, the immune system, and cancer. Lancet Oncol 5:617–625, 2004

Richards S, Umbreit JN, Fanucchi MP: Selective serotonin reuptake inhibitor-induced rhabdomyolysis associated with irinotecan. South Med J 96:1031–1033, 2003

Rodin G, Lloyd N, Katz M, et al: The treatment of depression in cancer patients: a systematic review. Support Care Cancer 15:123–136, 2007

Roscoe JA, Morrow GR, Hickok JT, et al: Effect of paroxetine hydrochloride (Paxil) on fatigue and depression in breast cancer patients receiving chemotherapy. Breast Cancer Res Treat 89:243–249, 2005

Saarto T, Wiffen PJ: Antidepressants for neuropathic pain. Cochrane Database of Systematic Reviews 2007, Issue 4. Art. No.: CD005454. DOI: 10.1002/14651858.CD005454.pub2.

Tahir TA, Eeles E, Karapareddy V: A randomized controlled trial of quetiapine versus placebo in the treatment of delirium. J Psychosom Res 69:485–490, 2010

Tan T, Barry P, Reken S, Baker M: Pharmacological management of neuropathic pain in non-specialist settings: summary of NICE guidance. BMJ 340:C1079, 2010

Theobald DE, Kirsh KL, Holtsclaw E, et al: An open-label, crossover trial of mirtazapine (15 and 30 mg) in cancer patients with pain and other distressing symptoms. J Pain Symptom Manage 23:442–447, 2002

Thompson DS: Mirtazapine for the treatment of depression and nausea in breast and gynecological oncology. Psychosomatics 41:356–359, 2000

Torta R, Berra C, Binaschi L, et al: Amisulpride in the short-term treatment of depressive and physical symptoms in cancer patients during chemotherapies. Support Care Cancer 15:539–546, 2007

Trzepacz PT: Is there a final common neural pathway in delirium? Focus on acetylcholine and dopamine. Semin Clin Neuropsychiatry 5:132–148, 2000

Weinberger MI, Bruce ML, Roth AJ, et al: Depression and barriers to mental health care in older cancer patients. Int J Geriatr Psychiatry 26:21–26, 2011

CHAPTER 8

Advancing Medical Education in Existential Dimensions of Advanced Cancer and Palliative Care

Shannon R. Poppito, Ph.D.
Glendon R. Tait, M.D., M.Sc., F.R.C.P.C.

IT HAS BECOME increasingly clear that "healing" dying patients is complex and extends much beyond treating symptoms to include psychosocial, existential, and spiritual aspects. Although anxiety (Kerrihard et al. 1999) and depression (Breitbart et al. 1995) are common in dying patients, pervasive but historically less well-defined concerns revolve around the experience of suffering—specifically, psychosocial, existential, and spiritual distress. In recent years, studies have elucidated, from the patients' perspectives, what concerns factor most prominently in one's sense of well-being. Although palliative care historically was very focused on pain and symptom management, much evidence now supports that patients' concerns extend well beyond these domains to such existential concerns as avoiding prolongation of dying, relieving perceived sense of burden on others, sense of control, and strengthening relationships (Chochinov 2006).

One line of evidence that informed this perspective surrounds the frequently encountered request for hastened death. Interestingly, when empirically examined, the will to live in dying patients was least correlated with pain and most correlated with psychiatric and existential variables such as hopelessness, burden to others, and dignity (Chochinov et al. 2005b).

To provide care that is aligned with the evidence about the patient experience, health professionals must be trained in how to address domains beyond pain and physical symptom management. However, limited medical education research and development has been done in the areas of knowledge, skills, and attitudes that are core to providing end-of-life care, specifically those that arise in the existential domain. In the culture of medicine—in which "doing" and "curing" are often valued most and the "soft" aspects of medicine are seen as time-consuming—engendering attention to existential care requires intentional and well-planned efforts. This means that the field must be expanded to a point where care of the existential experience of patients is considered a standard of care, not a luxury to which only some patients have access.

In this chapter, we endeavor to provide the foundations required to move forward the clinical care of patients with advanced illness and those at the end of life. We believe the evidence suggests that such change would result in more whole-person care of the human with illness—a level of care that is all too often lost when a patient becomes identified not by his or her name but as patient number 10 with "end-stage lymphoma." In the first part of this chapter, we provide a review of the educational landscape in palliative and end-of-life care, the principles of which should be readily applicable to patients from the time of diagnosis of a life-limiting disease through to the end of life. We outline research that has examined the state of medical education in this area at the individual medical professional trainee level—including areas of deficit in perceived competency—and at the institutional and administrative level. Finally, we intentionally give special attention to examining the influences that prevent educational and clinical practice from really evolving. It is the space between the articulated objectives and curricula of educational programs and the development of attitudes in health professionals that ultimately determines how they will really *be* in practice. Although this area has been receiving increased attention, the evidence will show that this greater awareness has not translated into health professionals' feeling competent in many of the areas deemed critical by patients.

In the second part of the chapter, armed with a view of the educational landscape, we will aim to provide a tour of the core existential issues in palliative and end-of-life care. The descriptions will no doubt feel familiar to everyone who has been touched by the often moving stories of patients. However, we recognize that the nomenclature is sometimes intimidating and feel it is critical for us as professionals to all agree on saying what we mean and meaning what we say. We examine definitions and situate them in the origins and evolution of the existential transition, paying attention to both existential philosophy and its foundations within existential psychotherapy. By providing a scaffolding of key transition points for patients, from diagnosis to dying, we hope to help readers identify opportunities to be authentically present for the rich existential experiences of patients, and to recognize the various tasks that come with this presence at different transition points. Finally, having explained how to be better at identifying such issues, we outline how best to address them. We intend this discussion to provide a framework not only for clinically approaching the existential care of patients but also for scaffolding educational programs.

Overall, we hope that assumptions will be challenged and perspectives broadened in a way required to continually advance the care of patients. In particular, we hope that some readers will become more personally competent in identifying and addressing existential issues in palliative care. We hope too that some will situate this awareness within the educational principles outlined and use the synergy of the two topics to champion change in their learning, teaching, and institutions.

The Educational Landscape

The importance of palliative and end-of-life care education has been articulated by many medical boards. In fact, this type of care is increasingly being identified as a core competency to be assessed as part of physicians' demonstrating readiness to practice. However, rigorous educational research in the area of palliative and end-of-life care is in its relative infancy. Although a chapter such as this cannot be exhaustive, we do provide a critical examination of the literature that is core to the goals of this chapter.

Sullivan et al. (2003) completed the first large study to assess the status of medical education in end-of-life care and to identify opportunities for improvement. Incorporating data generated from students, residents, and faculty, the authors found attitudes to be very favorable, but there were notable trainee-reported deficits in such areas as addressing patients' thoughts and fears, addressing spiritual and cultural issues, managing one's own feelings about a patient's death, and helping families with bereavement. Sullivan et al. (2004) studied the perspective of medical education deans in the United States and found that although the majority found the topic "very important," most opposed required courses or clerkship rotations. Participating deans cited several barriers to incorporating more end-of-life care, including lack of time and lack of faculty expertise. These barriers were also identified in a study of educational administrators in Canada (Oneschuk et al. 2004).

Another important vantage point in assessing the state of education is that of trainees' perceived competence. Billings et al. (2009) examined how attitudes and perceived preparedness impact perceived competence in end-of-life care. The findings indicated high perceived competence in expressing empathy and discussing code status, but feelings of incompetence in break-ing bad news and discussing religious and spiritual issues. Interestingly, the authors did find that experience was a predictor of perceived competence, demonstrated by the fact that senior residents, who reported more fre-quently delivering bad news, felt more competent than juniors. From their findings, they argued that clinical experience with end-of-life care was the most important factor in feelings of competence, not personal characteris-tics or attitudes toward end-of-life care.

Another study examined preparedness and attitudes in a large sample of psychiatry residents, which—despite psychiatrists often being involved in the psychological, existential, and spiritual care of patients with cancer, and those at the end of life—is the only study to date to examine the prepared-ness of residents in this specialty (Tait and Hodges 2009). We examined 82 psychiatry trainees' attitudes toward end-of-life care and their perceived preparedness in various domains core to end-of-life care. They also exam-ined residents' experiences with dying and suggestions for changes needed in education. Attitudes toward end-of-life care were very favorable; 91% of residents agreed it was important for all residents to receive training. Com-petencies that reached statistical significance for preparedness included managing pain, recognizing opioid tolerance, discussing end-of-life deci-sions, talking about fears, and telling a patient he or she is dying. Competen-cies that were statistically significant on the unprepared end of the spectrum included addressing cultural and spiritual aspects, helping with reconcilia-tion and saying good-bye, and responding to requests for physician-assisted suicide. Among the participants, all of whom were psychiatry residents, only 12% felt they learned a lot from psychiatrists about end-of-life care, whereas 61% felt they learned a lot from palliative care specialists. Desired changes in education included more longitudinal exposure and integration into core psychiatry rotations such as consultation-liaison psychiatry and geriatrics. The following were the most frequently cited areas in which psychiatry trainees wanted more training: existential concerns, depression, anxiety, and family care. It is concerning that many of the areas in which psychiatry residents, at all levels, felt unprepared, including existential, spiritual, and cultural aspects, would seem to be ones that should reside fairly close to the competency set of a psychiatrist, if not all physicians. It is reassuring that physicians and health care providers do not seem to simply lack an aware-ness of the patient's perspective. Indeed, Tait and Hodges found that resi-dents did conceptualize dignified care in a way similar to patients; however, the residents did not feel competent in many of the areas they, and patients, saw as important. These findings were echoed by Browall et al. (2010), who reported that, indeed, health care staff were able to identify the existential issues that were important to patients.

Why, then, do educational experiences, positive attitudes, and an aware-ness of the patient's experience not necessarily translate into feeling compe-tent in providing the care that patients need? Exploring the educational experience of physicians and trainees at all levels requires careful attention not only to the formal, intended curriculum, but even more importantly to the so-called hidden curriculum. The *hidden curriculum,* a term coined by Hafferty (1998), refers to the commonly held "understandings, customs, rit-uals, and taken for granted aspects of what goes on in the life-space we call medical education" (p. 404). This concept acknowledges medical schools as "cultural entities and moral communities" that participate in constructing notions of "good" and "bad" medicine. Whatever is learned in the formal or intended curriculum can either be reinforced or dismissed by the learning that takes place "on the job" from supervisors who model attitudes and prac-tices that may be adopted in an attempt to conform to the "norm." In pallia-tive and end-of-life care, this hidden curriculum is a particularly muddied water because although teachers may identify certain areas as important, they may not model these well, sometimes due to their own discomfort with caring for dying patients and the reactions evoked. Attitudinal learning occurs to a large extent in the hidden curriculum. Ensuring that health pro-fessionals acquire the "right" attitudes is the most difficult aspect of medical education, relative to knowledge or skills.

A study by Tait and Hodges (2012) illustrates the powerful learning that occurs in the hidden curriculum. As part of a study examining an educa-tional intervention with first-year psychiatry and family medicine residents, a qualitative interview design was used to examine residents' experience with palliative care education. Again, findings confirmed that the residents did not feel the training was adequate. However, most striking were the powerful messages they heard within the hidden curriculum, and the inher-ent contrast between the cultures of general medicine training rotations and palliative care. They described palliative care as "whole-person" care, which integrates psychosocial and spiritual care and aims to know a patient's story—and even makes time to do so. According to one resident,

> The only part of medicine that is not about saving people is palliative care. That's the only time it's OK to have sort of failed people in a way. I can un-derstand how oncologists can feel like they have failed when a patient is dy-ing or couldn't cure them. In palliative care it's more like, let's concentrate now on the end of your life.

However, the messages the residents heard from rotations in general medicine were the principles of "diagnose and discharge"—that there "isn't time to talk." One resident said,

It's not like your attending is going to ask you to talk about the most meaningful time in your patient's life. They want you to know diagnoses 22
through 47 on the differential diagnosis.

Several residents said they had also learned in their medical education
that getting close enough to a patient to know his or her story might threaten
professional boundaries or that one should isolate one's emotion because
emotional reactions to a patient may somehow be harmful. This was well illustrated in one resident physician's comment:

When I was in my medicine rotation in fourth year, I had four patients die
one after another all in two days. It was a disaster. We were on call and my
senior said "if you want, you can go sleep for two hours because you have had
a lot to deal with lately." I would have sacrificed sleep to talk to the team
about what I was worried about with those four patients, about whether we
could have done something differently.

These findings were echoed in a study by Borgstrom et al. (2010), who
examined medical students' experience and interpretation of values in relation to confronting dying patients. The study showed that students felt they
were receiving mixed messages even in the formal curriculum. As an example, they felt they were being taught that it is important to be sensitive and
perhaps even emotional in front of patients, but simultaneously that one
should never break down in front of patients. This study also found that the
hidden curriculum was a source of even more conflict, because students saw
supervisors model the importance of "self-preservation." Another study of
medical students' first experiences of death similarly found this tension
between "emotional concern" and "professional detachment" (Kelly and
Nisker 2010). All the while, residents caring for dying patients experience
feelings of guilt and failure after a patient's death, yet without supervision as
an outlet to process such feelings (Schroder et al. 2009).

Clearly, although many health professionals receive educational experiences in palliative and end-of-life care, powerful cultural messages are being
taught through the hidden curriculum that set up key parts of palliative care—
including psychosocial, spiritual, and existential care, all areas that require a
level of intimate emotional engagement—as being in conflict with the role of
health care provider. Explanations for this situation reside at several levels,
including the health care provider, patient and family, and broader sociocultural views on dying. For patients, one common source of existential distress,
although not always expressed as such by them or identified as such by their
caregivers, is the clear discussion of prognosis, or lack thereof. Although
patients may be aware of their worsening condition, physicians caring for

patients with life-threatening illnesses report that they are reluctant to discuss prognosis out of concern for destroying hope (Curtis et al. 2008). In cancer care, physicians, patients, and families have been described as having a "profound ambivalence and vacillation" in the context of simultaneously "hoping for the best and preparing for the worst" (Back et al. 2003). This can sometimes result in the offering of interventions that are likely to be of limited benefit. Indeed, the term *collusion* has been used to refer to the association between physicians' "activism" and patients' adherence to the "recovery plot" (The et al. 2000). For health care providers, providing care that addresses the existential distress of patients, and helps patients to make meaning of advancing illness or nearing death, may represent defeat in a culture that rewards "cure" and "rescue." Additionally, those individuals who are authentically present with a patient at the end of life may become aware of their own mortality and may even experience "death anxiety" themselves.

Defending against this death anxiety is, we feel, a cardinal reason for both patients and physicians to propagate belief in this role of "rescuer." More broadly, the "ultimate rescuer" is one of the two main defenses against death anxiety described by Yalom (1980), the other one being "specialness." The ultimate rescuer, with roots in childhood, is essentially some higher force or person, or godlike figure that will protect one from adversity, and death. Specialness, the other defense against death anxiety, is the irrational idea that somehow the rules of natural law, such as life and death, apply to other people but not to the person appealing the defense. Ultimately, seeking more power and control equates to more specialness, and therefore more defense against mortality. In the physician-patient relationship, Yalom suggests, it is important to patients' belief that they can survive and that they have a rescuer, the physician. At the same time, the godlike role of rescuer is comfortable for a physician who needs to believe in his or her own specialness and, thus, exemption from being mortal. Add to these individual influences the heavily ingrained rescue culture of medicine as a whole, and one has the perfect recipe for avoiding the existential care of patients.

Without a forum to examine one's own emotional reactions to caring for patients with cancer, and particularly those nearing the end of life, care providers will be at risk of keeping their own death anxiety at bay by not engaging with the existential experience of patients, potentially worsening the distress of patients. Alternatively, authentically sitting with patients' experience, and awareness of one's own mortality, can make possible not only a better experience for patients, but a richer experience for health professionals. Regardless of health professionals' fears of engaging with the intimacy of dying, many patients describe the period from terminal diagnosis as the most alive they have felt. A terminal diagnosis, or the threat of death, acts as a "boundary situation" (Jaspers 1932) that propels the individual into a different mode of being, a more authentic mode, and thus can trigger personal change. Indeed, the death of others can stimulate awareness of one's own mortality. We would advocate that the shift from an automatic to an authentic, intentional mode of being is exactly the shift that should be sought in physicians and other health professionals—that is to authentically, and really, take the time to sit, and be, with the experience of a patient with advanced illness, and tolerate the proximity of the many emotions that can go with this. Fostering this ability means giving trainees and practicing health professionals the opportunity to wake up, and be awake for, the experience of patients, despite the many notions in place that seek to keep health professionals in an automatic mode, such as "time constraints," "professional distance," or the idea that such presence is someone else's job.

Health professionals do demonstrate a capacity for reflection on experiences with dying patients, including reflecting on how their practice was informed by such experiences (Tait and Hodges 2012). However, in an area often laden with much emotion, trainees caring for dying patients must be provided more formal opportunities to debrief about the experience and learn strategies for managing their own reactions. This could begin with encouraging dialogue about the experience of caring for dying patients, an experience which, as Susan Block (2001) eloquently said, "challenges the physician to be present in the face of suffering, to find ways of using one's self therapeutically when medicine's technical and curative limits have been exhausted…." (p. 2904).

Fostering reflective capacity is crucial to a health professional's ability to engage on the intimate level required to identify and make meaning of a patient's existential distress. This means building a robust understanding of one's own processing of one's mortality. However, we would argue that one of the core ways to foster the necessary reflective capacity and emotional competence is to facilitate narrative competence. Briefly, narrative competence is a "set of skills required to recognize, absorb, interpret, and be moved by the stories one hears or reads" (p. 862), to better understand the experiences of patients, and of caring for patients. This involves attention to the stories, representing what was witnessed, and building affiliation with patients through doing so (Charon 2004). Ultimately, this means building the capacity to reflect not only on patients' stories, but on one's part in the story through one's encounters with patients. For self-reflection, and ultimately narrative competence, to be given tread in medical education, it needs to be formally taught and assessed.

Indeed, medical schools are increasingly developing narrative and humanities programs, using literature to expose students to stories and hone the experience of witnessing and interpreting stories. Such reflective practice builds the metacognitive skills necessary to be able to engage at deep levels with patients, beyond the technical aspects of their care. While the act of writing about one's experience with patients can help one to make meaning of it, it is equally important that guided feedback be built in (Mann et al. 2009; Wald et al. 2009). There are helpful guidelines for helping one to provide feedback on another's reflections, as illustrated in one description of a guided narrative intervention with medical students processing the loss of elderly patients (Wald et al. 2010). Although it is beyond the scope of this chapter to fully explore the use and value of narrative in medical education, narrative competence is fast becoming considered a core competency. More to the point, it is increasingly being viewed as an essential vehicle to teach and assess professionalism, lifelong learning, and other nonmedical expert competencies of physicians. This is further supported by a markedly increasing emphasis on self-assessment and reflection as part of demonstrating ongoing competence as a physician.

For the setting of this education, based on the evidence, we suggest providing longitudinal exposure in various clinical contexts. Opportunities should extend beyond "psychiatry" training settings or rotations to other settings where the existential issues of advanced illness arise, such as general medicine settings. If the learning is not integrated within general medicine settings, existential care will be seen as something "different" to be done by "someone else." Training settings also need to afford opportunities for trainees to learn with colleagues from other disciplines, including spiritual care, nursing, and psychology, and other physicians, working together to address the psychological and existential experiences of dying patients.

Whatever methods are chosen (didactic lecture or small group) and at whatever level (faculty development or trainee level), improving end-of-life education will require careful attention to the hidden curriculum of medicine, and any educational efforts should explicitly address this. This can be accomplished by building in opportunities for reflecting, in writing or verbally, or ideally both, on experiences with patients with advanced illness and those at the end of life. Such opportunities need to expressly solicit from health professionals their own reactions, and attempt to make meaning of those. This is critical to being able to authentically witness the stories of one's patients, and to erode one's own barriers that are erected to keep the "emotional" nature of the work at bay. Further, it is essential that trainees have the opportunity to debrief on difficult conversations with patients and on the emotions triggered by such; this requires role models to create an environment that invites, values, and provides time for debriefing.

Existential Issues in Advanced Cancer and Palliative Care

Nowhere across the life cycle are existential issues more prevalent than in end-of-life care. Palliative practitioners often witness patients in existential distress at the end of life, but most have little or no training to effectively identify and treat this form of suffering in their work with dying patients. The American Medical Association's *Code of Medical Ethics* (Levine 2012) defines existential suffering "as the experience of agony and distress that results from living in an unbearable state of existence" (p. 3). The medical and palliative care literature offers various, yet often vague, descriptions of existential pain and suffering at the end of life, but it has yet to come to a shared consensus on this powerful concept. There are myriad, ostensibly interchangeable, terms that connote existential-spiritual suffering in palliative care literature: "psycho-existential suffering" (Murata et al. 2006), "existential distress" (Schuman-Olivier et al. 2008), "existential pain" (Strang et al. 2004), and "spiritual pain" (Mako et al. 2006). To date, there is no widely held operational definition for this particular *kind* of suffering that triggers deep sadness, anxiety, and fear at the end of life. When symptoms are medically managed and physiological pain is effectively controlled, how do health care professionals then contend with this seemingly ominous entity called *existential suffering* with no commonly shared language or direction?

When clinicians choose to work in the fields of hospice and palliative care, they are consciously choosing to work among the dying. Death punctuates the ultimate questions of life, for both the patient and the practitioner. Existential questions may emerge, either tacitly or blatantly, for both regarding one's sense of being (i.e., identity) in the face of nonbeing (i.e., death): Who am I? Why am I here? What is the meaning of my life? What is the reason for my being alive? Why must I suffer and die? Am I ultimately alone? Who will I be ... and become? What mark will I leave? Knowingly or unknowingly, both patient and practitioner are confronted with life's ultimate concerns related to the following omnipresent existential domains:

- *Death:* nonexistence, mortality and finiteness, life limitations
- *Choice:* awareness of personal agency and the tyranny of freedom
- *Responsibility:* the ability to authentically respond to life, self, and others
- *Meaning and legacy:* values and contributions to the greater whole

Existential Transitions in Palliative Care

Initial Palliative Phase

The moment a patient is told that his or her disease is "incurable," immediate shock, fear of the unknown, and dread of what is to follow may pervade his or her mind and spirit. This powerful news may set into motion sobering existential concerns a person never before pondered: the meaning of suffering, death, personal agency, control, and responsibility. The very words *incurable* and *palliative* can easily stir an existential/identity crisis, in the form of foreboding questions that may cause overwhelming panic:

- Who will I become? [an invalid? a burden? a scary shadow of myself?]
- Why must I suffer and die [at such a young age]? Why me and not others?
- I have been healthy all my life—why and how is this happening to me?
- Is this my fault? Is God punishing me for past indiscretions?

After the initial existential shock of a terminal prognosis dissipates, the normal routine of doctor appointments, family visits, chemotherapy, radiation, bone scans, MRIs, and so forth, very often, paradoxically, serves to distract patients from the existential urgency of their illness. This is an optimal period during which to connect palliative patients to psychosocial services, such as a social worker or clinical psychologist, depending on the level of psychological distress. Preemptive psychosocial care is often quite helpful for patient and family as a preparatory measure to bolster emotional and practical resources in preparation for the final phases toward hospice care. Preparatory expectation management often becomes an effective first-line defense to end-of-life existential distress. This may consist of routine monthly touch-base visits with a social worker related to practical concerns, or may require weekly or biweekly appointments with a clinical psychologist to work through more pressing psychosocial as well as existential-spiritual concerns. The importance of this preparatory psychosocial period cannot be overstated because it sets the tone for navigating and orienting the patient and family through the palliative care process toward the end of life. This establishes early trust in the multidisciplinary care team, thereby helping to mitigate or diminish potential existential distress at the end of life.

Final Hospice Phase

When the message arrives, be it directly or indirectly, that the end is near and hospice is recommended, yet another, final, existential crisis is brought to bear. At no other moment in one's life is Heidegger's (1927/1962) existential notion of *being-towards-death* more profoundly felt and embodied than when one hears the word *hospice*. Existential suffering, in the form of existential angst, isolation, and despair, may emerge as a person realizes there is nothing more to be done. There is no way out. The individual realizes, "No one can live my life or die my death—the bell ultimately tolls for me."

The definitive existential crisis in the face of being-towards-death often gives rise to urgent existential questions that may elicit heightened existential suffering:

- How will I die? [in pain? at peace? at home or in hospice?]
- What is my unfinished business—what have I left undone?
- Have I made peace with my life, myself, and my loved ones?
- What impact or mark will I leave? How will I be remembered?
- Will I be surrounded by loved ones—or will I slip away unnoticed?

While confronting imminent death, patients are also faced with ultimate choices and responsibility regarding how, where, and with whom they will choose to die. Not only do they have a responsibility to their loved ones, but at a deeply embodied level, they realize they have a responsibility to themselves. The days or weeks prior to death are pregnant with rich generative and therapeutic meaning and potential. This period could be a purposeful time to engage in meaningful preparatory grief and bereavement work both with patient and loved ones.

By engaging in preparatory grief work with a patient, the clinician may help the patient mourn lost possibilities and unmet dreams, while preparing for the end of life. Perhaps the patient is a young adult who always dreamed of traveling the world, then someday settling down, falling in love, getting married, eventually buying a home and having a family. Very sadly, this patient will not live to see the day these dreams or possibilities come to fruition. Existential suffering not only arises in the face of unmet possibilities and unfulfilled dreams, but also through not being able to express the deep sadness, resentment, and frustration inherent within them. There is great opportunity for spiritual and existential growth at the end of life, by asking simple questions to engage the patient in this grief.

Existential suffering may also be mediated and dissipated through offering family preparatory grief and bereavement counseling prior to a patient's death. Very often, patients' existential distress heightens in the face of feeling like a burden to loved ones or from witnessing heartbroken family members become burned out in caring for them. Preparatory grief work helps the patient know that family members are being taken care of, and therefore are being left in good hands. This is also a purposeful time to engage the patient and family members in sharing their mutual gratitude, forgiveness, and meaningful memories. The existential distress of end-of-life isolation, angst, and despair can be assuaged by existential care and equanimity, thereby creating a peaceful sense of wholeness in the face of imminent death.

Existential Suffering: An Umbrella Concept

Ultimately, existential suffering emerges as a deep and profound feeling of absence, disconnection, or disorientation in the face of life-limits, finitude, and specifically one's mortality. Such suffering presents multidimensionally in the dying patient. Physically, pain arises from progressive disease. Acute physical pain, shortness of breath, and nausea all send existential messages to the embodied patient that his or her very being is at issue. This unremitting physical pain often gives rise to an existential life-crisis, which, if left unresolved, may give rise to existential suffering.

Heidegger (1927/1962), in his work *Being and Time,* delineated three primary existential crises or callings: 1) existential angst, 2) existential guilt, and 3) existential care. All three existential crises may be best understood as *existential wake-up calls,* in that they serve to awaken individuals to their authentic truth by way of confronting life-limits (angst), awareness of unlived potential (guilt), and reconciling with wholeness (care). Throughout the existential literature, death is revealed as the ultimate boundary situation (Heidegger 1927/1962; Jaspers 1932; Kierkegaard 1844), which triggers the primary source of existential suffering. In actuality, it is not necessarily death that elicits the most fear and dread, but rather the knowledge that one must continue to live in the face of it.

Existential suffering may, therefore, be effectively understood as an umbrella concept (see Figure 8–1), which encompasses the myriad ways people struggle with absence and limits (e.g., disconnection, disillusionment, disorientation) in their lives. Such existential suffering may be more broadly defined, beyond mere death anxiety, to encompass how individuals experience ruptures in relatedness as embodied through angst, guilt, isolation, and despair.

To say that existential pain and suffering derive primarily from death anxiety greatly underestimates the power of existential guilt, isolation, and despair, which are equally present in end-of-life distress. Therefore, existential suffering can be better understood as encompassing all levels and features of existential concern that derive from existential crises. It is intricately conjoined with an existential crisis in the face of absence (e.g., traumatic life event or shift), which gives rise to existential angst (i.e., death anxiety) in the face of life-limits or boundary situations. This may then stir feelings of existential isolation, guilt, and potential existential despair (e.g., meaninglessness, demoralization) in the dying patient.

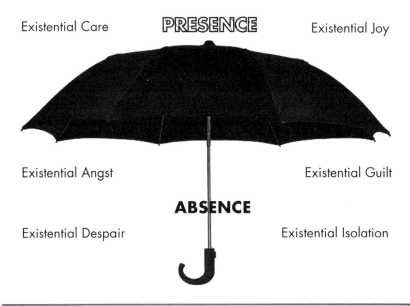

Existential Care   PRESENCE   Existential Joy

Existential Angst   Existential Guilt

ABSENCE

Existential Despair   Existential Isolation

FIGURE 8–1.   Existential suffering as an umbrella concept.

Existential Suffering: Ruptures in World-Relatedness

Existential suffering dialectically reflects ruptures in relatedness to self, others, and the world. For instance, while existential angst directly relates to the potential extinction of self, it dialectically reflects one's inherent dis-attachment from others and the world in general. Such knowledge of one's finitude or mortality may also ignite powerful feelings of existential isolation and despair in the face of dis-attachment from the self-other-world dialectic that often gives life meaning and purpose.

Van Deurzen (1998; van Deurzen and Arnold-Baker 2005) elucidates the existential quality and necessity of world-relatedness through revealing one's personhood as mirrored through interconnecting worlds (see Figure 8–2). She utilizes Heidegger's (1927/1962) concept of *being-in-the-world*, along with Binswanger's (1946) three intersecting worlds of being human: 1) *Umwelt*, the world of natural law and life-cycles; 2) *Mitwelt*, the world of so-cial relations; and 3) *Eigenwelt*, the world of self and individual identity. Van Deurzen further integrates the spiritual realm among these worlds, as de-rived from the existential works of Buber (1958), Jaspers (1932), and Tillich (1962), by adding the *Überwelt*, world of spirituality, to Binswanger's world-related repertoire. This spiritual realm not only connotes the world of reli-

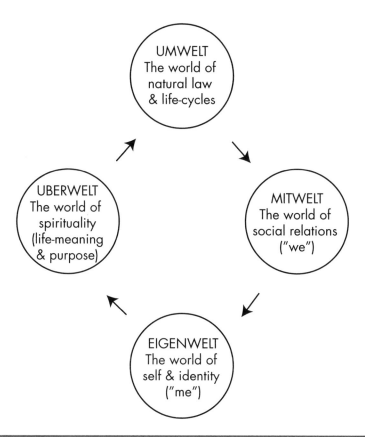

FIGURE 8–2. Existential isolation: ruptures in relational worlds.
Informed by the existential works of Binswanger (1946) and van Deurzen and Arnold-Baker (2005).

gious faith, but also is the realm whereby one finds and defines one's values, meaning, and purpose in life. This is precisely the realm where a patient's disconnection from meaning in life can lead to a sense of meaninglessness, futility, and, if left unattended, demoralization and eventually existential despair.

Likewise, when there is a rupture or disconnect in any one of these relational worlds, the individual may very likely experience existential suffering, most likely in the form of existential isolation. If this sense of disconnection from the natural, relational, personal, or spiritual world is left unattended and persists for too long, one may begin to experience existential despair. Much work has been done to disentangle the diagnostic criteria for depression at the end of life, to make room for terms like *demoralization* (Kissane and Clarke 2001, 2002) and *existential despair.* Existentially, in many ways, existential despair can be best understood by way of a prolongation of dis-connection (dis-pairing) in one or more realms of world-relatedness.

Similarly, Mako et al. (2006) describe a tripartite model of spiritual pain as experienced and expressed by 57 advanced cancer patients in palliative care. Patients described "spiritual pain" by way of emotional distress resulting from ruptures in three separate relational domains: 1) intrapsychic conflict related to self, 2) interpersonal conflict related to others, and 3) conflicts related to the divine or higher power. This tripartite model of end-of-life suffering can be quite helpful in palliative care education, because it identifies suffering beyond vague emotional distress to effectively target where or with whom the rela-tional rupture or disconnect has created such suffering. If practitioners are ef-fectively trained to probe deeper into the existential-spiritual end-of-life suffering, knowing that such distress potentially reflects a relational discon-nect between self and other(s) or a higher power, then better treatment and triage can be successfully established. For example, if an ordinarily religious el-derly patient has taken his rosary and Bible off his nightstand and begins to be-come emotionally and socially withdrawn, gentle therapeutic probing and a potential referral to chaplaincy might be in order.

The relevance of understanding existential-spiritual suffering as multi-dimensional in nature, and not strictly related to death anxiety, is of key im-portance here. The specter of potential death (i.e., disattachment from life) hitherto punctuates and prioritizes the power of relatedness to self, others, the world, and a higher power. The visceral pain related to terminal disease triggers an awakening to these powerful lifelong relations. If there is an ob-struction or rupture in any realm of relatedness, the dying patient may feel it most profoundly as existential anxiety, isolation, guilt, and eventually despair at the end of life.

Existentially, if physical pain and emotional-spiritual distress become too much to bear for the palliative patient, life may ultimately feel futile and meaningless. When patients can no longer tolerate the ultimate ambiguity of living in the face of death, they may succumb to feeling hopeless or help-less about continued existence. Viktor Frankl (1992) described the experi-ence of an *existential vacuum* as a profound state of emptiness that lies at the heart of human suffering, which serves to suck the meaning and purpose out of life itself. Racked with physical, mental, and spiritual suffering, patients question the value of continued existence. Feelings of despair, grief, rage, and resentment result from this extreme state of suffering.

Tillich (1962) described three modes in which humans were threatened by nonexistence: objectively through *death,* spiritually through *meaningless-ness,* and morally through *self-condemnation.* Seminal themes such as personal freedom, choice, and responsibility despite ultimate aloneness were further examined by Jean-Paul Sartre (1943). He believed the random nature of life and death punctuates each person's freedom to define his or her existence. The powerful paradox between meaning and futility amid life's capriciousness became the primary impetus for Sartre's notion of death denial (*bad faith*), and also the fertile ground for finding one's reason for being alive (*raison d'être*).

Many of the great existential philosophers emphasized the human capacity for self-transcendence in the face of death, adversity, or *boundary situations* (Jaspers 1932). Nietzsche's (1910/1968) "will to power," or the essence of his *Übermensch,* underscored this existential power to overcome life's limits and ultimately death. Frankl's (1970) "will to meaning" emphasized similar notions of self-transcendence in the face of death anxiety, by choosing to find meaning in suffering.

Case Vignette

Grace was a 34-year-old mother of four (ages 2–18 years), struggling with end-stage breast cancer and highly invasive metastatic bone pain. She presented in marked physical, mental, and emotional distress, while tearfully expressing, "I'm suffering from the inside out." During her intake evaluation, she shared stories of an extremely impoverished and abusive upbringing, which she "escaped by getting pregnant" as a teenager. Still quite young, Grace suffered from the knowledge that she would soon die and leave her small children "alone in the world without a mother." While exploring the theme of being motherless, Grace was given permission to delve deeper into her own impoverished relationship with her chronically mentally ill and suicidal mother. She shared how the profound loneliness she felt early in her life reflected the [existential] isolation she felt at the present moment preparing for her own death. Although she was surrounded by adoring children and family, her terminal illness brought her back to an earlier time when she felt "utterly vulnerable and defenseless" in a highly dysfunctional home. Early [existential] despair in the face of a "meaningless and futile life" gave rise to a very destructive eating disorder and self-injuring behavior, in order to maintain some modicum of control during her early traumatic years. At presentation, she was tearfully struggling to learn how to authentically take care of herself and her life, as if for the very first time, before dying. Although she was physically suffering from unremitting, often excruciating, metastatic bone pain, her deeper existential suffering became increasingly evident as she faced an early death. Grace tearfully shared the deep-seated grief and suffering she experienced with the painful knowledge that "I will probably die before I figure out how to actually take care of myself." Her premature death not only signaled a traumatic end of motherhood to her beloved children, but an equally devastating end to her childlike longing to be maternally cared for before she left the world.

Existential Anxiety: Being-Towards-Death and Being-Towards-Possibilities

> The idea of death, the fear of it, haunts the human animal like nothing else; it is a mainspring of human activity—activity designed largely to avoid the fatality of death, to overcome it by denying in some way that it is the final destiny for man.
>
> Ernest Becker (1973)

A powerful force under the umbrella of existential suffering is existential angst, or death anxiety. Yalom (1980) delineated the colloquial uses of existential angst through the concepts of "death anxiety," "mortal terror," and "fear of finitude" (p. 42). Kierkegaard (1844) understood such death anxiety as *dread* in the face of non-being. He delineated the colloquial terms of *fear* as being afraid of an identifiable *some-thing* in the world, and *dread* as a vague internal foreboding in the face of *no-thing* or nothingness. Heidegger (1927/1962) also distinguished between the fear of an identifiable object in the world (e.g., needle phobia) and an embodied existential *angst* directed at *being-towards-death* (e.g., receiving a terminal prognosis). Heidegger noted, "Anxiety 'does not know' what that in the face of which it is anxious is…that which threatens cannot bring itself close from a definite direction…it is already there, yet nowhere, it is so close that it is oppressive and stifles one's breath, and yet it is nowhere" (p. 231). For some individuals, the process of dying is frightening; for others, the state of nonexistence and annihilation threatens much more. Death anxiety, whatever its form, can be best understood as an embodied wake-up call in the face of confronting a real or perceived threat to one's being, identity, or mortality.

Paradoxically, most equate existential angst with death anxiety. By delving deeper into Heidegger's (1927/1962) definition, one finds that anxiety is reflective not only of *being-towards-death* but more pervasively in terms of *being-towards-possibilities.* Heidegger stated that "anxiety makes manifest *Being towards* [one's] ownmost potentiality-for-Being…Anxiety brings [one] face to face with its *Being-free* for the authenticity of its Being" (p. 232). This may prove most salient in palliative education, in that practitioners can be taught that end-of-life anxiety may derive not only from facing one's mortality, but also from having to face the possibility of choosing how to authentically live before one dies. If palliative care is understood as focusing solely on comforting (i.e., reducing physical and existential suffering), rather than curing, then palliative care practitioners may be able to help patients focus less on the one solitary, inevitable possibility of death—and more on the plethora of authentic possibilities (e.g., meaning making, legacy building, forgiveness, gratitude, reconciliation) that are available to patients before they die.

Angst: Not-Being-At-Home

The etymological root meaning of the German word *angst* derives from the Latin *angustia* (meaning "tension, tightness") and *angor* or *angere* (meaning "choking, clogging")—that is, to be engulfed in a tight or narrowed passage, to be restricted or suffocated (Merriam-Webster 1994). Heidegger (1927/1962) used the term *angst* interchangeably with *anxiety,* revealing it as feeling "uncanny" or "not-being-at-home" (p. 233). Interestingly, the words *angst, anger,* and *anguish* all derive from similar roots, thereby reflecting similar experiences of being gripped or trapped by an intense sense of anxiety, agitation, or agony. In all three cases patients are often overcome by a powerful sense of intensity—as if they are being gripped or choked by panic, rage, or grief. Angst, anger, and anguish all similarly reveal a feeling of "not-being-at-home," in that they reflect being summoned or awakened by life in the wake of an existential crisis. Heidegger revealed that existential angst derived from the lived-embodied sense of being "wrenched" out of everyday existence by a striking individualized consciousness that "I am someone who will someday die."

Case Vignette

Paul was a 37-year-old single Caucasian graphic artist, dying of acute lymphoblastic leukemia after two failed attempts at a matched unrelated allogeneic bone marrow transplant. He presented in acute pain and heightened anxiety, with chronic graft-versus-host disease covering the majority of his body, accompanied by painful oozing sores. His deer-in-headlights stare revealed that he was scared to death of his imminent terminal condition. The urgency in his tone of voice revealed an inner knowing that the end was near but that he would have to suffer with this knowledge for days or weeks to come. Having to live in the face of imminent death, isolated in his hospital bed and covered in painful sores, triggered unrelenting existential angst. Like many bone marrow transplant patients, Paul began to suffer from intense claustrophobia and panic attacks, where he felt an overwhelming sense of being "trapped" and "suffocated." It became increasingly evident that this had less to do with being confined to isolation in his hospital room than with the overwhelming angst he was experiencing in consciously confronting his own death. Paul would express his terminal condition as "a runaway train...heading off the tracks and off a cliff!" His intense death anxiety could hardly be quelled by lorazepam or olanzapine. Paul eventually found moments of respite while exploring meaningful events of his life and sharing unfinished business related to unfulfilled goals as a graphic artist and unmet dreams in finding love, getting married, and having children. It was as if meaningful dialogue and authentic self-expression allowed him to momentarily break free from his existential crisis of imminent death and partake in a nostalgic, peaceful space for a time.

Existential Guilt: Being Indebted to Life

> We feel ourselves guilty on account of the unused life,
> the unlived life within us.
>
> Otto Rank (1936)

Less often the medical focus of end-of-life distress is on the experience of existential guilt, which factors heavily into how a dying person reflects on life in the face of death. Existential guilt is best understood as an existential wake-up call that awakens the individual to take meaningful inventory and ownership for his or her life. Whereas neurotic guilt derives from moral, familial, or religious dictates that make a person feel indebted to an outside force, existential guilt can be understood as a calling to take responsibility for one's own life. One of the hallmark tenets of existentialism is to find the courage to live truthfully and authentically by overcoming obstacles that keep an individual from freely living true potential for being alive. When patients are racked with guilt at the end of life, it may have less to do with past mistakes and indiscretions than with the awareness that they did not fulfill their true potential for existing.

Interestingly, the German word for guilt (*Schuldig*) is used synonymously with the term *responsibility*. The ability to authentically awaken and respond to life by accepting responsibility for one's life, even in one's final days, allows a person to come to terms with one's past, present, and future as a cohesive whole and take meaningful ownership for it. Owning one's actions, one's choices, one's life as "mine" can be quite scary for the dying patient, yet ultimately very powerful and liberating. The power of self-possession—this is *me*; this is *my life*—offers a sense of authentic agency and authorship over one's existence. Frankl (1992), in his book *Man's Search for Meaning*, articulates this life-calling in the following terms:

> Ultimately, man should not ask what the meaning of his life is, but rather he must recognize that it is *he* who is asked. In a word, each man is questioned by life; and he can only answer to life by *answering for* his own life; to life he can only respond by being responsible. (pp. 113–114)

Likewise, Paul Tillich (1962), in his book *The Courage to Be*, similarly suggests that it takes great courage to authentically respond to life in order to ultimately fulfill one's reason for being alive:

> Man's being is not only given to him but also demanded of him. He is responsible for it; literally, he is required to answer [for] what he has made of his life. He who asks him is his judge, namely he himself.… Man is asked to make of himself what he is supposed to become to fulfill his destiny. (pp. 51–52)

Neurotic Versus Authentic Guilt

Very often, in end-of-life care, practitioners focus on the symptom level of neurotic guilt (e.g., exploring personal mistakes, faults, regrets, unfinished business) and fail to delve deeper to allow for authentic guilt to take shape and have voice. It is quite easy to give credence to neurotic guilt because it is a powerfully primitive and palpable force based on early neurotic attachments. Early psychic absences, insults, losses, or trauma often breed hardwired, lifelong neurotic attachments to pivotal people, moments, or events of the past. This keeps the person in a vicious "white-knuckled" vice grip to these past attachments—trying desperately to right the wrong or undo the damage of the past.

The developmental foundations of guilt are found in Erik Erikson's (1995) third stage of psychosocial development, and are marked by a developmental crisis between *initiative and guilt.* The developmental virtue and outcome of initiating one's life is precisely found in attaining meaning and purpose in it. In contrast, the developmental challenge of not achieving initiative, and eventual individuation, is found in neurotic guilt. The key distinction between neurotic guilt and authentic guilt is that neurotic guilt is a *fear-based reaction* to a threat upon one's sense of identity and others' expectations (e.g., "Who will I be if…I fail, disappoint, don't measure up?"), whereas authentic guilt is a *care-based response* to taking ownership and responsibility for one's own life (e.g., "This is *my* life and I need to take care of it"). Neurotic guilt is focused on repaying a debt to others (i.e., what I owe the world). Authentic guilt centers on repaying the debt to *my* life (i.e., what I owe myself and my potential for being alive). Sartre's (1943) term *raison d'être* speaks to this existential calling to fulfill one's *reason for being* alive. Patients are often racked with existential guilt at the end of life in the face of reflecting on this unlived potential and unlived life within. It is up to the palliative care practitioner to learn how to identify the subtle nuances between fear-based neurotic guilt and care-based authentic guilt, in order to allay the existential burdens that weigh heavy on patients at the end of life.

Case Vignette

Jim, a 52-year-old father of two, was dying of end-stage pancreatic cancer and was referred due to "acute psychological distress." He had survived a grueling Whipple surgery 6 months prior, and his acute unremitting abdominal pain was being effectively controlled and managed via a hydromorphone (Dilaudid) patient-controlled analgesia pump and fentanyl patches. Yet he was curiously still struggling with what he termed "aggressive pain and discomfort." Knowing that Jim suffered from lifelong bouts of severe depression and recurrent suicidality, the therapist chose to delve deeper into the particular discomfort he was experiencing.

At the outset, Jim made it clear he did not wish to focus on "the cancer," but instead on his relationship with his beloved father who had died of a massive heart attack when Jim was 15 years old. He proudly spoke of his father as a first-generation chicken farmer. Jim became quite tearful as he described his father's early impoverished upbringing and said, "I desperately wanted to make him proud!" Because his father died at such an early age, when Jim was filled with adolescent angst and rage, he described being on a "lifelong mission" to undo the wrong and repay the debt to his father by trying to fulfill his (imagined) expectations by becoming a successful lawyer. Although his true calling was to be a teacher, he gave up this authentic dream to repay a lifelong debt to his deceased father. In many ways, this indebtedness kept him ever-close to father's memory. Yet his lifelong depression was a clear indication of the ongoing neglect of his own reason for being alive for the sake of fulfilling what he imagined to be his father's expectations. In working with the therapist, Jim eventually learned to let go of the neurotic guilt that kept him clinging to his father, enabling himself to explore ways he could incorporate his father's legacy as a "great builder" by "building into" the lives of his children before he died. The following therapeutic excerpts reflect Jim's narrative transformation from neurotic to authentic guilt.

Neurotic Guilt: In Debt to Dad, "Paying Back Larry"

"My father, Larry, died of a massive heart attack when I was 15.… That's extremely important. [tears] He was the most important person in my life—my best friend.… It was just awful! I've never recovered from it. [tears] I felt like I killed him by my horrible anger at that age. All kinds of Oedipal crap! He was getting in my way…He wouldn't let me play basketball or go out with girls, and it really pissed me off!" [tears]

"I didn't really think I killed my dad, but I think I did have that energy, that anger toward him at that time, and that felt close enough. The guilt was enough! The guilt was tremendous…after he died I had to punish myself hard, and really be self-destructive for a long time afterwards. I felt like I had to do bad stuff to myself, like law school—I had to make myself get beaten up by a bunch of horrible lawyers for many years.… I figured since I killed my father, I had to pay the debt."

Authentic Guilt: Paying Back Life "Brick by Brick"

"My father was an incredible builder. We built all sorts of things together while I was growing up.… The only way I can allow myself to hold onto the soulfulness of my relationship with him is to constantly be tearing my house apart and building it back up again. I've pulled this damn house apart in so many different ways, it's ridiculous. It's the only way I can keep him close." [tears]

"I've really tried to build into my children's lives.… I tore down our patio to build my son an immense basketball court.… He's now a basketball radio announcer! Funny how that happened!" [knowing smile]

"Just before my Whipple surgery, my daughter and I went on a nonstop 50-hour cross-country trip to hike in Oregon.… Afterwards, Abby drew this picture of us hiking over this Olympic rainforest 7,500-foot glacier. [tears] She called it 'Brick by Brick.' [tears] I just can't get over that! [tears] She knew just what to name the story of my life."

Existential Care as an Answer to Existential Suffering

Existential suffering can best be understood as the pathway home to existential care. That is, by authentically responding to life, we learn to authentically take care of ourselves and their lives as a whole. It is through facing the ultimate limit of death that palliative patients are awakened to existential angst (i.e., *not-being-at-home-in-the-world*), which challenges them to live more authentically. From this initial wake-up call, these patients may be further awakened to existential guilt that challenges them to actualize their given potential for being alive.

When we authentically respond to life, even in the face of death, and begin to take ownership and care of our lives, we then return home to existential care, which Heidegger (1927/1962) reveals as *being-at-home-in-the-world.* Thus, all existential roads do not necessarily lead to death; rather, if navigated authentically, they often lead home to Care. Likewise, Heidegger states, "*Along with the sober anxiety which brings us face to face with our individualized ability-to-be, there goes an unshakable joy.*"

Very often we hear dying patients speak of how they spent their entire lives living for and taking care of others. Only when faced with their own mortality are they awakened to the need to finally take care of themselves. For instance, a 68-year-old mother of three and grandmother of 10, who is dying of metastatic lung cancer, may not necessarily be anguished at separating from her loved ones. Rather, when the therapeutic dialogue probes deeper, she may express profound suffering from the inner knowledge that she never truly lived the life she thought she was meant to live. She was raised in an era in which she was "supposed" to marry early and have a family, yet this was not necessarily her heart's desire. She painfully reveals she never wanted to marry and have children, but always longed to travel and be adventurous, unencumbered by familial obligations.

As this dying patient faces her mortality, she begins to awaken to the ache of this unrealized, deep-seated longing that never came to fruition. She also carries a heavy burden of guilt and shame for imagining a life beyond her family. Life has given this patient the ultimate gift of life, and in return it demands that she respond by being authentically responsible for her life. In responding to this authentic call to actualize her true potential (*raison d'être*), she must then commit to the task of authentically taking care of herself. Herein lies the crux of existential suffering. The distress of facing her mortality ignites existential angst in the face of the knowledge that she is running out of time. This angst then awakens existential guilt, via unlived potential, that ultimately demands reconciliation through existential care before death.

Enhancing existential care in this patient would derive from offering witnessed significance and allowing the patient to explore unrealized dreams and potential in the face of death. The palliative care practitioner would do well to authentically sit with this patient's story of suffering, without attempting to avoid, evade, or cover over the suffering with niceties that may serve to invalidate or infantilize. As Dettmore and Gabriele (2011) powerfully state in reference to responding to unrelieved patient suffering, "Don't just do something, stand there." Very often dying patients need someone to simply be there and bear witness to their suffering without judgment or critique.

Existential Care in Palliative Care: The Return Home

It is not enough to define domains of existential suffering without identifying a way to overcome such end-of-life distress. To this end, we have identified and defined the domains of existential absence (e.g., existential angst, isolation, guilt, and despair) experienced as ruptures in world-relatedness to self, others, and the world. If we return to the image of the umbrella covering the existential domains of suffering, we also see that it reveals the way beyond absence and suffering through the domains of presence and care. Likewise, if we understand Heidegger's (1927/1962) definition of existential angst as "not-being-at-home," then we may find the answer to angst through existential care, which he defined as "being-at-home-in-the-world-as-a-whole" (pp. 348–349). This existential wholeness reflects the etymological root of *healing,* derived from the Old English *haelan* and High Old German *heilen,* meaning "to make whole" (Merriam-Webster 1994).

Very often palliative practitioners ask how they can help give a dying patient hope, courage, meaning, dignity, or a will to live at the end of life. The good news is no one has the power to give courage or dignity—we as clinicians can only help the patient discover and find what is already there. Tillich (1962) states that courage lies at the heart of one's essential ontological structure and being. The root of courage, the French *coeur,* is the heart itself. Although we cannot give patients courage, we can allow them to tell their stories to help them realize, perhaps for the first time, that courage has been there all along. Likewise, Frankl (1970, 1992) challenged that when all else has been stripped away physically, mentally, spiritually, and existentially, patients still have the last vestige of human freedom to choose meaning in their suffering and in their life up to the very last moment and to their very last breath.

Navigating patients out of existential distress toward existential care requires palliative practitioners to authentically bear witness to the dying patient's story of suffering. If palliative practitioners can be taught to listen for the ruptures in dimensions of world-relatedness—targeting the cracks, the old wounds, the unmet needs—they may well learn how to help guide a dying patient home toward healing and wholeness before he or she dies. To learn this skill, palliative practitioners need to be offered a veritable existential road map across the temporal horizons of a patient's life review, exploring his or her past, present, and future. First, practitioners must learn to readily identify the multi-faceted nature of existential distress in their dying patient. Then, they must learn to utilize simple life-review probes that will allow them to listen for themes of existential angst and/or existential guilt in and through patients' life narratives.

Charon (2004), White and Epstein (1990), and Viederman and Perry (1980) all endorse the use and efficacy of patient life narratives and storytelling not only to collect salient historical data, but also to promote reciprocal dialogue between patient and practitioner to enhance relational trust and diminish distress. Tait et al. (2011) went one step further to integrate a structured dignity-conserving interview (Chochinov 2002; Chochinov et al. 2005a, 2011) into palliative care resident training. This dignity training allowed residents to witness firsthand how initiating a simple structured life review with dying patients could open purposeful therapeutic dialogue. This shifts the ordinarily technical psychiatric history taking toward a more relational meaning-making endeavor.

In the palliative care literature, several end-of-life therapeutic interventions offer some semblance of life review to promote age-old medical methods of storytelling to enhance terminally ill patients' quality of life and well-being. Breitbart et al. (2004) offer an overview of such psychotherapeutic interventions focusing on the existential domains of enhancing meaning making and legacy building at the end of life. Likewise, Spiegel and colleagues (Spiegel and Cordova 2001; Spiegel et al. 1981) developed supportive-expressive group therapy, integrating existential themes and patient life review in their work with metastatic breast cancer patients in order to bolster overall well-being. Chochinov and colleagues (Chochinov 2002; Chochinov et al. 2005a, 2011) developed Dignity therapy as a single-session narrative life review to enhance dignity at the end of life. This 1-hour audio-taped life review is then edited and offered back to the patient and family as a generativity document, effectively promoting meaning making and legacy building at the end of life. Breitbart and colleagues (Breitbart 2002, 2003; Breitbart and Poppito 2005; Brietbart et al. 2010) developed group and individual formats of meaning-centered psychotherapy, also focused primarily on bolstering meaning making and legacy building through narrative life-review activities, to enhance overall spiritual well-being in advanced cancer patients.

The question then arises that if narrative life review is recognized as having therapeutic efficacy, by enhancing meaning and legacy at the end of life, why are palliative practitioners not being actively trained to use these modalities to help promote healthy life completion with their patients?

When palliative practitioners (i.e., oncologists, nurses, psychiatrists, psychologists) are trained in these life-narrative techniques, all will have the shared interest and opportunity to potentially guide a dying patient out of existential distress toward existential care. This life review then becomes a fully dynamic and dialectical life-completion process, whereby the entire multidisciplinary team carries a shared incentive and authentic responsibility to build into the lives of their dying patients. Heidegger (1927/1962) challenges that we all, as human beings, are the shepherds of being. By tracking patients' lived stories of suffering to what lies *behind* them in their past and *between* life and death in the present, practitioners may help shepherd patients *beyond* their existential distress toward making peace with life. This can help patients make sense of the nonsense of their lives, so they may create a sense of closure with what is and what has been. Thus, palliative practitioners may initiate purposeful legacy-building dialogue to engage patients in exploring what mark they will leave that will live on beyond them.

Each time dying patients are given the opportunity to share another dimension of their life story and be offered witnessed significance from their care provider, they are given evidence that their life mattered in the eyes of another. This serves to fulfill existential absence with meaningful presence. The inherent value of this palliative education process is that all practitioners are given the opportunity to return back to why they chose to work with dying patients in the first place. End-of-life care reveals a sacred passage for all involved. No one enters this field to cure patients of their diseases and save them from death. They enter palliative medicine to relieve suffering and compassionately care for those who are leaving this world. There is no higher calling than to help guide a human being out of existential suffering into the light of existential care—returning back home to wholeness with life in the face of death.

> The kingdom of illness is designed on forgetting.
> So, if I take you to my forgetting, my sickness,
> and you bring yourself as practitioner and guide,
> once more I come home,
> and see that I have been home all along.
>   Diane Connelly (1993)

Conclusion

Given the paucity of palliative literature covering existential issues at the end of life, along with the myriad, ostensibly interchangeable yet nebulous definitions of existential suffering, it would seem plausible that palliative education does not yet include well-defined existential domains. However, there is no other place in medical education or medical practice where these existential dimensions are more prominent or more demanding of inclusion in standard of care practice than in palliative and hospice care. The goal of this chapter was not only to show the need to evolve palliative education in the direction of including existential domains, but also to help identify and define the most salient existential issues that dying patients may be experiencing. Existential suffering is merely one point on the existential spectrum in end-of-life care. If we understand existential suffering to be a distressful wake-up call in the face of one's mortality, than we must envision that this calling has an ultimate telos and potential. Thus, we cannot speak of existential domains in palliative care without showing that the absence of existential suffering is answered by the presence of existential care. By teaching palliative practitioners how first to identify existential suffering in their dying patients, and then to offer ways to navigate patients through the process of narrative life review and life-completion, we will help give agency and responsibility back to both patient and practitioner at the end of life.

Advancing medical education in the existential dimensions of end-of-life care shares many of the same challenges of integrating palliative care education in general, as well as some additional ones. We would like to suggest a road map for the journey ahead. At a broad level, the educational landscape of the country where one resides is important. That is, one must establish what are the core competencies for health professional training in the given discipline and setting, and which ones map onto existential aspects of end-of-life care. This step is important for getting institutional support for the education, including curricular time and resources. If the stated core competencies in a given country or setting do not include the nonphysical aspects of palliative care, including existential aspects, then the first step is to advocate, based on the evidence, for this to be included. However, individuals, and indeed institutions, may be well defended against addressing aspects of care and education that are "too emotional" for the reasons discussed earlier. Once the topic is identified as important, including allocation of time and resources, developing the actual curricula can proceed.

We suggest that the advancing of medical education in existential dimensions of end-of-life care is best situated within a narrative framework. This means soliciting, attending to, and witnessing the narratives of ourselves, our patients, and our colleagues. Educational experiences must be provided that require and allow providers to sit with and process the experience and emotions that go with end-of-life illness. Tait and Hodges (2012) argue that this is only possible when providers have the opportunity to solicit the patient's illness and life story, as distinguished from the medical history. Indeed, the palliative care setting, with less focus on curing, is the ideal setting in which to build skill in just being with our patients' experience, as well as story-skills essential to building humanism in physicians of any kind. Complementing narrative practice with reflective practice is crucial to processing the experience and learning from it.

Although physicians feel well prepared in many of the physical aspects of palliative care, they feel less competent and desire more training in areas such as existential, psychosocial, and spiritual care. Meanwhile, there are powerful cultural messages being taught in the hidden curriculum of medical education that have physicians and trainees feeling conflicted about whether they should get close enough to patients that they might be able to address these concerns.

Finally, from this chapter we trust that some readers will become more personally competent in identifying and addressing existential issues in palliative care. Some, we hope, will also situate this within the educational principles outlined and use the synergy of the two topics to champion change in their learning, teaching, and institutions. Either way, we hope assumptions will be challenged and perspectives broadened in a way required to continually advance the care of palliative patients.

Key Clinical Points

- The literature concerning existential issues at the end of life is scarce in the field of palliative care, as well as in psychiatry and psychology. Existential dimensions, however, are prominent and demand inclusion in the practice of palliative care and hospice programs.

- Physicians feel well prepared in many of the physical aspects of palliative care but less competent in areas such as existential, psychosocial, and spiritual care, in which they desire more training. The educational landscape of the country where one resides is important, too.

- Increasingly, medical schools are developing narrative and humanities programs, and using literature to expose students to stories, thereby stimulating reflective practice. Narrative competency is becoming considered a core competency.

- Longitudinal exposure to patients with advanced illness is needed in various clinical contexts—beyond psychiatry training settings and including general medical settings.

- Death, choice, responsibility, meaning, and legacy are the main existential domains for both patients and practitioners, from the initial palliative phase to the final hospice phase.

- Some examples of interventions that shift from ordinarily technical psychiatric history taking toward a more relational meaning-making endeavor include supportive-expressive group psychotherapy, meaning-centered psychotherapy, and dignity therapy.

References

Back AL, Arnold RM, Quil TE: Hope for the best, and prepare for the worst. Ann Intern Med 138:439–443, 2003

Becker E: The Denial of Death. New York, Free Press Paperbacks, 1973

Billings ME, Curtis JR, Engelberg RA: Medicine residents' self-perceived competence in end-of-life care. Acad Med 84:1533–1539, 2009

Binswanger L: The existential analysis school of thought (1946), in Existence: A New Dimension in Psychiatry and Psychology. Edited by May R, Angel E, Ellenberger HF. New York, Basic Books, 1958, pp 191–213

Block SD: Psychological considerations, growth, and transcendence at the end of life: the art of the possible. JAMA 285:2898–2905, 2001

Borgstrom E, Cohn S, Barclay S: Medical professionalism: conflicting values for tomorrow's doctors. J Gen Intern Med 25:1330–1336, 2010

Breitbart W: Spirituality and meaning in supportive care: spirituality- and meaning-centered group psychotherapy interventions in advanced cancer. Support Care Cancer 10:272–280, 2002

Breitbart W: Reframing hope: meaning-centered care for patients near the end of life. Interview by Karen S. Heller. J Palliat Med 6:979–988, 2003

Breitbart W, Poppito S: Individual Meaning-Centered Psychotherapy Treatment Manual. New York, Memorial Sloan-Kettering Cancer Center, unpublished document, 2005

Breitbart W, Bruera E, Chochinov H, et al: Neuropsychiatric syndromes and psychological symptoms in patients with advanced cancer. J Pain Symptom Manage 10:131–141, 1995

Breitbart W, Gibson C, Poppito S, et al: Psychotherapeutic interventions at the end of life: a focus on meaning and spirituality. Can J Psychiatry 49:366–372, 2004

Breitbart W, Rosenfeld B, Gibson C, et al: Meaning-centered group psychotherapy for patients with advanced cancer: a pilot randomized controlled trial. Psychooncology 19:21–28, 2010

Browall M, Melin-Johansson C, Strang S, et al: Health care staff's opinions about existential issues among patients with cancer. Palliat Support Care 8:59–68, 2010

Buber M: I and Thou. Translated by Kaufmann W. New York, Scribner, 1958

Charon R: Narrative and medicine. N Engl J Med 350:862–864, 2004

Chochinov H: Dignity-conserving care—a new model for palliative care. JAMA 17:2253–2260, 2002

Chochinov HM: Dying, dignity, and new horizons in palliative end-of-life care. CA Cancer J Clin 56:84–105, 2006

Chochinov HM, Hack T, Hassard T, et al: Dignity therapy: a novel psychotherapeutic intervention for patients near the end of life. J Clin Oncol 23:5520–5525, 2005a

Chochinov HM, Hack T, Hassard T, et al: Understanding the will to live in patients nearing death. Psychosomatics 46:7–10, 2005b

Chochinov HM, Kristjanson LJ, Breitbart W, et al: Effect of dignity therapy on distress and end-of-life experience in terminally ill patients: a randomised controlled trial. Lancet Oncol 12:753–762, 2011

Connelly D: All Sickness is Homesickness. Columbia, MD, Maryland Centre for Traditional Acupuncture, 1993

Curtis JR, Treece PD, Nielsen EL, et al: Integrating palliative and critical care: evaluation of a quality-improvement intervention. Am J Respir Crit Care Med 178:269–275, 2008

Dettmore D, Gabriele LC: Don't just do something, stand there: responding to unrelieved patient suffering. J Psychosoc Nurs Ment Health Serv 49:34–38, 2011

Erikson EH: Childhood and Society. London, Vintage, 1995

Frankl VE: The Will to Meaning: Foundations and Applications of Logotherapy. New York, New American Library, 1970

Frankl VE: Man's Search for Meaning: An Introduction to Logotherapy. Boston, MA, Beacon Press, 1992

Hafferty FW: Beyond curriculum reform: confronting medicine's hidden curriculum. Acad Med 73:403–407, 1998

Heidegger M: Being and Time (1927). Translated by Macquarrie J, Robinson ES. New York, Harper & Row, 1962

Jaspers K: Boundary situations, in Philosophy, Vol 2. Translated by Ashton EB. Chicago, IL, University of Chicago Press, 1932

Kelly E, Nisker J: Medical students' first clinical experiences of death. Med Educ 44:421–428, 2010

Kerrihard T, Breitbart W, Dent K, et al: Anxiety in patients with cancer and human immunodeficiency virus. Semin Clin Neuropsychiatry 4:114–132, 1999

Kierkegaard S: The Concept of Dread. Translated by Lowrie W. Princeton, NJ, Princeton University Press, 1844

Kissane DW, Clarke DM: Demoralization syndrome—a relevant psychiatric diagnosis for palliative care. J Palliat Care 17:12–21, 2001

Kissane DW, Clarke DM: Demoralization: its phenomenology and importance. Aust NZ J Psychiatry 36:733–742, 2002

Levine MA: Sedation to unconsciousness in end-of-life care. Report of the Council on Ethical and Judicial Affairs. CEJA Report 5-A-08. Available at: http://www.ama-assn.org/resources/doc/code-medical-ethics/2201a.pdf. Accessed July 29, 2012.

Mako C, Galek K, Poppito SR: Spiritual pain among patients with advanced cancer in palliative care. J Palliat Med 9:1106–1113, 2006

Mann K, Gordon J, MacLeod A: Reflection and reflective practice in health professions education: a systematic review. Adv Health Sci Educ Theory Pract 14:595–621, 2009

Merriam-Webster: Merriam-Webster Collegiate Dictionary, 10th Edition. Springfield, MA, Merriam-Webster, 1994

Murata H, Morita T, Japanese Task Force: Conceptualization of psycho-existential suffering by the Japanese Task Force: the first step of a nationwide project. Palliat Support Care 4:279–285, 2006

Nietzsche F: The Will to Power (1910). Translated by Kaufmann W. New York, Vintage Books, 1968

Oneschuk D, Moloughney B, Jones-McLean E, et al: The status of undergraduate palliative medicine education in Canada: a 2001 survey. J Palliat Care 20:32–37, 2004

Sartre JP: Being and Nothingness: An Essay on Phenomenological Ontology. Translated by Barnes H. New York, Philosophical Library, 1943

Schroder C, Heyland D, Jiang X, et al: Educating medical residents in end-of-life care: insights from a multicenter survey. J Palliat Med 12:459–470, 2009

Schuman-Olivier Z, Brendel DH, Forstein M, et al: The use of palliative sedation for existential distress: a psychiatric perspective. Harv Rev Psychiatry 16: 339–351, 2008

Spiegel D, Cordova M: Supportive-expressive group therapy and life extension of breast cancer patients: Spiegel et al. (1989). Adv Mind Body Med 17:38–41, 2001

Spiegel D, Bloom JR, Yalom I: Group support for patients with metastatic cancer. A randomized outcome study. Arch Gen Psychiatry 38:527–533, 1981

Strang, P, Strang, S, Hultborn, R, et al: Existential pain—an entity, a provocation, or a challenge? J Pain Symptom Manage 27:241–250, 2004

Sullivan AM, Lakoma MD, Block SD: The status of medical education in end-of-life care: a national report. J Gen Intern Med 18:685–695, 2003

Sullivan AM, Warren AG, Lakoma MD, et al: End-of-life care in the curriculum: a national study of medical education deans. Acad Med 79:760–768, 2004

Tait GR, Hodges BD: End of life care education for psychiatric residents: attitudes, preparedness, and conceptualizations of dignity. Acad Psychiatry 33:451–456, 2009

Tait GR, Hodges B: Residents learning from a narrative experience with dying patients: a qualitative study. Adv Health Sci Educ Theory Pract Oct 6, 2012 [E-pub ahead of print]. doi: 10.1007/s10459-012-9411-y

Tait GR, Schryer C, McDougall A, et al: Exploring the therapeutic power of narrative at the end of life: a qualitative analysis of narratives emerging in dignity therapy. BMJ Supportive and Palliative Care, 1:296–300, 2011. Available at: http://spcare.bmj.com. Accessed July 30, 2012.

The AM, Hak T, Koeter G, et al: Collusion in doctor-patient communication about imminent death: an ethnographic study. BMJ 321:1376–1381, 2000

Tillich P: The Courage to Be. The Fontana Library. London, Collins, 1962

van Deurzen E: Paradox and Passion in Psychotherapy: An Existential Approach to Therapy and Counselling. Chichester, UK, Wiley, 1998

van Deurzen E, Arnold-Baker C: Existential Perspectives on Human Issues: A Handbook for Therapeutic Practice. New York, Palgrave MacMillan, 2005

Viederman M, Perry SW 3rd: Use of a psychodynamic life narrative in the treatment of depression in the physically ill. Gen Hosp Psychiatry 2:177–185, 1980

Wald HS, Davis SW, Reis SP: Reflecting on reflections: enhancement of medical education curriculum with structured field notes and guided feedback. Acad Med 84:830–837, 2009

Wald HS, Reis SP, Monroe AD, et al: The loss of my elderly patient: interactive reflective writing to support medical students' rites of passage. Med Teach 32:178–184, 2010

White M, Epstein D: Narrative Means to Therapeutic Ends. New York, Norton, 1990

Yalom ID: Existential Psychotherapy. New York, Basic Books, 1980

CHAPTER 9

Rapid Psychometric Assessment of Distress and Depression

Alex J. Mitchell, M.B.B.S., B.Med.Sci., M.Sc., M.R.C.Psych.

IMPROVEMENTS IN survival in an aging population are bringing about a dramatic increase in the number of people living with the long-term consequences of cancer. It is estimated that in the United States the prevalence of cancer will increase from 13.8 million in 2010 to 18.2 million in 2020 (Mariotto et al. 2011). Many, perhaps most, of these individuals will suffer emotional complications that necessitate psychometric assessment. Recent studies have offered precise estimates of the proportion of people with cancer who suffer emotional complications that are of clinical significance. The point prevalence of major depression at any time in the first 2 years following a cancer diagnosis is 15% (Mitchell et al. 2011a). Major depression, diagnosed using DSM-IV criteria (American Psychiatric Association 1994), is the most studied complication, although its validity in cancer has not been adequately examined (Akechi et al. 2003). Notably, the clause excluding depression due to a medical disorder is often conveniently overlooked. It is important to realize that major depression is only one of several important mental health complications. Minor depression, anxiety disorders, and adjustment disorders are at least equally common. Indeed, a clinically relevant mood disorder of some type can be anticipated in 4 in 10 patients early in their disease course (Mitchell et al. 2011a). Less clear is the prevalence of depression in long-term survivors who are 3 or more years postdiagnosis. In an unpublished meta-analysis, a group at Leicester Royal Infirmary, of which

I am a part, found that approximately 10% of long-term survivors suffer depression, a rate not appreciably different from that seen in primary care attendees. This finding suggests that most long-term survivors will have a good outcome, but clinicians should be careful not to overlook the substantial minority who still need help with unmet needs.

Clinicians are aware that many patients who struggle emotionally after a cancer diagnosis do not meet standard criteria for DSM-IV major depression. In fact, at least half of those with a clinically significant mental health complication do not suffer from depression. Many may be labeled with an adjustment disorder, but this category lacks meaningful criteria and is poorly understood by patients. This has led to popularity of the concept of distress, to be measured as the sixth vital sign, the other five being temperature, blood pressure, pulse, respiratory rate, and pain (Holland and Bultz 2007). Estimates regarding prevalence of distress have been informed by early studies using the Brief Symptom Inventory (BSI; Derogatis 1993) and more recent research involving the Distress Thermometer (DT; Roth et al. 1998). Pooled BSI data from two studies involving over 7,000 patients illustrate that about 4 in 10 cancer patients report significant distress (Carlson et al. 2004; Zabora et al. 2001). This is reasonably consistent with studies that have employed other instruments, such as the General Health Questionnaire–12 (GHQ-12; Goldberg and Williams 1991). Although studies of prevalence are helpful, clinicians want to know who is at particular risk of distress following cancer. Individuals with certain cancers, such as lung, brain, and pancreatic cancer, are more likely to be distressed, but differences by cancer type are generally modest. Much more powerful predictors of distress include low quality of life, disability (e.g., low Karnofsky Performance scores), and ongoing unmet needs (Banks et al. 2010; Carlson et al. 2004). These considerations should therefore be included in clinical assessment. Surprisingly, the influence of disease stage is subject to considerable debate.

Both distress and depression are important not only for mental health professionals but also for cancer clinicians. The presence of distress is also linked with reduced health-related quality of life (Shim et al. 2006), poor satisfaction with medical care (Von Essen et al. 2002), and possibly reduced survival (Faller et al. 1999). Depression is one of the strongest determinants of health-related quality of life, and it also influences care and participation in treatment (Kennard et al. 2004; Steginga et al. 2008). A meta-analysis of 25 observational studies showed a 39% higher all-cause mortality rate in cancer patients diagnosed with major or minor depression (risk ratio 1.39; 95% CI, 1.10–1.89) (Satin et al. 2009). An important question, particularly in relation to distress, is when does it become serious enough to be clinically important. It is advisable to use duration (longer than 2 weeks) and, where possible, the clinical significance criterion that is a cornerstone of DSM-IV-TR

(American Psychiatric Association 2000), and likely to have even more prominence in DSM-5. The criteria for clinical significance are that "symptoms cause clinically important distress or impair work, social, or personal functioning" (p. 327). Clinical work at Leicester Royal Infirmary suggests that eight out of 10 people with major depression suffer both distress and dysfunction.

Rapid Clinical Assessment

Several national guidelines promote the need for integrated psychosocial care, and several recommend psychometric assessment to help clinicians detect emotional problems (Adler and Page 2007; Holland and Bultz 2007; Patrick et al. 2004). Most endorse routine universal screening, although no studies exist comparing the screening of every individual with the screening of only high-risk groups (Figure 9–1). The purpose of psychometric assessment is threefold:

1. To rule out patients without emotional complications who do not need professional help at this time. When conducted systematically in routine practice, this assessment can be called *screening,* and it can be measured by the negative predictive value (NPV) (Mitchell 2008b) (Figure 9–2).
2. To confirm the presence of a treatable emotional disorder. In epidemiological terminology, this assessment is often called *case-finding* and is crudely measured by the positive predictive value (PPV) (Mitchell 2008b) (see Figure 9–2).
3. To quantify the severity of the disorder, usually for the purpose of monitoring the response to treatment. Cancer clinicians, primary care clinicians, and mental health specialists each have a role in psychometric assessment, but cancer clinicians (physicians, nurses, treatment radiographers, and allied staff) are usually in a position to make the important first assessment.

Several informative surveys have examined rates of routine clinical inquiry regarding psychological issues. Only a minority of patients recall being asked about "mental stress, worry, or mood changes" (Butt et al. 2008). In self-report surveys, about one-third of clinicians report asking about emotional problems only occasionally; many prefer to rely on patients mentioning a problem first (Mitchell et al. 2008). Less than 15% of clinicians use a screening instrument; most prefer their own clinical judgment (Mitchell et al. 2008; Pirl et al. 2007). Observed interview studies confirm these findings. In discussing health-related quality of life, clinicians typically men-

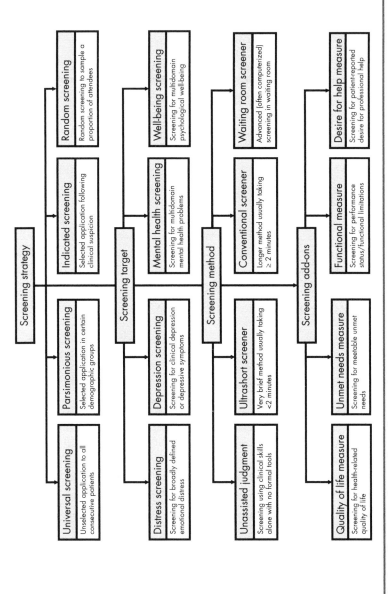

FIGURE 9–1. Conceptual overview of screening.

	Gold Standard Disorder	Gold Standard No disorder	
Test positive	A	B	A/(A + B) PPV
Test negative	C	D	D/(C + D) NPV
Total	A/(A + C) Se	D/(B + D) Sp	

FIGURE 9–2. Basic definitions of diagnostic accuracy.

Se (sensitivity)=the proportion of patients with disease in whom the test result is positive; Sp (specificity) = the proportion of patients without disease in whom the test result is negative; PPV (positive predictive value) = the proportion of true positives in those who screen positive; NPV (negative predictive value)=the proportion of true negatives in those who screen negative.

tion psychological aspects in less than 10% of interviews (Rodriguez et al. 2010). In general, emotional issues are discussed in about 15%–40% of consultations (Anderson et al. 2008; Detmar et al. 2001; Taylor et al. 2011). Interestingly, patients, not clinicians, initiate these discussions in most instances, because physicians gravitate toward medical issues (Pollak et al. 2007; Taylor et al. 2011). The main barriers to thorough assessment and formal screening appear to be perceived lack of time, lack of training, low personal skills, low confidence about diagnosis, and lack of availability of mental health services (Jones and Doebbeling 2007; Mitchell et al. 2008).

Given that cancer clinicians typically use their own clinical judgments to diagnose depression, an important question is how accurate that professional judgment is. Although several studies have examined the unassisted ability of cancer clinicians to identify depression or distress, only a minority have measured detection sensitivity as well as detection specificity (i.e., the ability to rule in and rule out cases) (Keller et al. 2004; Passik et al. 1998; Söllner et al. 2001). Söllner et al. (2001) examined the accuracy of eight oncologists who had evaluated 298 cancer patients against moderate or severe distress on the Hospital Anxiety and Depression Scale—Total score (HADS-T) (a 12v13 cutoff); the oncologists' sensitivity was 80% but specificity was only 33%. Using a HADS-T cutoff of 18 to represent severe distress, sensitivity was only 37% and specificity increased to 88%. These findings suggest that oncologists are likely to identify only a minority of those with severe distress. Fallowfield et al. (2001) compared cancer clinicians' ratings using visual analogue scales with an independent GHQ-12 score (at a cutoff ≥ 4). In this high-prevalence sample, detection sensitivity was only 29%. Patients given more time with clinicians were less likely to be missed. In a study of 400 patients, Mitchell et al. (2010b) looked at identification of distress by chemotherapy cancer nurses using distress defined by the DT. Nurse practitioners had a detection sensitivity of 50% and specificity of 80%. Interestingly, those clinicians with high self-rated confidence had higher sensitivity but lower specificity. It is rarely appreciated that low sensitivity and modest specificity can translate into a significant number of false-positive errors as well as false-negative errors. Assuming that distress is present in 40% of cancer patients (using data from Mitchell et al. 2010b), clinicians would probably miss 20 patients and misidentify 12 patients for every 100 people seen in routine care. The rate of false positives increases further when looking for depression where the prevalence of the index condition is low. There are many possible reasons for detection error, including both patient and provider factors. Not all patients want to talk about their problems (Kvåle 2007). Clinician-related factors linked with low detection include the willingness to look for emotional problems, clinical confidence/skills, and consultation time. Patient factors include confidence in the clinician, willingness to discuss personal difficulties, and belief that help is available. To address this limitation, the use of short, clinically acceptable tools is being extensively investigated.

Rapid Psychometric Assessment

In the past, researchers studying psychometrics in cancer settings looked simply at accuracy, leading to recommendations for the use of rather lengthy tools that were unpopular in busy clinical practice. The major innovation in the last 10 years has been to give equal consideration to acceptability. Acceptability is usually the rate-determining step underlying implementation of a screening program.

Numerous tools have been developed, varying from 1 item to 90 items (Vodermaier et al. 2009). The complexity of a tool is governed not simply by the item count but also by its completion time and difficulty of scoring. In this chapter I consider tools that take no more than 10 minutes to complete and consist of fewer than 15 items (Table 9–1). However, in clinical practice there is a strong case to focus on tools taking only 1–2 minutes. Tools can be divided into self-report, structured verbal, and computerized delivery. Rarely have the same stems been tested head-to-head using different methods of delivery. Clinicians are currently faced with a large number of rating scales of varying degrees of accuracy, acceptability, and evidence (Luckett et al. 2010; Vodermaier et al. 2009). Very few tools have been tested with a large sample and subjected to independent replication. The best known conventional self-report mood scale is the HADS (Zigmond and Snaith 1983). The HADS serves as a useful starting point in the development of rapid screening tools because it is considered reasonably accurate in its 14-item version (HADS-T) but too long for routine use (Mitchell et al. 2010b). That said, some groups have used computerized waiting room versions of the HADS in large clinically representative samples (Walker and Sharpe 2009). The accuracy of the HADS-T in terms of sensitivity and specificity is approximately 80%. A sensitivity of 80% and a specificity of 80% could be considered to be a minimum, but in clinical practice this will depend on prevalence. Varying sensitivity or varying specificity have very different effects on false-positive or false-negative errors, as can be seen from a plot of posttest probability tests with a variety of accuracies (Figure 9–3). At low prevalence settings that are typical when looking for depression tools, accuracy makes little difference in terms of false negatives but a big difference in terms of false positives. For screening (which is only the first step), higher sensitivities are preferred because these will favor the negative predictive value.

Simple structured verbal methods are perhaps the simplest and quickest of all screening modalities, and these can be memorized by clinicians (e.g., asking the patient, "Are you depressed?" or "How distressed have you been in the previous week?") (Lloyd-Williams et al. 2004). A meta-analysis of verbal stem questions against interview-defined depression found that a single "depression" question has a sensitivity of 72% and specificity of 83%, slightly inferior to a "loss-of-interest" question, which had a sensitivity of 83% and specificity of 86% (Mitchell 2008a). Despite the low sensitivity, where the prevalence of depression is low, negative predictive value is reasonably maintained, allowing the "are you depressed" question to be used as an initial first step. That said, the loss-of-interest question is preferred. Combining the two questions (low mood and low interest, where only one positive answer is required) is better, with a sensitivity of 91% and specificity of 86%, and perhaps offers the optimal balance between accuracy and length of methods tested to date. These data cannot be extrapolated to the detection of distress because of the significant difference in prevalence between depression and distress. Validation studies against distress must be conducted, ideally using a robust gold standard. Unfortunately, a gold standard

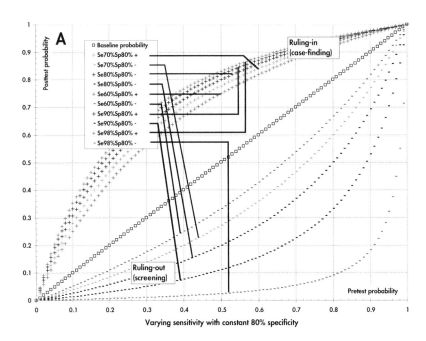

Varying sensitivity with constant 80% specificity

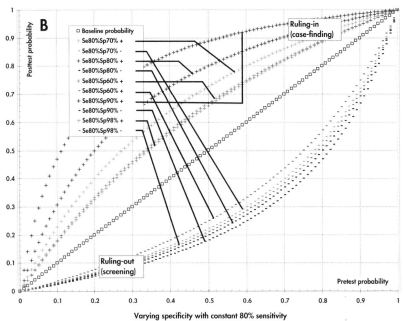

Varying specificity with constant 80% sensitivity

FIGURE 9–3. Conditional probability plots with varying sensitivity or specificity.

Graphs show rule-in (case-finding) and rule-out (screening) success of six methods used to identify cancer-related distress. Bayesian conditional probability plot illustrates posttest probability (y axis) according to pretest probability prevalence (x axis). (*A*) Varying sensitivity (Se) with constant 80% specificity (Sp). (*B*) Varying specificity with constant 80% sensitivity.

Added key lines connecting probabilities to plotted curves indicate color coding in original.

for distress defined by interview is in dispute, and adjustment disorder or any affective disorder may be a close approximation. A meta-analysis of the verbal stem questions measured against broadly defined distress found less adequate performance when looking for distress than when looking for depression, raising a question about reliance on one simple verbal question (Table 9–2) (Mitchell 2010). Accuracy can be improved using two questions (sensitivity 68% and specificity 93%), but this is based on data from one study alone.

These issues regarding longer questionnaires and low accuracy of the verbal stem questions led several groups to reexamine visual-analogue scales (VASs) that had been introduced in the 1970s for evaluation of mood, suicidal thoughts, pain, and quality of life (Folstein 1973). Chochinov et al. (1997) examined a VAS ranging from "worst possible mood" to "best possible mood." In 1998, however, the Distress Thermometer was introduced (Roth et al. 1998). The DT has done much to revitalize interest from cancer clinicians looking for a rapid method of screening for emotional complications of cancer without recourse to complex scoring or algorithms. The DT was developed by a panel of 23 health professionals and a patient representative working in collaboration with the National Comprehensive Cancer Network and is currently royalty free (National Comprehensive Cancer Network 2007). The DT is a simple pencil-and-paper measure consisting of a 0–10 scale anchored at zero with "no distress" and at 10 with "extreme distress." Patients are asked to answer the question, "How distressed have you been during the past week on a scale of 0 to 10?" A revised cutoff of 4 or above is recommended as significant but generally mild distress, whereas 6 or 7 denotes moderate distress and 8 or higher indicates severe distress. An important addition is a problem checklist that highlights potential unmet needs for a patient that may be linked with perceived distress. Diagnostic validity studies of the DT against an interview-based standard suggest that the DT has reasonable sensitivity but lower than ideal specificity. In the real world, assuming a 40% prevalence of distress, then clinicians relying on the DT (at ≥4) would miss 9 patients and misidentify 20 patients for every 100

TABLE 9–1. Summary of rapid psychometric assessment methods for emotional disorder

Number of items	Scale	Abbreviation	Primary focus	Diagnostic validity study in cancer	Replication study in cancer	Randomized implementation study
14	Hospital Anxiety and Depression Scale—Total score	HADS-T	Distress	Yes	Yes	Yes
13	Beck Depression Inventory Short Form	BDI-SF	Depression	Yes	No	No
13	Psychological Distress Inventory	PDI	Distress	Yes	No	No
12	General Health Questionnaire–12	GHQ-12	Distress	Yes	No	No
11	Bech-Rafaelsen Melancholia Scale	MES	Depression	No	No	No
10	Center for Epidemiologic Studies Depression Scale–10	CESD-10	Depression	No	No	No
10	Depression Scale	DEPS-10	Depression	No	No	No

TABLE 9–1. Summary of rapid psychometric assessment methods for emotional disorder *(continued)*

Number of items	Scale	Abbreviation	Primary focus	Diagnostic validity study in cancer	Replication study in cancer	Randomized implementation study
10	Edinburgh Postnatal Depression Scale	EPDS	Depression	Yes	Yes	No
10	Montgomery-Åsberg Depression Rating Scale	MADRS	Depression	No	No	No
10	Zung Self-Rating Depression Scale—Short	SDS-10	Depression	No	No	No
9	Hornheide Short Form	—	Depression	Yes	No	No
9	Patient Health Questionnaire–9	PHQ-9	Depression	No	No	No
8	Edinburgh Postnatal Depression Scale 8	EPDS-8	Depression	No	No	No
8	Even Briefer Assessment Scale for Depression	EBAS DEP	Depression	No	No	No

TABLE 9–1. Summary of rapid psychometric assessment methods for emotional disorder (*continued*)

Scale	Abbreviation	Primary focus	Diagnostic validity study in cancer	Replication study in cancer	Randomized implementation study
Number of items					
8 Medical Outcomes Scale 8	MOS-8	Depression	No	No	No
8 Patient Health Questionnaire–8	PHQ-8	Depression	No	Yes	No
7 Beck Depression Inventory–7	BDI-7	Depression	No	No	No
7 Duke Anxiety-Depression Scale	DADS-7	Depression	No	No	No
7 Edinburgh Postnatal Depression Scale—depression items	EPDS-7	Depression	No	No	No
7 Hamilton Depression Scale–7	HAMD-7	Depression	No	No	No
7 Hornheide Screening Instrument	HSI	Depression	Yes	No	No
7 Hospital Anxiety and Depression scale—Anxiety subscale	HADS-A	Anxiety	Yes	No	No

TABLE 9–1. Summary of rapid psychometric assessment methods for emotional disorder (*continued*)

Number of items	Scale	Abbreviation	Primary focus	Diagnostic validity study in cancer	Replication study in cancer	Randomized implementation study
7	Hospital Anxiety and Depression Scale—Depression subscale	HADS-D	Depression	Yes	Yes	No
6	Brief Edinburgh Postnatal Depression Scale	BEDS	Depression	Yes	No	No
6	Center for Epidemiologic Studies Depression Scale–6	CESD-6	Depression	No	No	No
6	Hamilton Depression Scale–6	HAMD-6	Depression	No	No	No
5	Edinburgh Postnatal Depression Scale–5	EPDS-5	Depression	No	No	No
5	Emotion Thermometers	ET	Multiple domains	Yes	No	No
5	Geriatric Depression Scale–5	GDS-5	Depression	No	No	No

TABLE 9–1. Summary of rapid psychometric assessment methods for emotional disorder (*continued*)

Number of items	Scale	Abbreviation	Primary focus	Diagnostic validity study in cancer	Replication study in cancer	Randomized implementation study
5	World Health Organization 5-item screen (Well-Being Index)	WHO-5	Multiple domains	No	No	No
4	Brief Case-Find for Depression	BCFD	Depression	Yes	No	No
4	Geriatric Depression Scale–4	GDS-4	Depression	No	No	No
3	Edinburgh Postnatal Depression Scale— anxiety subscale	EPDS-3	Depression	No	No	No
3	Patient Health Questionnaire– 2+help question	PHQ-2+help question	Depression	Yes	No	No
2	Any two verbal questions	—	Depression	Yes	Yes	No
2	Beck Depression Inventory—2	BDI-2	Depression	No	No	No

TABLE 9–1.	Summary of rapid psychometric assessment methods for emotional disorder *(continued)*				
Number of items	Scale	Abbreviation	Primary focus	Diagnostic validity study in cancer	Replication study in cancer	Randomized implementation study
2	Distress Thermometer and Impact Thermometer (combined)	DT/IT	Distress	Yes	No	No
2	Patient Health Questionnaire–2	PHQ-2	Depression	Yes	No	No
1	Any single verbal item	—	Depression	Yes	Yes	No
1	Distress Thermometer	DT	Distress	Yes	Yes	Yes
1	Help Thermometer	HelpT	Desire for help	Yes	No	No
1	Impact Thermometer	IT	Distress	Yes	No	No
1	Geriatric Depression Scale 1	GDS1	Depression	No	No	No
1	Patient Health Questionnaire Q1	PHQ Q1	Depression	Yes	No	No
1	Patient Health Questionnaire Q2	PHQ Q2	Depression	Yes	No	No

TABLE 9–2.   Updated summary of meta-analyses in detection of distress or depression

Tool	Acceptability of tool	Weighted sensitivity	Weighted specificity	Case-finding clinical utility[a]	Screening clinical utility[a]	Number of studies
Distress @ 40%						
Distress Thermometer (1 item)	High	78.5% (95% CI, 69.8–86.1)	67.4% (95% CI, 60.1–74.3)	Poor	Average	4
Single verbal question (1 item)	High	67.3% (95% CI, 51.0–81.6)	78.9% (95% CI, 58.3%–93.7)	Poor	Average	4
HADS-T (14 items)	Low-Moderate	70.4% (95% CI, 56.1–82.9)	80.6% (95% CI, 72.8–87.4)	Average	Good	13
Depression @ 15%						
Single verbal question (1 item)	High	68.3% (95% CI, 52.9–81.8)	88.1% (95% CI, 80.4–94.1)	Poor	Excellent	9
Two verbal questions (2 items)	High	95.6% (95% CI, 88.9–99.3)	88.9% (95% CI, 79.0–96.0)	Average	Excellent	4
Distress Thermometer (1 item)	High	81.8% (95% CI, 0.768–0.865)	70.9% (95% CI, 63.7–77.6)	Poor	Good	5

TABLE 9–2. Updated summary of meta-analyses in detection of distress or depression (*continued*)

Tool	Acceptability of tool	Weighted sensitivity	Weighted specificity	Case-finding clinical utility[a]	Screening clinical utility[a]	Number of studies
EPDS (10 items)	Moderate	66.9% (95% CI, 51.7–80.4)	84.5% (95% CI, 78.3–89.9)	Poor	Good	4
HADS-A (7 items)	Moderate	77.1% (95% CI, 0.689–0.844)	84.2% (95% CI, 72.1–93.4)	Poor	Good	4
HADS-D (7 items)	Moderate	66.6% (95% CI, 54.5–77.7)	83.4% (95% CI, 75.6–89.9)	Poor	Good	18
HADS-T (14 items)	Low–Moderate	76.4% (95% CI, 69.9–82.2)	79.4% (95% CI, 59.9–93.5)	Poor	Good	8

Note. Summary updated from Mitchell 2010. DT = Distress Thermometer; EPDS = Edinburgh Postnatal Depression Scale; HADS-A = Hospital Anxiety and Depression Scale—Anxiety subscale; HADS-D = Hospital Anxiety and Depression Scale—Depression subscale; HADS-T = Hospital Anxiety and Depression Scale—Total score

[a]Calculated from clinical utility index assuming 40% prevalence of distress and 15% prevalence of depression.

people seen in routine care. This represents a gain of 3 fewer false negatives but at a cost of 8 additional false positives compared with clinicians using their own unassisted judgment. This high false-positive risk is why all patients who screen positive on the DT require a second-step assessment.

Several other methods of measuring distress have been proposed. The Psychological Distress Inventory (PDI) is a 13-item scale first proposed to measure distress in breast cancer patients (Morasso et al. 1996). The developers tested the PDI against a structured clinical interview as the criterion, and a cutoff of 28 or 29 is considered clinically significant. Several variants on the thermometer format have also been developed. Lees and Lloyd-Williams (1999) tested a VAS anchored with a sad face and a happy face. They reported a high correlation with the HADS-T but did not report sensitivity or specificity. Gil et al. (2005) conducted a multicenter study in Europe to assess the value of both the DT and a custom Mood Thermometer, using the HADS as the comparator. Interestingly, the DT was more highly associated with HADS Anxiety scores than Depression scores, whereas the Mood Thermometer was related to both HADS Anxiety and Depression scores. Mitchell et al. (2010a) developed a five-item Emotion Thermometer designed to measure multidomain emotional complications of cancer. It had good validity against DSM-IV-TR–defined depression and HADS-T in early cancer, but studies are awaited regarding interview-defined distress (Mitchell et al. 2010a). In addition to these custom scales, abbreviated versions of every major mood scale have been published using factor analysis or Rasch analysis. An important caveat is that often the abbreviated version is untested in an independent sample, making interpretation difficult.

Implementation of Rapid Psychometric Assessment

The availability of accurate and acceptable tools does not guarantee an improvement in patient outcomes. Any newly proposed tool or test should be compared with existing standards, even if the standard is unassisted clinical skills. Following diagnostic validity testing, a randomized controlled trial should be performed in which relevant outcomes are measured with and without the tool. Researchers may or may not also allocate dedicated treatment to the randomized group; however, as a minimum standard, usual care is offered to those in the control condition. Randomized implementation studies have shown mixed success to date (Bidstrup et al. 2011) and have yet to fulfill the promise of nonrandomized studies.

McLachlan et al. (2001) examined the effect of a coordinated psychosocial intervention that included assessment of quality of life in a group with cancers at various sites. Physicians in contact with 10 consecutive patients were randomly assigned to either a control group, in which the screening results were not made available to patients or staff, or an intervention group, in which the information was available to the staff. Midway through the study, the physicians changed intervention status. A significant decrease in depression was found in the intervention group, but only in the subgroup of patients who were depressed at baseline. In a crossover design in a study of patients with cancers at various sites who were undergoing palliative chemotherapy, Detmar et al. (2002) investigated the effect of assessment of quality of life on staff-patient discussions of related issues. Patients were randomly assigned to a control group with normal care or to an intervention group in which they were screened and the result was made available to the staff. Significantly more patients in the intervention group improved with respect to mental health and role functioning over time, which was included as a secondary outcome. Velikova et al. (2004) examined the effect of routine measurements on level of quality of life and management of quality of life in patients randomly assigned to one of three conditions: not screened, screened but with the results not available to the oncologist, or screened with the results available to the oncologist. Both screened groups had significantly improved quality of life when compared with the unscreened group. Carlson et al. (2010) examined the effect of screening on the level of psychological distress in lung and breast cancer patients randomized to minimal screening (results not available to patient or physician), full screening (results available to patient and physician), or full screening with optional triage and referral. In the last group, 20% fewer patients had continued high distress. Accepting a referral was the best predictor of improvement in this group. Other outcomes of interest from screening implementation studies include participation rates, effect on staff-patient communication, and effect on frontline intervention and referral. More long-term studies looking at these outcomes are urgently needed.

Discussion

Emotional disorders are important and treatable complications of cancer. Depression is a well-defined concept favored by clinicians, and distress is a broad, all-encompassing concept favored by patients. Frontline cancer clinicians who are not experts in mental health have varying levels of confidence and skills in the detection of depression and distress. Unassisted, they are likely to miss about half of those with clinically significant disorders and make a misidentification (false-positive judgment) in 10%–20% of cases. Clinicians who do not have access to screening tools are advised to make a repeat clinical assessment in cases of diagnostic uncertainty. A large number of tools are now available to help with identification of emotional disorders, including many that are royalty free and several that can be used simply and quickly by nonspecialists. Unfortunately, the evidence base supporting these methods is inadequate. In fact, only seven rapid methods have been examined in diagnostic validity studies (see Table 9–2).

Comparing the three validated methods (HADS-T, DT, and single verbal question) side by side (see Table 9–2) for the detection of distress suggests that in a screening capacity, there is currently no clear-cut best tool. The HADS-T has the highest clinical utility in screening but it is relatively long, difficult to score, and subject to copyright restrictions. The HADS-T is also the only method that could be considered as a confirmatory (rule-in or case-finding) test. The DT and single verbal question are acceptable but suffer from considerable inaccuracy. This can be partly overcome by incorporating a mandatory follow-up assessment for those who screen positive. This follow-up assessment should itself have good psychometric properties but also may require some compromise in duration. An example would be an assessment by an experienced mental health professional (where available). However, it should be noted that this two-step algorithm is most effective when the prevalence of the condition is low (i.e., for depression not for distress). Comparing the seven validated methods side by side (see Table 9–2) for the identification of depression shows the inadequate clinical utility of any tool for confirming a diagnosis of depression. This means that even in centers using screening tools, there is no substitute for skilled clinical assessment. However, in a screening capacity, most options offer reasonable accuracy. Most are flattered by the low prevalence of major depression when judged cross-sectionally (Figure 9–3). The performance of tools over multiple applications over the course of a year or more has yet to be examined.

Issues of acceptability (and cost) are likely to guide implementation as much as or more than accuracy alone. Lessons from studies with the Edmonton Symptom Assessment Scale (ESAS) show that completion rates vary by increasing age, higher opioid dose, and the presence of confusion (Chang et al. 2000). In attempts to tease out the optimal tool, a limited number of head-to-head studies have been conduced, but these are restricted to clinical depression. For example, Mitchell et al. (2008) examined several screening tools in a sample of 217 chemotherapy attendees who had early cancer (Mitchell et al. 2010a). In a comparison of the accuracy of the two-item Patient Health Questionnaire (PHQ-2), nine-item Patient Health Questionnaire (PHQ-9), HADS-T, and HADS–Depression subscale, the PHQ-2 was revealed to be the optimal strategy for detection of DSM-IV–

defined major or minor depression. Akizuki et al. (2003) found the HADS superior to either the Distress Thermometer or one verbal question. Grassi et al. (2009) also showed superiority of the HADS over ultra-short methods, with an overall accuracy for ICD-10 cases, but this did not reach statistical significance. In the most extensive comparison to date, Singer et al. (2008) compared six scales in 250 individuals diagnosed according to DSM-IV. Against the HADS, the Emotional Functioning subscale of the European Organization for Research and Treatment of Cancer Quality of Life Core Questionnaire (EORTC QLQ-C30) and a single-item VAS were highly accurate (Singer et al. 2008).

In summary, in spite of many worthwhile developments, it must be acknowledged that the accuracy of short and ultra-short tools is modest and no tool should be relied upon in isolation. Although the appropriate use of screening tools almost certainly enhances recognition of distress and depression in clinical practice, further assessment and treatment are warranted to capitalize on this enhanced identification. Rapid psychometric assessment can be used as part of a package of assessment that is augmented by measurement of quality of life, impairment, unmet needs (e.g., in a problem list), or desire for help (Hoffman et al. 2004; Marrit et al. 2008; Vachon 2006). Although screening has been extensively researched, further work is needed to compare screening strategies, screening targets, and screening methods.

Key Clinical Points

- Rapid psychometric assessment aims to take into account both acceptability and accuracy.

- Identification of depression alone is not sufficient; clinicians must also consider broader emotional issues such as anxiety or distress.

- The evidence base supporting current tools remains inadequate, and tools may perform differently when helping with the detection of depression compared with distress.

- Clinicians without access to tools should be prepared for repeating assessments where diagnoses are uncertain.

- Tools should not be relied upon alone but should be part of a holistic assessment that may include assessing unmet needs, disability, suicidal thoughts, quality of life, and desire for further support.

- Further research is needed, particularly regarding implementation of screening, use of longitudinal screening, and assessment of multiple emotional domains.

References

Adler NE, Page AEK (ed): Cancer Care for the Whole Patient: Meeting Psychosocial Health Needs. Washington, DC, National Academies Press, 2007

Akechi T, Nakano T, Akizuki N, et al: Somatic symptoms for diagnosing major depression in cancer patients. Psychosomatics 44:244–248, 2003

Akizuki N, Akechi T, Nakanishi T, et al: Development of a brief screening interview for adjustment disorders and major depression in patients with cancer. Cancer 97:2605–2613, 2003

American Psychiatric Association: Diagnostic and Statistical Manual of Mental Disorders, 4th Edition. Washington, DC, American Psychiatric Association, 1994

American Psychiatric Association: Diagnostic and Statistical Manual of Mental Disorders, 4th Edition, Text Revision. Washington, DC, American Psychiatric Association, 2000

Anderson WG, Alexander SC, Rodriguez KL, et al: "What concerns me is…" Expression of emotion by advanced cancer patients during outpatient visits. Support Care Cancer 16:803–811, 2008

Banks E, Byles JE, Gibson RE, et al: Is psychological distress in people living with cancer related to the fact of diagnosis, current treatment or level of disability? Findings from a large Australian study. Med J Aust 193(suppl):S62–S67, 2010

Bidstrup PE, Johansen C, Mitchell AJ: Screening for cancer-related distress: summary of evidence from tools to programmes. Acta Oncol 50:194–204, 2011

Butt Z, Wagner LI, Beaumont JL, et al: Longitudinal screening and management of fatigue, pain, and emotional distress associated with cancer therapy. Support Care Cancer 16:151–159, 2008

Carlson LE, Angen M, Cullum J, et al: High levels of untreated distress and fatigue in cancer patients. Br J Cancer 90:2297–2304, 2004

Carlson LE, Groff SL, Maciejewski O, et al: Screening for distress in lung and breast cancer outpatients: a randomized controlled trial. J Clin Oncol 28:4884–4891, 2010

Chang VT, Hwang SS, Feuerman M: Validation of the Edmonton Symptom Assessment Scale. Cancer 88:2164–2171, 2000

Chochinov HM, Wilson KG, Enns M, et al: "Are you depressed?" Screening for depression in the terminally ill. Am J Psychiatry 154:674–676, 1997

Derogatis LR: Brief Symptom Inventory (BSI): Administration, Scoring, and Procedures Manual, 3rd Edition. Minneapolis, MN, National Computer Systems, 1993

Detmar SB, Muller MJ, Wever LD, et al: The patient–physician relationship. Patient-physician communication during outpatient palliative treatment visits: an observational study. JAMA 285:1351–1357, 2001

Detmar SB, Muller MJ, Schornagel JH, et al: Health-related quality-of-life assessments and patient-physician communication: a randomized controlled trial. JAMA 288:3027–3034, 2002

Faller H, Bulzebruck H, Drings P, et al: Coping, distress, and survival among patients with lung cancer. Arch Gen Psychiatry 56:756–762, 1999

Fallowfield L, Ratcliffe D, Jenkins V, et al: Psychiatric morbidity and its recognition by doctors in patients with cancer. Br J Cancer 84:1011–1015, 2001

Folstein MF: Reliability, validity, and clinical application of Visual Analog Mood Scale. Psychol Med 3:479–486, 1973

Gil F, Grassi L, Travado L, et al: Southern European Psycho-Oncology Study Group. Use of distress and depression thermometers to measure psychosocial morbidity among Southern European cancer patients. Support Care Cancer 13:600–606, 2005

Grassi L, Sabato S, Rossi E, et al: Affective syndromes and their screening in cancer patients with early and stable disease: Italian ICD-10 data and performance of the Distress Thermometer from the Southern European Psycho-Oncology Study (SEPOS). J Affect Disord 114:193–199, 2009

Goldberg D, Williams P: A User's Guide to the General Health Questionnaire. Berkshire, England, Nfer-Nelson, 1991

Hoffman BM, Zevon MA, D'Arrigo MC, et al: Screening for distress in cancer patients: the NCCN rapid-screening measure. Psychooncology 13:792–799, 2004

Holland JC, Bultz BD; National Comprehensive Cancer Network (NCCN): The NCCN guideline for distress management: a case for making distress the sixth vital sign. J Natl Compr Canc Netw 5:3–7, 2007

Jones LE, Doebbeling CC: Suboptimal depression screening following cancer diagnosis. Gen Hosp Psychiatry 29:547–554, 2007

Keller M, Sommerfeldt S, Fischer C, et al: Recognition of distress and psychiatric morbidity in cancer patients: a multi-method approach. Ann Oncol 15:1243–1249, 2004

Kennard BD, Smith SM, Olvera R, et al: Nonadherence in adolescent oncology patients: preliminary data on psychological risk factors and relationships to outcome. J Clin Psychol Med Settings 11:30–39, 2004

Kvåle K: Do cancer patients always want to talk about difficult emotions? A qualitative study of cancer inpatients communication needs. Eur J Oncol Nurs 11:320–327, 2007

Lees N, Lloyd-Williams M: Assessing depression in palliative care patients using the visual analogue scale: a pilot study. Eur J Cancer Care (Engl) 8:220–223, 1999

Lloyd-Williams M, Dennis M, Taylor F: A prospective study to compare three depression screening tools in patients who are terminally ill. Gen Hosp Psychiatry 26:384–389, 2004

Luckett T, Butow PN, King MT, et al: A review and recommendations for optimal outcome measures of anxiety, depression and general distress in studies evaluating psychosocial interventions for English-speaking adults with heterogeneous cancer diagnoses. Support Care Cancer 18:1241–1262, 2010

Mariotto AB, Yabroff KR, Shao Y, et al: Projections of the cost of cancer care in the United States: 2010–2020. J Natl Cancer Inst 103:117–128, 2011

Marrit A, Tuinman MA, Gazendam-Donofrio SM, et al: Screening and referral for psychosocial distress in oncologic practice use of the distress thermometer. Cancer 113:870–878, 2008

McLachlan SA, Allenby A, Matthews J, et al: Randomized trial of coordinated psychosocial interventions based on patient self-assessments versus standard care to improve the psychosocial functioning of patients with cancer. J Clin Oncol 19:4117–4125, 2001

Mitchell AJ: Are one or two simple questions sufficient to detect depression in cancer and palliative care? A Bayesian meta-analysis. Br J Cancer 98:1934–1943, 2008a

Mitchell AJ: How to design and implement screening studies, in Psycho-Oncology 2nd Edition. Edited by Holland JC, Brietbart WS, Jacobsen PB. New York, Oxford University Press, 2008b, pp 648–654

Mitchell AJ: Short screening tools for cancer-related distress: a review and diagnostic validity meta-analysis. J Natl Compr Canc Netw 8:487–494, 2010

Mitchell AJ, Kaar S, Coggan C, et al: Acceptability of common screening methods used to detect distress and related mood disorders-preferences of cancer specialists and non-specialists. Psychooncology 17:226–236, 2008

Mitchell AJ, Baker-Glenn E, Symonds P: Can the distress thermometer be improved by additional mood domains? Part I: validation of the emotion thermometer tool. Psychooncology 19:125–133, 2010a

Mitchell AJ, Meader N, Symonds P: Diagnostic validity of the Hospital Anxiety and Depression Scale (HADS) in cancer and palliative settings: a meta-analysis. J Affect Disord 126:335–348, 2010b

Mitchell AJ, Chan M, Bhatti H, et al: Prevalence of depression, anxiety, and adjustment disorder in oncological, haematological, and palliative-care settings: a meta-analysis of 94 interview-based studies. Lancet Oncol 12:160–174, 2011a

Mitchell AJ, Hussain N, Grainger L, et al: Identification of patient-reported distress by clinical nurse specialists in routine oncology practice: a multicentre UK study. Psychooncology 20:1076–1083, 2011b

Morasso G, Costantini M, Baracco G, et al: Assessing psychological distress in cancer patients: validation of a self-administered questionnaire. Oncology 53:295–302, 1996

National Comprehensive Cancer Network: NCCN Clinical Practice Guidelines in Oncology Distress Management V.1.2007. 2007. Available at: http://www.nccn.org/professionals/physician_gls/PDF/distress.pdf. Accessed July 30, 2012.

Passik SD, Dugan W, McDonald MV, et al: Oncologists' recognition of depression in their patients with cancer. J Clin Oncol 16:1594–1600, 1998

Patrick DL, Ferketich SL, Frame PS: National Institutes of Health State-of-the-Science Conference Statement. Symptom management in cancer: pain, depression, and fatigue. July 15–17, 2002. J Natl Cancer Inst 32:9–16, 2004

Pirl W, Muriel A, Hwang V, et al: Screening for psychosocial distress: a national survey of oncologists. J Support Oncol 5:499–504, 2007

Pollak KI, Arnold RM, Jeffreys AS, et al: Oncologist communication about emotion during visits with patients with advanced cancer. J Clin Oncol 25:5748–5752, 2007

Rodriguez KL, Bayliss N, Alexander SC, et al: How oncologists and their patients with advanced cancer communicate about health-related quality of life. Psychooncology 19:490–499, 2010

Roth AJ, Kornblith AB, Batel-Copel L, et al: Rapid screening for psychologic distress in men with prostate carcinoma: a pilot study. Cancer 82:1904–1908, 1998

Satin JR, Linden W, Phillips MJ: Depression as a predictor of disease progression and mortality in cancer patients: a meta-analysis. Cancer 115:5349–5361, 2009

Shim EJ, Mehnert A, Koyama A, et al: Health-related quality of life in breast cancer: cross-cultural survey of German, Japanese, and South Korean patients. Breast Cancer Res Treat 99:341–350, 2006

Singer S, Danker H, Dietz A, et al: Screening for mental disorders in laryngeal cancer patients: a comparison of 6 methods. Psychooncology 17:280–286, 2008

Söllner W, DeVries A, Steixner E, et al: How successful are oncologists in identifying patient distress, perceived social support, and need for psychosocial counselling? Br J Cancer 84:179–185, 2001

Steginga SK, Campbell A, Ferguson M, et al: Socio-demographic, psychosocial and attitudinal predictors of help seeking after cancer diagnosis. Psychooncology 17:997–1005, 2008

Taylor S, Harley C, Campbell LJ, et al: Discussion of emotional and social impact of cancer during outpatient oncology consultations. Psychooncology 20:242–251, 2011

Vachon M: Psychosocial distress and coping after cancer treatment. Cancer Nurs 29(suppl):26–31, 2006

Velikova G, Booth L, Smith AB, et al: Measuring quality of life in routine oncology practice improves communication and patient well-being: a randomized controlled trial. J Clin Oncol 22:714–724, 2004

Vodermaier A, Linden W, Siu C: Screening for emotional distress in cancer patients: a systematic review of assessment instruments. J Natl Cancer Inst 101:1464–1488, 2009

Von Essen L, Larsson G, Oberg K, et al: Satisfaction with care: associations with health-related quality of life and psychosocial function among Swedish patients with endocrine gastrointestinal tumors. Eur J Cancer Care 11:91–99, 2002

Walker J, Sharpe M: Depression care for people with cancer: a collaborative care intervention. Gen Hosp Psychiatry 31:436–441, 2009

Zabora J, BrintzenhofeSzoc K, Curbow B, et al: The prevalence of psychological distress by cancer site. Psychooncology 10:19–28, 2001

Zigmond AS, Snaith RP: The Hospital Anxiety and Depression Scale. Acta Psychiatr Scand 67:361–370, 1983

CHAPTER 10

The Value of Quality of Life Assessment in Cancer Patients

Bernhard Holzner, Ph.D.
Johannes Giesinger, Ph.D.
Fabio Efficace, Ph.D.

PATIENTS' HEALTH STATUS has traditionally been assessed by physicians' ratings, but this practice is now acknowledged to underestimate the severity of symptoms (Pakhomov et al. 2008; Weingart et al. 2005) and to lack sensitivity to change (Basch et al. 2009). Furthermore, patients' self-reports frequently identify symptoms earlier than clinicians do (Basch 2009), or even capture side effects that clinicians completely miss (Pakhomov et al. 2008; Weingart et al. 2005). Good examples of such underrecognized and poorly studied chemotherapy side effects are taste alterations (Bernhardson et al. 2008; Hong et al. 2009; Zabernigg et al. 2010) and peripheral neuropathy (Farquhar-Smith 2011), which are frequently reported by patients but rarely asked about by physicians. Symptoms that may not be volunteered by patients include sexual issues (Stead et al. 2003) and emotional difficulties (Fallowfield et al. 2001). Detmar et al. (2000) report that a high percentage of patients want to talk about emotional and social issues with their treating physician but expect these issues to be raised by physicians, who in turn are often too pressed for time to adequately inquire about patient distress (Holland 1999). As a consequence, clinically significant distress often goes unrecognized by medical staff members in clinical oncology settings (Holland 1999; Payne et al. 1999) and is underreferred to mental health professionals (Newport and Nemeroff 1998; Sharpe et al. 2004).

Hence, in the last two decades there has been growing awareness of the importance of incorporating patient-reported outcomes (PROs) into oncology research.[1] This development is reflected in the "Guidance for Industry" by the U.S. Food and Drug Administration (FDA; 2009), which recommends including PROs in studies for medical product development. Similarly, the European Medicines Agency has encouraged the use of PROs to assess outcomes in clinical trials (European Medicines Agency, Committee for Medicinal Products for Human Use 2005).

Within PRO research, a major concept is quality of life (QOL), a term that is often used synonymously with PRO and that refers to a number of physical and psychosocial symptoms as well as to functioning domains. To assess PROs (or QOL) in cancer patients, a number of valid and reliable measures have been developed (Fayers and Machin 2000). The main use of these questionnaires has been in clinical trials to provide an additional outcome measure to compare oncological treatment regimens, with the questionnaires usually being administered at different stages of the disease and at various times in the course of treatment. However, QOL is also assessed in daily clinical routines (Erharter et al. 2010; Luckett et al. 2009; Taenzer et al. 2000; Velikova et al. 2004), where PROs may enhance symptom management and contribute to clinical decision making. Thus, aside from measuring adverse events[2] and physical symptoms, PROs also address psychosocial issues, such as anxiety or depression, providing valuable information on patients' health status and therewith are able to contribute to improving symptom management in oncology.

---

[1]According to the U.S. Food and Drug Administration (2009), *patient-reported outcomes* are defined as a "measurement based on a report that comes directly from the patient (i.e., study subject) about the status of a patient's health condition without amendment or interpretation of the patient's response by a clinician or anyone else. A PRO can be measured by self-report or by interview provided that the interviewer records only the patient's response" (p. 32).

[2]According to the U.S. National Cancer Institute (2010a), *adverse events* are defined as "any unfavorable and unintended sign (including an abnormal laboratory finding), symptom, or disease temporally associated with the use of a medical treatment or procedure that may or may *not* be considered related to the medical treatment or procedure" (p. 1).

Assessment Instruments

A number of QOL instruments have been developed for use in oncology; these range from generic QOL measures to cancer-specific ones (see Table 10–1). Generic measures can be particularly suitable for health policy research and are not devised for any specific cancer population. Cancer-specific measures have the advantage of addressing problems specific to a given cancer population. These latter measures can be a valuable source of information, particularly in clinical trials when comparing different types of treatments. However, there is no gold standard; that is, no measure is the most accurate and generally accepted, and no measure is useful in all different settings. Indeed, choosing among the most appropriate measures depends on a number of issues, including the clinical setting (research or routine practice), the purpose of the QOL assessment, and the specific cancer population being evaluated. Furthermore, specific information on psychometric properties of the measure (e.g., reliability, validity, responsiveness[3]) must be taken into account when selecting a measure for a specific purpose. Additionally, when choosing an instrument for a given setting, one should select a robust psychometric measure, with proven evidence of the development process and published data of the psychometric characteristics.

European Organisation for Research and Treatment of Cancer Measurement System

The European Organisation for Research and Treatment of Cancer (EORTC) Quality of Life Group has developed a measurement system including questionnaires for general cancer-specific issues, specific patient groups, or specific symptoms. All of these measures have been developed cross-culturally (i.e., including patients and researchers from various countries in all development stages) and are available in a large number of languages. Recently, the EORTC Quality of Life Group published the first computer-adaptive test (CAT) measures for its PRO scales. The EORTC measures are available at www.eortc.be/qol.

---

[3]*Reliability* refers to the consistency of multiple measurements. *Validity* denotes that an instrument measures what it intends to measure. *Responsiveness* describes an instrument's ability to capture change in the measured construct.

TABLE 10–1.   Some frequently used quality of life measures

Instrument	Target population	Number of items	Time recall period	Domains evaluated (number of items)
Functional Assessment of Cancer Therapy—General (FACT-G; Cella et al. 1993)	Cancer-specific	27	Past 7 days	Emotional well-being (6 items); functional well-being (7); physical well-being (7); social/family well-being (7)
Functional Living Index—Cancer (FLIC; Schipper et al. 1984)	Cancer-specific	22	Times range from today to past month	Physical well-being and ability (9 items); psychological well-being (6); social well-being (2); nausea (2); hardship due to cancer (3)
EORTC QLQ-C30 (Aaronson et al. 1993)	Cancer-specific	30 (revised from 36 items in initial validation study)	Past week	Functioning domains: physical (5 items); role (2); emotional (4); cognitive (2); social (2); global QOL (2) Symptom domains/items: 3 fatigue; 2 nausea/vomiting; 2 pain; 1 each dyspnea, sleep disturbance, appetite loss, constipation, diarrhea, financial impact

TABLE 10–1. Some frequently used quality of life measures (*continued*)

Instrument	Target population	Number of items	Time recall period	Domains evaluated (number of items)
Rotterdam Symptom Check List (RSCL; de Haes et al. 1996)	Cancer-specific	38 (30 symptoms, 8 activity items)	Past week	Activity (8 items); response options range from "unable" to "with difficulty without help" Symptoms: psychological distress (8 items); physical distress (19); disease-specific symptoms (3)
Short-Form 36-Item Health Survey (SF-36; Ware et al. 1992)	Generic	36	Last week or last 4 weeks	Physical and mental component summary scales Subscales: physical functioning (10 items), role-physical functioning (4), bodily pain (2), general health (5), vitality (4), social functioning (2), role-emotional functioning (3), mental health (5)
EQ-5D (EuroQol Group 1990)	Generic	5 items and global health state visual-analog scale	Today	Mobility (1 item), self-care (1), usual activities (1), pain/discomfort (1), depression/anxiety (1), global health state (1)

EORTC QLQ-C30

The EORTC QLQ-C30 (Aaronson et al. 1993), an internationally validated and widely used cancer-targeted QOL instrument, assesses various aspects of QOL. This 30-item questionnaire contains five functioning scales, a scale for global QOL, and nine symptom scales (see Table 10–1). For palliative care patients, a 15-item short form is available (QLQ-C15-PAL). This short form is limited to those symptoms and functioning domains that are of specific relevance in palliative care patients.

Specific EORTC Questionnaire Modules

In addition to the QLQ-C30 core questionnaire, the EORTC measurement system provides disease-specific questionnaire modules as add-ons. These so-called modules have been developed for a wide range of diagnostic groups (e.g., breast cancer, colorectal cancer, lung cancer, testicular cancer), for specific symptoms (e.g., fatigue, peripheral neuropathy), for specific treatments (e.g., high-dose chemotherapy), and for other important cancer-related issues (e.g., patient information, patient satisfaction, spiritual well-being, quality of life in elderly patients).

EORTC CAT Measures

Within an ongoing project of the EORTC Quality of Life Group, CAT measures for the QLQ-C30 scales are currently being developed. These new CAT measures are conceptualized to reflect the same constructs as the QLQ-C30 scales (Petersen et al. 2010). At this writing, the EORTC CAT measures for Physical Functioning (Petersen et al. 2011) and Fatigue (Giesinger et al. 2011) are available, with the other constructs of the QLQ-C30 to follow in the foreseeable future.

When completing a CAT, a patient does not fill in a fixed set of items as in traditional questionnaires, but instead obtains an individually tailored item set. For this purpose, each CAT comprises an item bank (i.e., a set of items with their psychometric characteristics) and an algorithm for selecting the most informative items to be administered to a certain patient. This selection is based on the patient's responses to the previous items. CAT measures significantly reduce the number of items administered to a patient and increases measurement precision. Therefore, patient burden is limited not only due to the shorter test length, but also through omitting items that are not relevant to a patient's health status.

Functional Assessment of Chronic Illness Therapy

In the United States, Cella et al. (1993) developed the Functional Assessment of Chronic Illness Therapy (FACIT). This includes the widely used Functional Assessment of Cancer Therapy—General (FACT-G), which comprises 27 items covering physical, social, emotional, and functional well-being. To supplement the FACT-G, a wide range of disease- or symptom-specific questionnaires are available within the FACIT measurement system, including versions in numerous languages that have been validated cross-culturally. For further details see Table 10–1. The FACIT measures are available at www.facit.org.

Patient Reported Outcomes Measurement Information System

The Patient Reported Outcomes Measurement Information System (PROMIS; www.nihpromis.org), supported by the U.S. National Institutes of Health (NIH), has been developing item banks for major PRO constructs (e.g., pain, depression, fatigue, sexual functioning). Item banks contain items for a certain construct and their respective psychometric characteristics. Thus, item banks are the basis for CATs and also allow the creation of questionnaires with a fixed item set for all patients (i.e., traditional questionnaires). Development of the PROMIS item banks is done in the United States only, although translations of the measures are planned. The PROMIS measures are available via www.nihpromis.org.

PRO Version of the Common Terminology Criteria for Adverse Events

In a collaborative U.S. project, the NIH, the National Cancer Institute, and the Memorial Sloan-Kettering Cancer Center have recently started to develop PRO measures for the Common Terminology Criteria for Adverse Events (CTCAE). This project, called the Patient-Reported Outcomes version of the Common Terminology Criteria for Adverse Events (PRO-CTCAE), has created items assessing symptom severity, frequency, and impact for those adverse events for which self-report is reasonable (excluding, e.g., symptoms requiring laboratory tests to determine). To date, these items have been evaluated within interviews with cancer patients and are about to undergo validation in a large cancer patient sample (National Cancer Institute 2010b). Additional details are available at http://outcomes.cancer.gov/tools/pro-ctcae.html.

Interpretation of Quality of Life Scores

Minimal Important Differences and Changes in QOL Scores

To improve interpretation of QOL data collected within clinical trials, research efforts have focused on minimal important differences (MIDs) and minimal important changes (MICs) over time. An MID or MIC is the smallest difference in PRO score points that is of clinical relevance.

MIDs are of special importance to clinical trials investigating the impact of specific interventions, because they are required to assess whether or not the size of an observed impact is of clinical relevance. In general, two different methodological approaches to defining MIDs have been employed, using anchor-based and distribution-based criteria. Anchor-based criteria relate differences in QOL scores to additional parameters such as global patient or physician ratings on relevance of change in health status, or clinical parameters (e.g., treatment phase, response to treatment). This allows calculating score differences for patients indicating relevant change or not, for patients responding to treatment or not, and so forth. Probably the most cited study on MICs for the EORTC QLQ-C30 was conducted by Osoba et al. (1998) using an anchor-based approach. As anchors for the QOL scales, the authors used single items asking for change of the respective symptom with seven response categories ranging from "very much worse" to "very much better." Based on this anchor item, a change of 5–10 score points on a QLQ-C30 was considered "a little" change, 10–20 points as "moderate" change, and >20 points as "very much" change. A more recent study from Maringwa et al. (2011) used World Health Organization performance status and weight change as anchors for a sample of lung cancer patients. Based on an anchor-based study including a range of QOL instruments, Ringash et al. (2007) proposed 10% of scale range as a rule of thumb for determining MIDs.

Distribution-based methodology employs distribution of QOL scores in certain patient groups using standard deviation units to indicate MIDs. Analyses referring to the standard measurement error of a QOL scale (e.g., Terwee et al. 2009) are as well classified as being distribution based.

A study by Eton et al. (2004) combined distribution- and anchor-based criteria for MIDs for the Functional Assessment of Cancer Therapy—Breast (FACT-B) in breast cancer patients. Distribution-based criteria included standard deviation and standard error of measurement, whereas anchor-based criteria included Eastern Cooperative Oncology Group (ECOG) performance status, current pain, and response to treatment. The authors found congruency of both methods, resulting in MIDs of 5–6 points for the Functional Assessment of Cancer Therapy—General (FACT-G) and 7–8 points for the FACT-B.

Thresholds for Absolute QOL Scores

Whereas the MIDs and MICs help to interpret the impact of disease and treatment in a relative manner by comparison to previous assessments or patient groups, these thresholds do not allow calculating symptom prevalences, and MIDs are not sufficient for screening patients for treatment needs and symptom burden. Therefore, researchers have increasingly started to introduce cutoff scores to define absolute thresholds for clinically relevant symptom burden or impairment. This allows the interpretation of absolute scores, the calculation of prevalence rates, and symptom screening within clinical routine.

Some studies have dichotomized PRO data using different types of cut-off scores—for example, to calculate symptom prevalences or to flag relevant symptom burden in studies using QOL data for symptom screening or monitoring within clinical routine. This is mostly done based on rather arbitrary thresholds defined ad hoc, because little research has been done so far on establishing cutoff scores empirically. Current approaches are either referring to the wording of the response categories, to percentiles of score distributions (in particular percentiles from general population), or to external criteria.

Cutoff Scores Based on Wording of Response Categories

Johnsen et al. (2009) calculated symptom prevalences for hematological patients based on the QLQ-C30 using a cutoff related to wording of the response categories of the questionnaire ("not at all," "a little," "quite a bit," "very much"). According to the authors, a patient had a symptom or problem if the score corresponded to at least "a little" and had a severe symptom or problem if the score corresponded to "quite a bit" or "very much." A similar approach to calculating toxicity rates was taken by Oberguggenberger et al. (2011) in breast cancer patients receiving endocrine therapy with aromatase inhibitors.

Distribution-Based Cutoff Scores

In a study by Velikova et al. (2004) on the impact of routine QOL monitoring on a range of PROs, relevant symptom burden was indicated by flagging patients exceeding mean general population scores on the QLQ-C30. In their study on symptom monitoring within daily clinical routine, Erharter et al. (2010) suggested the use of the 75th or 90th percentiles of the PRO score distribution in patients with the same diagnosis and treatment phase. Fayers (2001) suggested percentiles from QOL score distribution in the general population as possible cutoff scores for determining clinically relevant symptom burden.

Criterion-Based Cutoff Scores

For developing cutoff scores, some researchers have used different external criteria, including, for example, other QOL measures or patient ratings. Snyder et al. (2010) established cutoff scores for the QLQ-C30 using unmet needs defined by dichotomized scores from the Supportive Care Needs Survey (SCNS) as external criteria. For six QLQ-C30 scales, sensitivity was above 0.85 and specificity was above 0.50 with regard to unmet care needs. A more detailed analysis on congruency of classifications based on these two instruments was given in a previous paper (Snyder et al. 2009a).

Another recent study from Snyder et al. (2011) used different external criteria for the QLQ-C30—namely, patient ratings of their two most bothersome issues. For prediction of these most bothersome issues, sensitivity was 0.75 for aspects of functioning (specificity 0.64), whereas for symptoms, prediction was somewhat more accurate (sensitivity = 0.83; specificity = 0.76). The authors also found that diagnostic performance of change scores (i.e., score difference from previous assessment) was lower than that of absolute scores.

Hwang et al. (2002) developed cutoff scores for a single-item fatigue measure with a score range from 0 to 10. The authors categorized the scale range into four categories ("none," "mild," "moderate," and "severe fatigue") separately for usual and worst fatigue. To define these cutoff scores, they used further fatigue measures, QOL measures, and distress measures, plus Karnofsky performance status and survival, as criteria in multiple analyses of variance. Based on this methodology, they concluded that for screening purposes fatigue levels exceeding a score of 3 for usual fatigue or of 4 for worst may require further assessment.

Adjusting Thresholds to Sociodemographic and Clinical Patient Characteristics

Related to the development of cutoff scores for QOL measures is the question regarding to what sociodemographic or clinical patient characteristics the cutoff scores should be adjusted. So far, this question has not been investigated sufficiently. A common approach is to adjust QOL scores to sex and age (Hjermstad et al. 1998; Schwarz and Hinz 2001), which might be useful for some symptoms but rather problematic for others because it may disguise important differences. Adjusting, for example, physical functioning to age is reasonable because in general, young persons are expected to have better physical functioning than old persons. In contrast, it is more difficult to decide whether or not to adjust distress or depression scores to age, because this may even out true age-related differences. Also, women tend to report higher somatic symptom levels than men (Giesinger et al. 2009; Schwarz and Hinz 2001); in adjusting the respective cutoff scores to sex, discrepancies in symptom prevalences disappear, and in the context of symptom screening, symptoms may be underrecognized in women. With regard to pain, this might be especially difficult because current evidence (Greenspan et al. 2007) suggests that higher pain levels in women may be related to physiological factors (e.g., estrogen level; Aloisi 2003) as well as to response behavior. Thus, whereas differences in pain reporting (e.g., due to sex-related differential item functioning) lend support to the adjustment of pain cutoff scores to sex, differences in physiology may preclude such adjustment. Future research on PRO cutoff scores should therefore also address the matter of adjusting cutoff scores to patient characteristics for each PRO domain separately.

Overview of Clinical Applications of Quality of Life Data

Outcome Measure in Clinical Trials

Although the main focus of this chapter is to outline the use of QOL assessment in clinical practice, a paragraph needs to be dedicated to the historical use of QOL as an outcome measure in the context of clinical trials. In 1996 the American Society of Clinical Oncology pointed to the key role that QOL _assessment plays in cancer research. Indeed, major research organizations routinely consider inclusion of such outcomes in randomized controlled trials (Osoba 1992). Some of these QOL data have also served as a basis for (or in support of) drug approval by the FDA (Rock et al. 2007). Notably, however, in rare examples, QOL data from clinical trials have also served as the only source of information for drug approvals by the FDA (Johnson et al. 2003).

We emphasize that the implementation of a QOL assessment in a clinical trial setting should follow rigorous methodological rules to provide meaningful data to better inform clinical decisions (Efficace et al. 2003). Actually, a number of previous works have suggested that if such QOL assessment is not performed by following a number of methodological criteria, it is unlikely to provide informative data to be used to improve patient care (Efficace et al. 2004a).

The need to collect QOL data in a clinical trial setting can be more pronounced in specific trial contexts, such as when the prognosis of the patients under study is unfavorable, when the expected impact on clinical effectiveness is small, or when the expected impact on QOL is large. QOL can also be the main end point in equivalence studies when the treatments are expected to be equivalent in clinical efficacy; in this case, a new treatment would be deemed preferable if it confers some QOL benefit. Several randomized controlled trials in oncology have successfully implemented QOL or other types of PROs and have provided additional robust data to better understand overall treatment effectiveness from the patients' perspective. The inclusion of QOL evaluation in cancer clinical trials has been informative, providing useful additional data, for example, regarding brain, breast, and prostate cancer patients (de Haes et al. 2003; Osoba et al. 1999; Taphoorn et al. 2005).

QOL Monitoring in Daily Clinical Routine

QOL studies historically have been conducted with the expectation that in time health care providers would routinely incorporate measurements of QOL into clinical practice. Now, advanced computer technology widely available at medical institutions allows a reduction of required human resources, making the routine collection of data feasible in busy clinical practices. Furthermore, technology enables real-time QOL assessments and immediate presentation of results to clinicians. To extend QOL assessments beyond the clinical setting, Web-based data collection applications can be used. Such tools allow monitoring of QOL and symptoms at time points that may be important for the patients' well-being, even when they are away from the hospital.

Interestingly, a number of studies have shown that patients' self-reported QOL parameters provide independent prognostic information about survival in advanced diseases (Efficace et al. 2008; Gotay et al. 2008). Potentially, this finding could have crucial clinical implications, for example, by allowing clinicians using QOL information in routine practice to have additional prognostic information concerning survival or disease progression for a particular patient. Although this is potentially another added value of collecting QOL data in routine practice, ways of actually using this information have to be explored in future studies.

QOL Parameters as Prognostic Factors

What is the role of patient-related factors as concerns prognosis? Do they add helpful information beyond strong clinical or laboratory data? In considering these questions, it is important to distinguish between two broad areas of research. Given the heterogeneity of concepts that have been considered in the scientific literature, a brief introduction on the topic is necessary. First, interest in the psychosocial aspects of cancer patients, as related to clinical outcomes, has a long history (Derogatis et al. 1979). Within this broad area of research, it is important to distinguish between studies stemming from behavioral research, which have used psychosocial theory–driven constructs, and studies that have exclusively focused on "QOL parameters." For example, the former studies have focused on social support, psychosocial distress, and mental adjustment, whereas the latter studies have examined the somewhat limited QOL aspects, such as pain, fatigue, or emotional and physical functioning (de Graeff et al. 2001). Studies that have investigated the link between psychosocial factors and clinical outcomes have often been plagued by methodological shortcomings, including relatively small cohorts and inadequate control of biomedical factors, which have hampered clear conclusions (Mulder et al. 1992). Although some studies that evaluated the relationships between psychosocial variables and survival have noted positive results (Butow et al. 1999; Spiegel et al. 1989), more recent work provides little consistent evidence that psychological coping styles or psychosocial/psychotherapy interventions are related to survival in cancer patients (Chow et al. 2004; Coyne et al. 2007; Petticrew et al. 2002).

Along with this historical line of psychosocial research, a second, more recent, line of study has focused on investigating the predictive power of patients' QOL parameters for length of survival. This is actually one of the most interesting findings of the last decade in QOL research. These studies have used methodologically sound QOL instruments, such as the EORTC QLQ-C30. The prognostic value of QOL parameters has been shown in a wide range of specific cancer populations, including breast (Kramer et al. 2000), colorectal (Maisey et al. 2002), lung (Eton et al. 2003), melanoma (Chiarion-Sileni et al. 2003), and esophageal (Blazeby et al. 2001), as well as in large cohorts of patients with varied malignancies (Dancey et al. 1997). Interestingly, some authors have also validated their findings on independent samples. Efficace et al. (2006), for example, found that patients' self-reported "social functioning" was an independent prognostic factor for survival in advanced colorectal cancer patients beyond a number of key traditional prognostic indicators and also validated this finding in an independent sample of colorectal cancer patients, thus lending further support that this QOL aspect indeed provides unique prognostic information in this population (Efficace et al. 2008). For more extensive discussion on the topic, readers can consult the review by Montazeri (2009).

We emphasize, however, that the large majority of studies investigating the prognostic value of QOL parameters for survival have been conducted with advanced metastatic cancer populations, and this finding was not replicated in patients with earlier stages of the disease (Efficace et al. 2004b). What is the reason for the association between QOL parameters and length of survival in advanced disease? Some hypotheses have been proposed to explain the mechanisms underlying the association between health-related QOL data and survival (Coates et al. 1992, 2000). At the current stage of research in this area, the most plausible explanation is that patients' QOL ratings on QOL questionnaires might reflect an early perception of the severity of the disease in a more accurate way than conventional prognostic indices. Therefore, patients who report worse QOL are the ones with a worse underlying disease. This hypothesis does not imply a true causative relationship between QOL parameters and survival but indeed underscores that patients themselves are better judges of their own health status than are other traditionally known clinical prognostic indicators.

Regardless of the potential clinical implications of the association between QOL parameters and length of survival in advanced disease, the main scientific value of this area of research is to point out that what patients are reporting, through the use of standardized QOL questionnaires, provides clinically meaningful information about prognosis that often goes beyond traditional prognostic indicators. This evidence could have crucial clinical implications, for example, by allowing clinicians using QOL information in routine practice to have additional prognostic information on a particular patient. In this scenario, the physician could simply ask the patient to complete a given questionnaire and then could interpret the patient's score for prognostic purposes. In advanced-disease settings, this information could further assist physicians to optimize the use of palliative care and to make more informed and tailor-made treatment decisions.

Electronic QOL Data Capture

Several studies have shown that the use of computer technology is an acceptable and efficient method for obtaining self-reported information on physical and psychosocial symptoms. These data are highly comparable to those collected by paper-and-pencil approaches (Coons et al. 2009; Velikova et al. 1999). Touch-screen computer surveys are also acceptable for older patients, even though these individuals may lack computer experience (Buxton et al. 1998; Taenzer et al. 1997).

For the incorporation of PROs in clinical routines, the use of computer technology is indispensable. Computer-based testing provides an innovative methodology for PRO data collection that makes symptom assessment more "clinic friendly" (Cella and Lloyd 1994). Data collection is done electronically, in particular using tablet PCs or touch-screen computers.

A number of software packages for electronic PRO data capture have been developed (Evaluation Software Development 2011; Velikova et al. 2004; Verdonck-de Leeuw et al. 2009). The following software examples serve as an overview of common features required for PRO data collection:

the Computer-based Health Evaluation System (CHES) has a strong focus on PRO data collection within clinical routines, including graphical presentation of results, whereas the PROMIS Assessment Center focuses more on multicenter PRO data collection for research purposes.

Computer-based Health Evaluation System

CHES (Evaluation Software Development 2011; www.ches.at) allows the assessment of PROs in daily oncological routine and research. The software allows implementation of all common types of questionnaires (depending on copyright issues) and presents results graphically to clinicians and researchers. (For an example, see Figure 10–1.) For research purposes, the software contains interfaces for data export to statistical programs and for data import from clinical information systems. Within an ongoing collaborative project with the EORTC Quality of Life Group, the software is being further developed in regard to multilingualism, Web-based PRO assessments, and the administration of CAT measures.

Patients respond to items via touch-screen computers. Additional clinical and sociodemographic data can easily be added by the medical staff.

In detail, the software application comprises the following features:

- Graphical presentation of results: Results are presented as eye-catching multicolored graphs in real time. The graphical output links PRO scores to the course of disease and treatment, and specific medical interventions can be easily incorporated and displayed. Optionally, results can be shown in cross-sectional or longitudinal format.
- Flag system: Based on reference values from the literature or previously collected data, a flag system indicates patients with clinically relevant problems.
- Clinical report generator: Clinical reports on current questionnaire results can be generated as PDF files. These contain graphical charts as well as automatically generated text reports of relevant results.
- Data export/import module: Export and import of sociodemographic, clinical, and questionnaire data are possible for Statistical Package for the Social Sciences (SPSS) or Microsoft Excel files. Furthermore, tables containing reference values and specific program configurations can be transferred.
- Interface to clinical information systems (Health Level 7 [HL7]): To exchange data between CHES and various other databases in use as clinical information systems, an HL7 interface was integrated.
- Study monitoring module: For management of clinical studies including medical as well as PRO data collection, a module was incorporated in

CHES. The clinician or researcher can define which medical data need to be collected and which questionnaires have to be completed at certain time points. For missing data, warnings are displayed, and a log file of these warnings can be printed.

- Web-based data collection/home monitoring: To extend data collection beyond hospital settings, a Web interface for CHES has been programmed and is currently under testing.
- Multilingual version: The application allows changing languages at start-up (without reinstallation). English and Italian beta versions of CHES are available; further languages are planned.

PROMIS Assessment Center

Within the PROMIS project, not only PRO measures are being developed. The Assessment Center also is available online (www.assessmentcenter.net), enabling Web-based PRO data assessment. The software is available for free under a license agreement and comprises a researcher front-end and a patient-front end. The Web site offers a wide range of PROMIS measures covering major QOL issues and symptoms, and it allows clinicians and researchers to implement, for example, electronic case report forms and informed consent forms. Besides these preconfigured features, the Web site provides the possibility to add researcher-created questions and forms. For research purposes, it provides convenient data export features and enables the implementation of complex study designs (e.g., branching, multiple arms, repeated assessments) (Gershon et al. 2010).

Symptom Management and Screening Within Clinical Routines

For clinical practice, the clear and user-friendly presentation of PRO results is regarded to be essential. Velikova et al. (2004), for example, designed and used multiple small graphs presenting all results on a single page, making it easy to identify PRO changes of cancer patients over time. Studies in which routine computer-based assessment of QOL in clinical practice was evaluated suggest some important benefits for the physicians, as well as for patients and their treatment: screening for and prioritizing potential health and/or psychosocial problems, facilitating communication and shared clinical decision making, monitoring changes or response to treatment, and improving patient management (Higginson and Carr 2001).

With regard to fatigue, electronic data capture allows screening for fatigue in inpatient and outpatient settings, to optimize detection of patients in need of fatigue interventions. In addition, the impact of such interventions can be monitored through longitudinal assessments.

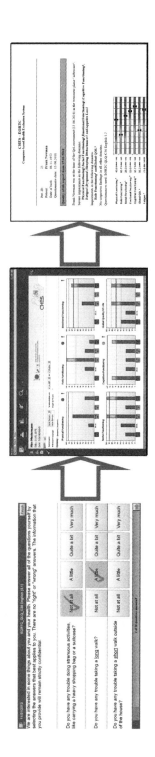

FIGURE 10–1. Patient-reported outcome (PRO) data flow; from data entry on the tablet PC (*left*), to graphical presentation within the Computer-based Health Evaluation System (CHES) (*middle*), to a printout of a clinical PRO report (*right*).

PRO monitoring in general has gained importance in the last decade, and a small number of randomized controlled trials have been conducted to investigate the impact of PRO monitoring on patient-physician communication, medical treatment, and health outcome. An article by Luckett et al. (2009) reviewing these studies found limited evidence for such an impact. The authors identified six randomized controlled trials evaluating the impact of PRO monitoring (Boyes et al. 2006; Detmar et al. 2002; McLachlan et al. 2001; Rosenbloom et al. 2007; Trowbridge et al. 1997; Velikova et al. 2004). The overall conclusion was that no solid evidence showed that PRO monitoring had an impact on patient outcomes but that this monitoring did have an effect on physician-patient communication. A major finding from this review was that physicians used PRO data only intermittently and for undetermined purpose. This finding is of crucial importance for the implementation of PRO monitoring because it highlights the need for comprehensive training of physicians with regard to use and interpretation of PRO data. Such training contributes also to their motivation for including these data in medical decision making. Identified barriers to the use of PRO data included time and resource constraints, the absence of suitable instruments, and the physicians' belief that their subjective evaluation was sufficient.

In a study on the impact of routine PRO monitoring, Detmar et al. (2002) analyzed patient-physician communication in detail. The authors found that physicians spent two-thirds of the conversation on medical or technical issues and one-fourth on QOL issues. In contrast, patients' communication was focused one-half on medical or technical issues and one-half on QOL. About one-third of the patients with serious QOL impairments did not discuss these problems, and the most likely issues to remain undiscussed were emotional functioning and fatigue.

Patients' willingness to participate in routine PRO monitoring is generally found to be high (Basch et al. 2007; Carlson et al. 2001), and a large proportion of patients would recommend the use of electronic PRO monitoring (Abernethy et al. 2009).

Patient Example for PRO Monitoring in Daily Clinical Routine

Figures 10–2 and 10–3 are examples of the graphical presentation of EORTC QLQ-C30 scales within the software CHES, which is used for QOL monitoring at Innsbruck Medical University in Austria. The QOL scores were collected from a male patient born in 1959 and diagnosed with rectal cancer in 2010. He received chemotherapy after initial surgery.

Figure 10–2 shows the cross-sectional report for the patient's assessment at the third chemotherapy cycle. Coloring of the bars (shown here by labeling) is based on percentiles of score distribution in the Austrian general population. The center-right (originally red) area reflects the score range below the 10th percentile for functioning scales (for which high scores indicate a good health status) and above the 90th percentile for symptom scales (for which low scores indicate a low symptom burden). The center-left (yellow) area reflects the score range above the 75th and below the 25th percentile, respectively, whereas the left (green) area reflects "normal" scores. The coloring of bars facilitates interpretation by indicating scale direction and by relating individual scores to reference values. At the third chemotherapy cycle, the patient had major problems with physical functioning, fatigue, and diarrhea, whereas cognitive functioning, dyspnea, sleeping disturbances, and constipation did not differ relevantly from general population scores. These findings can be detailed within patient-physician contact and may be a basis for initiating medical interventions.

Figure 10–3 shows longitudinal results for the QLQ-C30 scales Fatigue and Global QOL. After the end of chemotherapy (CT)—that is, in the aftercare phase (AC)—the patient's fatigue level decreased to that of the general population, resulting in an increase in global QOL.

In general, the comprehensive graphical presentation of the QOL results (cross-sectional and longitudinal) allows quick and easy symptom screening, tracking of symptom trajectories, and an appraisal of the patient's health status. In relation to patient-physician communication, the QOL results can provide a basis for focused communication and collection of more information about symptoms exceeding certain thresholds.

Telemonitoring

Especially with regard to chemotherapy, side effects and related symptom burden are known to be most severe a few days after application of cytostatic drugs (Hawkins and Grunberg 2009). Therefore, a major drawback of traditional or even computer-based PRO assessment in clinical routines is the tendency to neglect patients' health status outside of the hospital, which may lead to an underestimation of the actual symptom burden. This shortcoming can be overcome by a Web-based assessment tool for home monitoring. Measuring QOL frequently enough may increase longitudinal information and potentially enable clinicians to identify early signs of adverse events and thus intervene prospectively to minimize complications. Web-based data capture allows assessment of symptoms at time points that are crucial for patients' well-being, even when they are not in the hospital.

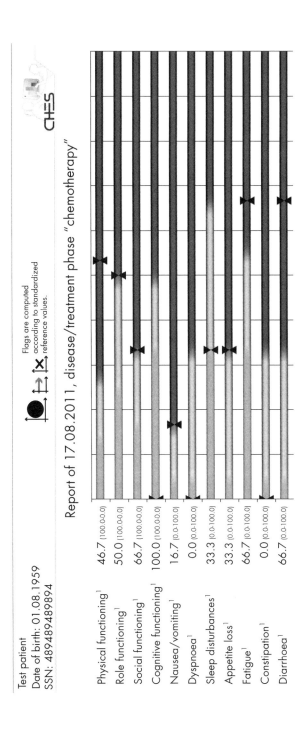

FIGURE 10–2. Cross-sectional presentation of individual quality of life (QOL) patient data within the Computer-based Health Evaluation System (CHES).

See text for discussion of color-coding. Here, green area is shown as medium-gray at left; yellow as light gray, left-center; red as dark gray, center-right.

[1]Reference group: cancer patients receiving chemotherapy.

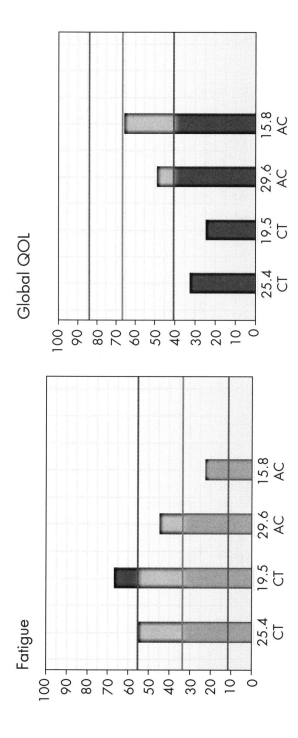

FIGURE 10–3. Longitudinal presentation of individual quality of life (QOL) patient data within the Computer-based Health Evaluation System (CHES). CT=chemotherapy; AC=aftercare phase.

Although Web-based PRO assessment is still in its infancy, its benefits within oncological care have been documented in a few studies (Basch et al. 2005; Kroenke et al. 2010; Snyder et al. 2009b; Vickers et al. 2010). An outstanding example of Web-based symptom monitoring in cancer patients was developed and implemented by Bush et al. (2005) to measure short-term (dynamic) changes in QOL by employing frequent, brief, online QOL assessments and more extensive, monthly online assessments. This study showed high feasibility of the Web-based methodology and yielded good patient compliance and high user satisfaction.

The assessment of patients' health and well-being during their stays at home will require additional administrative resources. The Internet, however, provides an inexpensive technology. Basch et al. (2005) suggest that administrative efficiency might even improve if patients report adverse events before clinical interactions and this information is subsequently shared with clinicians, saving time that investigators would otherwise have to spend eliciting that information.

Conclusion

Over the last two decades, the approach to the assessment of the patient's well-being has changed. Methodologically robust patient-reported questionnaires are now available for use in both clinical research and clinical practice. Health technology assessment has made tremendous progress, allowing the completion of such questionnaires in electronic formats and via the Web, further facilitating data collection. Although the use of QOL questionnaires in clinical research has a long-standing history, the use of such questionnaires in clinical practice is relatively new. Some important methodological issues still need to be resolved in the implementation of such measures in electronic formats, but several excellent examples of such measures are available (Basch and Abernethy 2011; Detmar et al. 2002; Velikova et al. 2004) that can be of great help in patients' management.

Key Clinical Points

- Quality of life (QOL) measurement is one dimension of patient-reported outcomes.
- QOL measures assess physical and psychosocial symptoms as well as functioning.
- QOL measures assess the impact of cancer on the patient and may identify previously undetected distress.

- Use of new technologies, such as computer-based administration of QOL inventories, allows measurements for routine clinical care.

- The burden of chemotherapy and its side effects can be effectively accessed via telemonitoring.

References

Aaronson NK, Ahmedzai S, Bergman B, et al: The European Organization for Research and Treatment of Cancer QLQ-C30: a quality-of-life instrument for use in international clinical trials in oncology. J Natl Cancer Inst 85:365–376, 1993

Abernethy AP, Herndon JE 2nd, Wheeler JL, et al: Feasibility and acceptability to patients of a longitudinal system for evaluating cancer-related symptoms and quality of life: pilot study of an e/Tablet data-collection system in academic oncology. J Pain Symptom Manage 37:1027–1038, 2009

Aloisi AM: Gonadal hormones and sex differences in pain reactivity. Clin J Pain 19:168–174, 2003

American Society of Clinical Oncology: Outcomes of cancer treatment for technology assessment and cancer treatment guidelines. American Society of Clinical Oncology. J Clin Oncol 14:671–679, 1996

Basch E: Patient-reported outcomes in drug safety evaluation. Ann Oncol 20:1905–1906, 2009

Basch E, Abernethy AP: Supporting clinical practice decisions with real-time patient-reported outcomes. J Clin Oncol 29:954–956, 2011

Basch E, Artz D, Dulko D, et al: Patient online self-reporting of toxicity symptoms during chemotherapy. J Clin Oncol 23:3552–3561, 2005

Basch E, Iasonos A, Barz A, et al: Long-term toxicity monitoring via electronic patient-reported outcomes in patients receiving chemotherapy. J Clin Oncol 25:5374–5380, 2007

Basch E, Jia X, Heller G, et al: Adverse symptom event reporting by patients vs clinicians: relationships with clinical outcomes. J Natl Cancer Inst 101:1624–1632, 2009

Bernhardson BM, Tishelman C, Rutqvist LE: Self-reported taste and smell changes during cancer chemotherapy. Support Care Cancer 16:275–283, 2008

Blazeby JM, Brookes ST, Alderson D: The prognostic value of quality of life scores during treatment for oesophageal cancer. Gut 49:227–230, 2001

Boyes A, Newell S, Girgis A, et al: Does routine assessment and real-time feedback improve cancer patients' psychosocial well-being? Eur J Cancer Care (Engl) 15:163–171, 2006

Bush N, Donaldson G, Moinpour C, et al: Development, feasibility and compliance of a web-based system for very frequent QOL and symptom home self-assessment after hematopoietic stem cell transplantation. Qual Life Res 14:77–93, 2005

Butow PN, Coates AS, Dunn SM: Psychosocial predictors of survival in metastatic melanoma. J Clin Oncol 17:2256–2263, 1999

Buxton J, White M, Osoba D: Patients' experiences using a computerized program with a touch-sensitive video monitor for the assessment of health-related quality of life. Qual Life Res 7:513–519, 1998

Carlson LE, Speca M, Hagen N, et al: Computerized quality-of-life screening in a cancer pain clinic. J Palliat Care 17:46–52, 2001

Cella DF, Lloyd SR: Data collection strategies for patient-reported information. Qual Manag Health Care 2:28–35, 1994

Cella DF, Tulsky DS, Gray G, et al: The Functional Assessment of Cancer Therapy scale: development and validation of the general measure. J Clin Oncol 11:570–579, 1993

Chiarion-Sileni V, Del Bianco P, De Salvo GL, et al: Quality of life evaluation in a randomised trial of chemotherapy versus bio-chemotherapy in advanced melanoma patients. Eur J Cancer 39:1577–1585, 2003

Chow E, Tsao MN, Harth T: Does psychosocial intervention improve survival in cancer? A meta-analysis. Palliat Med 18:25–31, 2004

Coates A, Gebski V, Signorini D, et al: Prognostic value of quality-of-life scores during chemotherapy for advanced breast cancer. Australian New Zealand Breast Cancer Trials Group. J Clin Oncol 10:1833–1838, 1992

Coates AS, Hurny C, Peterson HF, et al: Quality-of-life scores predict outcome in metastatic but not early breast cancer. International Breast Cancer Study Group. J Clin Oncol 18:3768–3774, 2000

Coons S, Gwaltney C, Hays R, et al: Recommendations on evidence needed to support measurement equivalence between electronic and paper-based patient-reported outcome (PRO) measures: ISPOR ePRO Good Research Practices Task Force report. Value Health 12:419–429, 2009

Coyne JC, Stefanek M, Palmer SC: Psychotherapy and survival in cancer: the conflict between hope and evidence. Psychol Bull 133:367–394, 2007

Dancey J, Zee B, Osoba D, et al: Quality of life scores: an independent prognostic variable in a general population of cancer patients receiving chemotherapy. The National Cancer Institute of Canada Clinical Trials Group. Qual Life Res 6:151–158, 1997

de Graeff A, de Leeuw JR, Ros WJ, et al: Sociodemographic factors and quality of life as prognostic indicators in head and neck cancer. Eur J Cancer 37:332–339, 2001

de Haes JC, Olschewski M, Fayers PM, et al: The Rotterdam Symptom Checklist. Groningen, Northern Centre for Health Care Research, University of Groningen, the Netherlands, 1996, pp 1–38

de Haes H, Olschewski M, Kaufmann M, et al: Quality of life in goserelin-treated versus cyclophosphamide + methotrexate + fluorouracil-treated premenopausal and perimenopausal patients with node-positive, early breast cancer: the Zoladex Early Breast Cancer Research Association Trialists Group. J Clin Oncol 21:4510–4516, 2003

Derogatis LR, Abeloff MD, Melisaratos N: Psychological coping mechanisms and survival time in metastatic breast cancer. JAMA 242:1504–1508, 1979

Detmar SB, Aaronson NK, Wever LD, et al: How are you feeling? Who wants to know? Patients' and oncologists' preferences for discussing health-related quality-of-life issues. J Clin Oncol 18:3295–3301, 2000

Detmar SB, Muller MJ, Schornagel JH, et al: Health-related quality-of-life assessments and patient-physician communication: a randomized controlled trial. JAMA 288:3027–3034, 2002

Efficace F, Bottomley A, Osoba D, et al: Beyond the development of health-related quality-of-life (HRQOL) measures: a checklist for evaluating HRQOL outcomes in cancer clinical trials—does HRQOL evaluation in prostate cancer research inform clinical decision making? J Clin Oncol 21:3502–3511, 2003

Efficace F, Bottomley A, Vanvoorden V, et al: Methodological issues in assessing health-related quality of life of colorectal cancer patients in randomised controlled trials. Eur J Cancer 40:187–197, 2004a

Efficace F, Therasse P, Piccart MJ, et al: Health-related quality of life parameters as prognostic factors in a nonmetastatic breast cancer population: an international multicenter study. J Clin Oncol 22:3381–3388, 2004b

Efficace F, Bottomley A, Coens C, et al: Does a patient's self-reported health-related quality of life predict survival beyond key biomedical data in advanced colorectal cancer? Eur J Cancer 42:42–49, 2006

Efficace F, Innominato PF, Bjarnason G, et al: Validation of patient's self-reported social functioning as an independent prognostic factor for survival in metastatic colorectal cancer patients: results of an international study by the Chronotherapy Group of the European Organisation for Research and Treatment of Cancer. J Clin Oncol 26:2020–2026, 2008

Erharter A, Giesinger J, Kemmler G, et al: Implementation of computer-based quality-of-life monitoring in brain tumor outpatients in routine clinical practice. J Pain Symptom Manage 39:219–229, 2010

Eton DT, Fairclough DL, Cella D, et al: Early change in patient-reported health during lung cancer chemotherapy predicts clinical outcomes beyond those predicted by baseline report: results from Eastern Cooperative Oncology Group Study 5592. J Clin Oncol 21:1536–1543, 2003

Eton DT, Cella D, Yost KJ, et al: A combination of distribution- and anchor-based approaches determined minimally important differences (MIDs) for four endpoints in a breast cancer scale. J Clin Epidemiol 57:898–910, 2004

European Medicines Agency, Committee for Medicinal Products for Human Use: Reflection paper on the regulatory guidance for the use of health-related quality of life (HRQL) measures in the evaluation of medicinal products. July 2005. Available at: http://www.ispor.org/workpaper/emea-hrql-guidance.pdf. Accessed July 30, 2012.

The EuroQol Group: EuroQol-a new facility for the measurement of health-related quality of life. Health Policy 16:199–208, 1990

Evaluation Software Development: ESD: Computer-Based Health Evaluation System (CHES) (software). Innsbruck, Austria, CHES, 2011

Fallowfield L, Ratcliffe D, Jenkins V, et al: Psychiatric morbidity and its recognition by doctors in patients with cancer. Br J Cancer 84:1011–1015, 2001

Farquhar-Smith P: Chemotherapy-induced neuropathic pain. Curr Opin Support Palliat Care, 5:1–7, 2011

Fayers PM: Interpreting quality of life data: population-based reference data for the EORTC QLQ-C30. Eur J Cancer 37:1331–1334, 2001

Fayers P, Machin D: Quality of Life: Assessment, Analysis, and Interpretation. Chichester, UK, Wiley, 2000

Gershon RC, Rothrock N, Hanrahan R, et al: The use of PROMIS and assessment center to deliver patient-reported outcome measures in clinical research. J Appl Meas 11:304–314, 2010

Giesinger J, Kemmler G, Mueller V, et al: Are gender-associated differences in quality of life in patients with colorectal cancer disease-specific? Qual Life Res 18: 547–555, 2009

Giesinger JM, Aa Petersen M, Groenvold M, et al: Cross-cultural development of an item list for computer-adaptive testing of fatigue in oncological patients. Health Qual Life Outcomes 9:19, 2011

Gotay CC, Kawamoto CT, Bottomley A, et al: The prognostic significance of patient-reported outcomes in cancer clinical trials. J Clin Oncol 26:1355–1363, 2008

Greenspan JD, Craft RM, LeResche L, et al: Studying sex and gender differences in pain and analgesia: a consensus report. Pain 132 (suppl 1):S26–S45, 2007

Hawkins R, Grunberg S: Chemotherapy-induced nausea and vomiting: challenges and opportunities for improved patient outcomes. Clin J Oncol Nurs 13:54–64, 2009

Higginson IJ, Carr AJ: Measuring quality of life: using quality of life measures in the clinical setting. BMJ 322:1297–1300, 2001

Hjermstad MJ, Fayers PM, Bjordal K, et al: Using reference data on quality of life—the importance of adjusting for age and gender, exemplified by the EORTC QLQ-C30 (+3). Eur J Cancer 34:1381–1389, 1998

Holland JC: Update: NCCN practice guidelines for the management of psychosocial distress. Oncology 13:459–507, 1999

Hong JH, Omur-Ozbek P, Stanek BT, et al: Taste and odor abnormalities in cancer patients. J Support Oncol 7:58–65, 2009

Hwang SS, Chang VT, Cogswell J, et al: Clinical relevance of fatigue levels in cancer patients at a Veterans Administration Medical Center. Cancer 94:2481–2489, 2002

Johnsen AT, Tholstrup D, Petersen MA, et al: Health related quality of life in a nationally representative sample of haematological patients. Eur J Haematol 83:139–148, 2009

Johnson JR, Williams G, Pazdur R: End points and United States Food and Drug Administration approval of oncology drugs. J Clin Oncol 21:1404–1411, 2003

Kramer JA, Curran D, Piccart M, et al: Identification and interpretation of clinical and quality of life prognostic factors for survival and response to treatment in first-line chemotherapy in advanced breast cancer. Eur J Cancer 36:1498–1506, 2000

Kroenke K, Theobald D, Wu J, et al: Effect of telecare management on pain and depression in patients with cancer: a randomized trial. JAMA 304:163–171, 2010

Luckett T, Butow JN, King MT: Improving patient outcomes through the routine use of patient-reported data in cancer clinics: future directions. Psychooncology 18:1129–1138, 2009

Maisey NR, Norman A, Watson M, et al: Baseline quality of life predicts survival in patients with advanced colorectal cancer. Eur J Cancer 38:1351–1357, 2002

Maringwa JT, Quinten C, King M, et al: Minimal important differences for interpreting health-related quality of life scores from the EORTC QLQ-C30 in lung cancer patients participating in randomized controlled trials. Support Care Cancer 19:1753–1760, 2011

McLachlan SA, Allenby A, Matthews J, et al: Randomized trial of coordinated psychosocial interventions based on patient self-assessments versus standard care to improve the psychosocial functioning of patients with cancer. J Clin Oncol 19:4117–4125, 2001

Montazeri A: Quality of life data as prognostic indicators of survival in cancer patients: an overview of the literature from 1982 to 2008. Health Qual Life Outcomes 7:102, 2009

Mulder C, Van Der Pompe G, Spiegel D, et al: Do psychosocial factors influence the course of breast cancer? A review of recent literature, methodological problems and future directions. Psychooncology 1:155–167, 1992

National Cancer Institute: Common Terminology Criteria for Adverse Events (CTCAE) and Common Toxicity Criteria (CTC), Version 4.0. December 2010a. Available at: http://ctep.cancer.gov/protocolDevelopment/electronic_applications/ctc.htm. Accessed July 30, 2012.

National Cancer Institute: Patient-Reported Outcomes version of the Common Terminology Criteria for Adverse Events (PRO-CTCAE). August 2010b. Available at: http://outcomes.cancer.gov/tools/pro-ctcae.html. Accessed July 30, 2012.

Newport DJ, Nemeroff CB: Assessment and treatment of depression in the cancer patient. J Psychosom Res 45:215–237, 1998

Oberguggenberger A, Hubalek M, Sztankay M, et al: Is the toxicity of adjuvant aromatase inhibitor therapy underestimated? Complementary information from patient-reported outcomes (PROs). Breast Cancer Res Treat 128:553–561, 2011

Osoba D: The Quality of Life Committee of the Clinical Trials Group of the National Cancer Institute of Canada: organization and functions. Qual Life Res 1:211–218, 1992

Osoba D, Rodrigues G, Myles J, et al: Interpreting the significance of changes in health-related quality-of-life scores. J Clin Oncol 16:139–144, 1998

Osoba D, Tannock IF, Ernst DS, et al: Health-related quality of life in men with metastatic prostate cancer treated with prednisone alone or mitoxantrone and prednisone. J Clin Oncol 17:1654–1663, 1999

Pakhomov SV, Jacobsen SJ, Chute CG, et al: Agreement between patient-reported symptoms and their documentation in the medical record. Am J Manag Care 14:530–539, 2008

Payne DK, Hoffman RG, Theodoulou M, et al: Screening for anxiety and depression in women with breast cancer. Psychiatry and medical oncology gear up for managed care. Psychosomatics 40:64–69, 1999

Petersen MA, Groenvold M, Aaronson NK, et al: Development of computerised adaptive testing (CAT) for the EORTC QLQ-C30 dimensions—general approach and initial results for physical functioning. Eur J Cancer 46:1352–1358, 2010

Petersen MA, Groenvold M, Aaronson NK, et al: Development of computerized adaptive testing (CAT) for the EORTC QLQ-C30 physical functioning dimension. Qual Life Res 20:479–490, 2011

Petticrew M, Bell R, Hunter D: Influence of psychological coping on survival and recurrence in people with cancer: systematic review. BMJ 325:1066, 2002

Ringash J, O'Sullivan B, Bezjak A, et al: Interpreting clinically significant changes in patient-reported outcomes. Cancer 110:196–202, 2007

Rock EP, Kennedy DL, Furness MH, et al: Patient-reported outcomes supporting anticancer product approvals. J Clin Oncol 25:5094–5099, 2007

Rosenbloom SK, Victorson DE, Hahn EA, et al: Assessment is not enough: a randomized controlled trial of the effects of HRQL assessment on quality of life and satisfaction in oncology clinical practice. Psychooncology 16:1069–1079, 2007

Schipper H, Clinch J, McMurray A, et al: Measuring the quality of life of cancer patients: the Functional Living Index–Cancer: development and validation. J Clin Oncol 2:472–83, 1994

Schwarz R, Hinz A: Reference data for the quality of life questionnaire EORTC QLQ-C30 in the general German population. Eur J Cancer 37:1345–1351, 2001

Sharpe M, Strong V, Allen K, et al: Major depression in outpatients attending a regional cancer centre: screening and unmet treatment needs. Br J Cancer 90:314–320, 2004

Snyder CF, Garrett-Mayer E, Blackford AL, et al: Concordance of cancer patients' function, symptoms, and supportive care needs. Qual Life Res 18:991–998, 2009a

Snyder CF, Jensen R, Courtin SO, et al: PatientViewpoint: a website for patient-reported outcomes assessment. Qual Life Res 18:793–800, 2009b

Snyder CF, Blackford AL, Brahmer JR, et al: Needs assessments can identify scores on HRQOL questionnaires that represent problems for patients: an illustration with the Supportive Care Needs Survey and the QLQ-C30. Qual Life Res 19:837–845, 2010

Snyder CF, Blackford AL, Aaronson NK, et al: Can patient-reported outcome measures identify cancer patients' most bothersome issues? J Clin Oncol 29:1216–1220, 2011

Spiegel D, Bloom JR, Kraemer HC, et al: Effect of psychosocial treatment on survival of patients with metastatic breast cancer. Lancet 2:888–891, 1989

Stead ML, Brown JM, Fallowfield L, et al: Lack of communication between healthcare professionals and women with ovarian cancer about sexual issues. Br J Cancer 88:666–671, 2003

Taenzer PA, Speca M, Atkinson MJ, et al: Computerized quality-of-life screening in an oncology clinic. Cancer Pract 5:168–175, 1997

Taenzer PA, Bultz BD, Carlson LE, et al: Impact of computerized quality of life screening on physician behaviour and patient satisfaction in lung cancer outpatients. Psychooncology 9:203–213, 2000

Taphoorn M, Stupp R, Coens C, et al: Health-related quality of life in patients with glioblastoma: a randomised controlled trial. Lancet Oncol 6:937–944, 2005

Terwee CB, Roorda LD, Knol DL, et al: Linking measurement error to minimal important change of patient-reported outcomes. J Clin Epidemiol 62:1062–1067, 2009

Trowbridge R, Dugan W, Jay SJ, et al: Determining the effectiveness of a clinical-practice intervention in improving the control of pain in outpatients with cancer. Acad Med 72:798–800, 1997

U.S. Food and Drug Administration: Guidance for industry—patient-reported outcome measures: use in medical product development to support labeling claims. 2009.
Available at: http://www.ispor.org/workpaper/FDA%20PRO%20Guidance.pdf. Accessed July 30, 2012.

Velikova G, Wright EP, Smith AB, et al: Automated collection of quality-of-life data: a comparison of paper and computer touch-screen questionnaires. J Clin Oncol 17:998–1007, 1999

Velikova G, Booth L, Smith AB, et al: Measuring quality of life in routine oncology practice improves communication and patient well-being: a randomized controlled trial. J Clin Oncol 22:714–724, 2004

Verdonck-de Leeuw IM, de Bree R, Keizer AL, et al: Computerized prospective screening for high levels of emotional distress in head and neck cancer patients and referral rate to psychosocial care. Oral Oncol 45:E129–E133, 2009

Vickers AJ, Savage CJ, Shouery M, et al: Validation study of a web-based assessment of functional recovery after radical prostatectomy. Health Qual Life Outcomes 8:82, 2010

Ware JE, Sherbourne CD: The MOS 36-item short-form health survey (SF-36), I: conceptual framework and item selection. Med Care 30:473–483, 1992

Weingart SN, Pagovich O, Sands DZ, et al: What can hospitalized patients tell us about adverse events? Learning from patient-reported incidents. J Gen Intern Med 20:830–836, 2005

Zabernigg A, Gamper EM, Giesinger JM, et al: Taste alterations in cancer patients receiving chemotherapy: a neglected side effect? Oncologist 15:913–920, 2010

CHAPTER 11

Support of the Dying Patient

Psychological Issues and Communication

Friedrich Stiefel, M.D.
Sonia Krenz, Ph.D.

IN THIS CHAPTER we discuss five key elements of the psychological support of the dying patient. We present an integrated model of adaptation to existential threat; describe the main psychological challenges that impending death represents for the patient; explain different psychotherapeutic interventions in palliative care; discuss how to support clinicians, which include physicians, nurses, and other health care professionals working with the dying patient; and identify communication challenges in palliative care and provide information about communication skills training (CST). This chapter is clinically oriented and based on our experiences as a liaison psychiatrist and a psychologist working in palliative care, and as teachers of CST.

An Integrated Model of Patients' Adjustment to Existential Threat

As illustrated in Figure 11–1, many factors contribute to the patient's adjustment to existential threat. Although these factors are interwoven and mutually influence each other, for didactic reasons they are described separately.

Facing Death

Impending death implies that a person is facing the limits of life, a situation that often invites the person to look back and to reflect about his or her past and to search for meaning. Although feelings of being fulfilled or dissatisfied emerge, depending on one's life trajectory, meaning is mainly related to relationships (family, friends, and encounters with significant persons). Separation and death also stimulate thoughts and emotions, which are closely linked to the patient's early development (was the person raised in loving, secure, and trustful relationships?), past experiences (was the person able to live life without major traumatizing events?), and current situation (does the person feel supported?). In other words, whether a patient faces death with serenity or with fear or denial depends to a large degree on the patient's relational attachment and his or her biography.

Personal Biography and Personality

A patient's personal biographical elements and personality are important sources of strength and adaptation but may also be sources of distress and psychiatric disturbance. The actual situation of existential threat and impending separation from loved ones may—in case of difficulties during development and major life events—reactivate unresolved issues of the past, such as major losses or other traumatic events. Although a patient may not be aware that the current distress is nourished by painful emotions of the past, clinicians may help the patient to establish links and thus understand, at least in part, his or her reaction and find meaning in his or her current experience. Therefore, knowing key elements of the patient's biography is crucial for the clinician 1) to evaluate the patient's strengths and vulnerabilities, 2) to reinforce the patient's identity as a person and not just as having a disease, 3) to establish a relationship and therapeutic alliance through narrativity, and 4) to link past and present and thus produce a sense of continuity and meaning in a moment of rupture with regard to the patient's biopsychosocial situation (Stiefel et al. 1998).

Personality, shaped by the patient's early development and biography, is another important factor with regard to adaptation to existential threat. Although personality is a rather static construct, it is important for the clinician to gain a general idea of how a patient's personality is organized. Personality traits should be taken into account because they shape communication with and care of the patient in the terminal phase of disease (Stiefel and Razavi 2006). The clinician should consider various questions: Does the patient show neuroticism—defined as a propensity for anxiety—and might the patient be appeased by detailed information? Does the patient demonstrate borderline traits that demand the treating team to exert a special

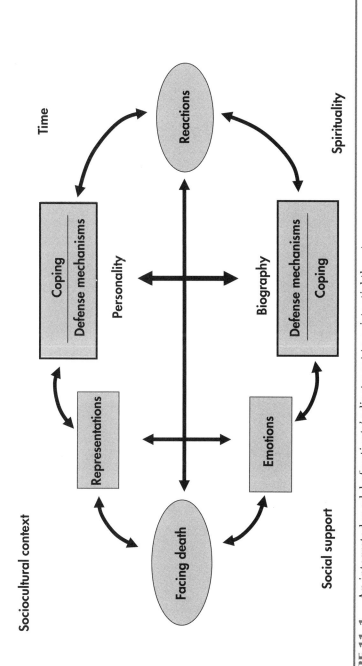

FIGURE 11–1. An integrated model of patients' adjustment to existential threat.

The contextual factors—including spirituality, which might be individual as well as contextual—are represented outside the individual factors.

effort when the patient is fighting against feelings of being not understood and abandoned? Does the patient show dependent traits, requiring more attention from staff than other patients do?

Representations and Emotions

Representations—defined as a combination of acquired factual information and fantasies and misperceptions—about stage of disease, prognosis, death and dying, and what is to be expected after death, influence the patient's emotions, and simultaneously his or her emotions are shaping these representations. Although threatening and/or erroneous representations can be (to a certain degree) clarified and confronted with the clinician's medical information, emotions do not call for medical explications; instead, emotions should be welcomed to be expressed, listened to, clarified with regard to their sources, responded to with empathy, and possibly understood. The clinician's understanding of representations and emotions fosters the therapeutic alliance and thus prevents the patient's feelings of isolation (Guex et al. 2000). The clinician's capacity to "simply" contain threatful representations and emotions is a most important therapeutic act, which at times may be completed by clarifications of the underlying reasons and of the contextual and biographical links. Finally, the clinician not only needs to identify, contain, and work with the patient's representations and emotions, but also needs to attempt to understand how the patient deals with them—that is, how the patient copes with and defends against them.

Coping and Defense Mechanisms

Coping strategies, which are conscious and modifiable through learning, can help to resolve problems or emotional tensions and must be distinguished from defense mechanisms (Weisman 1979). Defenses such as denial, which are unconscious, mediate between internal needs of the individual and external reality, and they emerge in situations of strong affective load (Bernard et al. 2010); they are triggered by external events, as well as by thoughts and emotions, such as anxiety, and aim to protect the individual and preserve psychological equilibrium.

Investigation of the patient's past coping strategies (information seeking, sharing of concerns, submitting to the inevitable, etc.) can reveal clues about the person's resources and remind the patient of strategies he or she has used successfully for facing adversity. Discussion about coping might also lead the patient to try new ways of dealing with reality. On the other hand, identification of a patient's defense mechanisms can guide the clinician in how to accompany the patient; these defenses should not—at the end of a patient's life—be challenged or interpreted.

Case Vignette

A 40-year-old mother of two small children who had advanced breast cancer coped with her situation by distraction (she reported that she consciously put her situation out of her mind, allowing her to sometimes have the impression of living an almost normal life with her kids). With regard to her defenses, she showed partial denial, recognizing that she had cancer but believing that "the treatment will cure me." The treating oncologist, worrying that the patient had not informed her children about the rapid progression of the disease, confronted the patient repeatedly with precise medical information, stating that he had no other treatment options. Despite the patient's increased nervousness and desire not to receive more information, the oncologist continued to confront her and also started to talk about death and dying. As a consequence, the patient's denial increased to a total denial of her illness. She reported that she had no reason to be hospitalized, said that she felt cured, and requested to be discharged. When she was again confronted with her medical situation, her defenses increased. The patient said that "patients are intoxicated and treated like prisoners in this hospital" (projection). Finally, the clinician responded to the patient's severe agitation by treating her with neuroleptics, with the effect that she was sedated during the final days of her life.

This example illustrates that patients coping with advanced disease should be respected and that challenging their defenses by confronting them with a reality they are not able to face is counterproductive. The careful observation of defenses allows the clinician to evaluate the patient's vulnerability. Immature defenses, such as projection, massive denial, or splitting, indicate a higher degree of vulnerability, and call for the adaptation of discussions about prognosis, death, and dying to the limited capacity of the patient. In addition, defenses might be partially or totally present; for example, total denial (denial of being ill) is an indicator of massive psychological vulnerability, whereas partial denial (denial of the severity of the disease, its implications, or prognosis) is prevalent and indicates a lesser degree of vulnerability. Identification of predominant defense mechanisms also allows the clinician to gain insight about how the patient reacts unconsciously toward threat and how he or she faces reality. This information will enable the clinician 1) to adapt to the patient's needs (e.g., a patient who is predominantly intellectualizing should not be confronted without great attention to the emotional aspects of his or her situation); 2) to increase understanding of the patient's reactions and thus foster empathy and the therapeutic alliance; and 3) to mediate between the patient and his or her significant others, who may operate with different defensive styles (e.g., by explaining to the family the significance and function of denial for a patient under existential threat) (Guex et al. 2000).

Although the defenses used by a patient with advanced disease have to be considered as protective—decreasing the patient's anxiety in a situation of existential threat—they can become dysfunctional if they lead the patient to actions that might harm self or significant others (e.g., if the patient in the case vignette above had left the hospital and tried to take her children to the family's house in the mountains while not in adequate physical condition to drive a car). In such a case, any measure—reassuring the patient, providing psychopharmacological treatment—that aims to decrease the patient's anxiety is indicated, allowing him or her to have a more adequate perception of reality. Dysfunctional denial is thus identified when the patient's denial is translated into a behavior or attitude that can harm self or others.

Social Support

Social support is known to be crucial for a patient's adjustment to disease, especially in times of progression of disease. At the same time, it has to be taken into account that dying patients often withdraw from relationships (or at least try to diminish their intensity), because establishing and maintaining relationships requires "psychological energy," which is often reduced at the end of life. Therefore, the challenge for significant others and clinicians is to find ways to be with the patient while taking into account and respecting the patient's limited capacities to engage in relationships. It is important to carefully "read" the patient from a psychological point of view and to adapt to his or her needs by 1) observing nonverbal behaviors indicating the desire for more closeness or distance; 2) respecting the person's defense mechanisms; 3) accepting that it is the patient who faces death and that the patient has the right to face it in his or her own way; and 4) showing tolerance toward, containing, and if possible understanding the patient's emotions. In other words, the goal is to meet the patient where he or she is, in terms of thoughts, emotions, and ways of dealing with them. Significant others, however, might sometimes have difficulty coming to terms with the discrepancy between their own needs (for closeness, for expressing feelings and thoughts) and the needs of the patient.

For example, if a patient who is unable to leave the hospital expresses the desire to take a trip to the countryside, a family member might respond, "We share this desire and hope that this might become possible; still, we have to take into account that your medical situation is now quite serious and does not allow you to take such an action." Or if a patient asks repeatedly if a more aggressive treatment could contribute to becoming healthy again, a simple answer addressing the limited treatment option may be medically correct, but may not be appropriate from a psychological perspective. In such a situation, the clinician might express that he understands the patient's desire, but that at the moment such a treatment is not indicated. Sometimes it might also be beneficial to clarify the question before answering it by providing medical information. This is illustrated by the following case vignette.

Case Vignette

A young palliative care physician reported during supervision that a 55-year-old former mathematician with a brain tumor had asked the physician during the daily visit if he could order another CT scan of his head. The physician answered that such an investigation would be useless because it would not be followed by a change in the therapeutic strategy, which was palliative. As a consequence, the patient refused to talk to him for several days. A more appropriate way to handle this situation would have been to cautiously try to clarify the underlying question (whether the patient still hoped to be cured, whether his intention was to perceive the extent of his brain tumor or to check if he was still "worthy" of being investigated) and to address the patient's underlying emotions (fear, self-deception, or sadness).

For a patient with psychological distress, the clinician is well advised to investigate the patient's social network and to evaluate whether differences in experiences between patients and significant others exist (Bernard et al. 2010). Sometimes, an explanation to relatives that a dying patient is experiencing rapid progression of disease, and suggestions about how the family can remain engaged, can be a great relief for the patient. Diverging views (e.g., the patient is in denial, and family members wish to discuss unresolved issues or say goodbye) should be discussed with significant others to increase their understanding, as well as their patient empathy and support.

Case Vignette

A 55-year-old man with advanced colon cancer reported to the nurses that he sometimes had the impression that his wife was more of a burden than was his suffering from cancer. Invited to elaborate on his thoughts, the patient reported that often his wife had outbursts of anger when they talked about his medical situation, but he did not understand what made her "get mad at him." With the patient's consent, a meeting between the treating physician, the head nurse, and the patient's wife was arranged, during which she explained that she had the impression that "he doesn't care about me and the long-standing relationship we had together," given the fact that when they spoke about the future, he would state, "There have been millions who died before me and millions who will die after me...." Her interpretation of this statement was that she just did not count for him, because the impending separation was "just a trivial and normal event" in his perception. The discussion with the medical staff allowed this woman to understand that his statement was only an expression of his personal way of facing death, and that his reference to the million others who die was his attempt to diminish his anxiety by referring to death as a natural process. Relieved by the discussion, the wife became able to react without feelings of being personally harmed by the patient's words. This discussion allowed the tensions between the couple to diminish, and the patient and his wife were again able to feel close and supportive.

This example illustrates that tensions between dying patients and significant others may be due to erroneous interpretations and difficulty allowing the patient to have a different perspective on the situation. Family members might feel sad or angered by a patient's attitude toward death. The clinician can help ease tension by informing significant others that there is no right or wrong way to face death and that individuals must be allowed to react in their own way to existential threat.

Sociocultural Context

Cultural context and cultural identity—which includes religious, educational, and socioeconomic factors that shape an individual—influence the experiences of the life cycles of humans (Erikson 1950), especially at the end of life. Respect for a patient, even if the clinician cannot fully understand the patient's cultural identity, also implies having "curiosity" (a word that has its roots in *curare*, meaning "to heal"). Curiosity implies the desire to invite the patient to express his or her values, convictions, and interrogations, and to allow the patient to feel respected and understood both in his or her "singularity" and "collectivity."

Cultural misunderstandings, however, can also arise between patients and carers of the same cultural context and can become sources of distress. For example, the still persisting myth of a good death in the "culture of palliative care" may conflict with the patient's experience and increase his or her feelings of isolation, or clinicians might respond with frank hostility to a patient's request for assisted suicide, leaving the patient with feelings of abandonment. What is needed in today's heterogeneous societies is not a detailed knowledge about different cultures, but more openness and genuine tolerance toward "the other."

Too often, carers feel that trying to understand a different point of view requires them to give up their own convictions and values, as if the patient's and carer's perspectives have to be superimposed in order for the individuals to "remain together."

Time

Time is another important variable when evaluating a patient's distress. Although in general Kübler-Ross's (1969) conceptualization of adjustment to disease and existential threat is useful, confusion still arises in patients, family members, and staff with regard to the different phases described (shock and denial, bargaining, mourning, etc.), and especially with regard to reaching the final stage of acceptance, as if death is an acceptable consequence of life for everyone. Much is gained when the insight prevails that it is more important to join the patient where he or she is than to expect the patient to make an effort toward acceptance; if this is understood, tensions between the patient and the family or staff diminish. Providing room for expression and allowing the patient to live the last phase of life in his or her own way, thus respecting the individual's singularity, contributes to allowing the patient to retain a sense of self.

Spirituality

Spiritual preoccupations may emerge at the end of life when a patient is facing uncertainty and the questions "Where do we come from?" and "Where do we go?" The clinician's thoughtless request for consultation by a spiritual (or religious) specialist before listening to what the patient has to say demonstrates the clinician's insecurity. Fear that clinicians will not be able to discuss issues related to spirituality hampers the patient's possibility of expressing his or her needs; it also hampers the encounter between patient and carers and the organization of specialized spiritual support when the latter is really indicated. Some clinicians who consider themselves atheists or have a complicated relationship with religion may respond negatively to patients' requests to discuss spiritual concerns. Although clinicians should be at ease before engaging in discussions about spiritual issues, they also should be able to reflect on their resistances and understand that they do not have to adhere to any belief system to invite the patient express spiritual concerns. Frequently, the patient does not seek specific answers but only wishes to express thoughts and be listened to. Because staff are commonly confronted with patients facing spiritual difficulties, discussions about how to respond to spiritual needs should be part of the postgraduate education within a team.

Case Vignette

An elderly former teacher with lung cancer who was often agitated during the night reported to the consulting psychiatrist that he sometimes felt anxious and tense, wondering how he "will be received above" when his time comes. He explained that he did not adhere to any church but believed in God and was quite concerned about what happens after death. During the discussions, the patient finally admitted that he had not been faithful to his wife, a fact that he hadn't told her, and that he therefore feared his end and the possibility of a final sanction. Although the psychiatrist did not feel really competent to discuss such matters, he also respected the patient's desire to speak with him—and him only, as the patient stated—about this issue. Confronted with the patient's repeated question, "How do you think God will react?" the psychiatrist finally spontaneously stated that he believes that "God knows that love and human relationship is a very complex issue" and that God might well be able to forgive the patient's behavior, which He understands as not having been guided by the intention to harm his wife. The patient felt markedly relieved by this discussion, and his agitation at night disappeared.

This example illustrates that the patient had great confidence in this young physician and felt more comfortable talking to him, whom he had known for several months, than to an unknown person from pastoral care. It also illustrates that some of the patient's spiritual concerns are issues that call for a human response that is nonjudgmental and free of any moralistic attitude. People's limitations can largely be explained by their development. The patient in this vignette, for example, was raised in a dysfunctional family with parents who were unable to provide him with a secure and stable relationship, thus influencing his later attachment style, which was characterized by a great fear of depending on a dyadic relationship and a need to secure himself by repeatedly engaging in extramarital love affairs.

Some patients, however, need specialized pastoral care. These patients include those who specifically demand specialized spiritual support, who are dealing with issues that surpass the experience and competence of the clinician, or who are in spiritual distress that is clearly not related to psychological suffering (e.g., depression).

Psychological Challenges of the Dying Patient

In this section, we discuss the main psychological challenges the dying patient has to face: coping with loss of control, facing uncertainty and separation, and dealing with unresolved issues from the past.

Loss of Control

Death is often less feared than the loss of control associated with rapid progression of disease. Despite the fact that impotence is part of the human condition and everyone knows "deep down" that man's destiny is not in his hands, this "knowledge" remains largely unconscious throughout life. The often unexpected, emerging limits of life therefore evoke a variety of emotions and reactions: anxiety, anger, despair, helplessness, shame, jealousy. These emotions influence the patient's thoughts, verbal expressions, and reactions, and may manifest themselves in different ways, such as a desire to hasten death or suicidal ideation, requests for further treatments, complaints or aggressiveness against family members and carers, social withdrawal, denial of the medical reality, or psychiatric disturbances (Razavi and Stiefel 1994; Stiefel and Razavi 1994).

Facing Uncertainty and Separation

Like impotence, uncertainty (e.g., about "where we come from and where we will go") is also part of the human condition, largely denied throughout life and often accentuated by impending death. Toward the unknown, the void, and the beyond, a person often projects what he or she "knows" or has experienced and learned during life. In other words, what is projected on death is often closely related to how a person has lived. For some people, appeasement and submission to the inevitable may become possible, whereas others may be haunted by profound anxieties leading to agitation and despair.

A patient who feels anchored in a secure relationship and surrounded by loved ones may feel sad about leaving them soon, but the fact that the person was and still is able to live with stable and comforting relationships usually provides a feeling of security that helps when facing separation and the unknown (Bowlby 1988). In contrast, patients who lacked close and secure relationships, especially in childhood, experience separation as abandonment or rejection and are possessed by the feeling of having to face uncertainty alone.

Facing the Future, Reflecting on the Past

Another challenge facing dying patients is that the approaching limits often oblige them to look back on their past and to consider the good and the bad: how they have given and how they have received, what they regret and what they are proud of, what has left them with shame and sorrow and what has provided them with confidence and joy. These reflections rarely concern material things, but mainly relate to human encounters and the relationships that were constructed during a lifetime; for most patients, it is the latter that accounts for the richness or poverty perceived at the end and that often leaves them with the impression of a meaningful or meaningless life (Stiefel et al. 2008). In other words, the patient is always contemplating current *and* past relationships and associated satisfaction, regrets, sadness, or despair.

Psychological and Psychotherapeutic Interventions in Palliative Care

Impending death and the associated loss of control and sense of powerlessness, uncertainty and separation, and search for meaning in life arouse archaic emotions and strong reactions. From a general point of view, and before we describe the specific psychotherapeutic interventions, we discuss the role of the clinician in helping the dying patient to deal with these issues.

Containing, Mentalization, and Narrative

The clinician's role in the care of the dying patient can be compared to the role that parents assume toward their child: to engage when he or she is subjected to painful emotions (containing) and to try to understand and reflect on his or her situation (mentalization). Containing is one of the nonspecific elements of any psychological or psychotherapeutic approach. It allows the patient to identify with the clinician's capacity to face and sustain painful emotions such as anxiety, anger, or sadness. For many patients, a containing environment is sufficient to help them feel comforted and able to cope with existential threat (Stiefel and Bernard 2008).

Mentalization refers to the parents' capacity to reflect on what their child experiences and why he or she experiences the situation that way. For example, although a young son may not yet be able to understand what happens to him in a given situation (e.g., he feels angry because he is tired or hungry), the parents' understanding of the child's experience allows them not only to react appropriately, but also to remind the child, without losing their minds, that he should now go to bed. Even if the child remains unable to fully understand what happens to him, he identifies with the parents' attitude, and he benefits—also on an emotional level—from their capacity to reflect. Similarly, patients who are cared for by clinicians who have the capacity to mentalize, by reflecting and understanding the patients' reactions and emotions, usually remain calm even if they do not totally understand what happens to them.

Some patients perceive that their current emotions are linked to similar emotions experienced in the past and they engage in a narrative process (i.e., they begin to tell their story), providing the elements that allow themselves and others to understand the present feelings, thoughts, and reactions. Establishing links and enhancing understanding become a powerful tool to regain control, to recognize oneself in an unexpected reaction, and to reestablish a sense of continuity.

Case Vignette

A 42-year-old woman, recently diagnosed with breast cancer and facing chemotherapy, consulted a psychologist. Angered and agitated, she complained about her cruel destiny: she, who had always lived correctly, who never smoked or abused alcohol, was now confronted with breast cancer. The first consultation was dedicated to the expression of her emotions, contained by the psychologist, who hypothesized 1) that the patient had a tendency to offer herself as a sacrifice, given the fact that she cared for years for her mother-in-law, who suffered from Alzheimer disease, while educating her children and working for her husband's business, and 2) that cancer represented a supplementary, unjust burden of her life that she could no longer tolerate and that interferes with her usual way of functioning by means of offering herself as a sacrifice (mentalization).

During the second consultation, the patient was even more agitated, stating that she was very close to an outburst of anger in front of her family or her husband's clients. Invited to speak about what happened since the last consultation, the patient reported that she informed her mother about the impending chemotherapy and that her mother's only reaction was to ask, "Who will now help me with my shopping?" Questioned about her life trajectory and her relationship with her mother, the patient explained that her father died when she was 3 years old and that she was raised in poor circumstances by her mother, who was a simple working-class woman trying to get the best out of her life (narrative). She reported that her mother never received any help from family or neighbors but was always complimented for her courage, and that she (the patient) as a child helped her mother and was called in the village "the brave little soldier."

Linking the past and the present, the psychologist stated 1) that the patient's angered reaction was quite understandable, given that she once again was in a situation of need, yet nobody, not even her mother, showed concern, and 2) that her anger may make her feel uncomfortable, because she always assumed the role of the "brave little soldier" without complaints. The patient felt relieved by this comment and was able to recognize that her unusual and thus frightening feelings of anger could be understood as a sign that she should modify her habit of caring for others and neglecting her own needs. A brief psychodynamic-oriented psychotherapy of 15 sessions complemented these first consultations, leading to an increase in the patient's autonomy and a decrease of guilt when she defended her own interests.

Psychodynamic Psychotherapy in Palliative Care

Psychodynamic interventions are intended to help patients develop self-understanding and insight into recurrent problems with others. During the therapeutic process, symptoms and interpersonal difficulties are identified and interpreted based on the concept that insight and experiences in the therapeutic relationship can be transferred to "the world outside the therapeutic setting" (Kaplan and Sadock 1998).

Psychodynamic interventions share some key assumptions (Stiefel and Bernard 2008): 1) the existence of an unconscious, which colors a person's thoughts, emotions, and behaviors; 2) the influence of early development on later stages of life; 3) the organization of the psyche by the ego, which has the capacity to reason and to anticipate, the id, which is a source of sexual and aggressive drives, and the superego, which dominates these drives and is generally called "guilty conscience"; 4) the protection of the individual's equilibrium by (unconscious) defense mechanisms, such as rationalization, projection, or denial, which are triggered by threatening emotions or thoughts; and 5) the observation that unresolved issues of the patient are reenacted in the therapeutic setting, where they can be interpreted, discussed, and thus modified. Table 11–1 summarizes these assumptions.

The different types of psychodynamic psychotherapy range from *insight-oriented psychotherapy*, which uncovers repressed, unconscious material to help a patient gain autonomy, to *supportive psychotherapy*, which, for more vulnerable patients, aims to suppress anxiety-provoking unconscious and conscious material and to foster ego functions and defenses that contribute to the patient's adjustment to disease (Lewin 2005). For dying patients, supportive psychotherapy is in most situations the treatment of choice.

A special form of psychodynamic psychotherapy is the psychodynamic life narrative, which can be used to conceptualize human responses to physical illness and to help the patient understand his or her current reactions by linking them to important elements of the patient's life trajectory. The therapist focuses primarily on the current crisis and symptoms, but also attempts to complete the narrative of the patient by specifically investigating his or her development and important elements of the patient's life trajectory, which usually contains information that may also in part explain his or her current reactions to illness. In the previous vignette on the "brave little soldier," the psychologist's intervention focused mainly on the patient's psychodynamic life narrative; the patient felt relieved because she could recognize that her feelings of anger, which were completely new for her, were an understandable consequence of her life trajectory and, as such, not a "bad" reaction but a sign to modify—at least momentarily—her "altruistic" attitude. In other words, she realized that her reaction "made sense," and she was no longer disturbed by an emotion she had never experienced in the past. This type of therapy offers the patient an opportunity to develop a sense of control and coherence in a situation that beforehand has been perceived as chaotic (Viederman 2000).

Systemic Psychotherapy in Palliative Care

Systemic psychotherapy is based on general systems theory, which understands a system, such as the family, as an organized system. The main goal is to understand not only the functions of the different elements of a system but also their interrelations. Systemic psychotherapy views the family or other forms of social coexistence as a complex and integrated whole, which is greater than the sum of its parts (Minuchin 1988; Sameroff 1983).

Any of the different forms of systemic therapy can be beneficial in the palliative care setting. An example of systemic therapy that has been scientifically evaluated is family-focused grief therapy, a preventive intervention for high-risk families that is based on the assumption that the family is the primary provider of care for the terminally ill patient and that the family's relational functioning affects the patient (Kissane et al. 1996a, 1996b). The aim of family-focused grief therapy is to optimize family functioning and to facilitate the sharing of grief in order to minimize psychosocial morbidity by

TABLE 11–1. Key assumptions of psychodynamic psychotherapy
The unconscious colors thoughts, emotions, and behavior.
Childhood development influences later stages of life.
The psyche is organized by the ego (executive functions), the id (drives), and the superego (guilty conscience).
Defense mechanisms preserve the psychological equilibrium.
Unresolved issues of the past can be reenacted and resolved in the therapeutic setting.

means of a time-limited intervention (four to eight sessions of 90 minutes each). In other words, amelioration of functioning of a family that is struggling with losses (e.g., loss of the health of a family member) and anticipating the future loss of the patient will ultimately also be of benefit for the patient.

Cognitive and Behavioral Psychotherapy in Palliative Care

Cognitive and behavioral interventions are based on the assumption that conscious thoughts and behaviors are most relevant in the etiology and maintenance of psychological disorders. The interventions, often completed by homework assignments, intend to reduce psychological distress and enhance adaptive coping by modifying maladaptive thoughts and behaviors, and by providing new skills (Hollon and Beck 2004).

According to cognitive theory (Beck 1991), maladaptive thoughts are part of an integrated knowledge structure (schema) that influences the way judgments are built. In cognitive therapy, patients are invited to systematically evaluate their beliefs, judgments, and information processes and to challenge them with alternative views provided by the therapist (Beck et al. 1979). Behavioral interventions focus on overt behaviors and strategies to modify them. These interventions are based on classical stimulus-response theory, founded by Pavlov and Gantt (1928).

Cognitive and behavioral interventions for medically ill patients are most often mentioned with regard to symptom control, such as control of pain (Turk and Feldman 2000). Although cognitive and behavioral techniques are optimal in a one-to-one professional-patient relationship, in most medical settings the lack of time requires that these methods be provided by means of written or audiotaped material.

Several studies confirmed that focusing on positive states of mind (Seligman and Csikszentmihalyi 2000) through the acquisition of stress management skills with cognitive and behavioral interventions can have a positive impact on improving quality of life in cancer patients (Penedo et al. 2004, 2006). Although these studies were not conducted in the palliative care setting, patients with advanced disease are challenged by different physical, psychological, and social stressors (pain, facing loss, dealing with financial questions) and therefore might also benefit from such skill improvements.

Existential Psychotherapy in Palliative Care

Humanistic psychology emerged in the 1950s in reaction to both behaviorism and psychoanalysis. The main principles of humanistic psychology are summarized by five postulates developed by Bugental (1964): 1) human beings cannot be reduced to components; 2) human beings belong to a unique human context; 3) human consciousness includes the awareness of oneself in the context of other people; 4) human beings have choices and responsibilities; and 5) human beings are intentional—they seek meaning, value, and creativity. These principles are reiterated in Table 11–2.

According to Richman (1995), existential psychotherapy—which is part of humanistic psychology—with the terminally ill should be based on the view that every life is worth living to the very end. Objectives of the treatment are to enrich the last days of life, to deal with unfinished business, to increase social and family cohesion, and to prepare for a "good" death. One of the most frequently used forms of existential therapy is Viktor Frankl's logotherapy, which is based on his experience as a prisoner in a Nazi concentration camp during World War II (Stiefel and Bernard 2008). This therapy is concerned with the search for meaning; Frankl considered that men perceive meaning in three main domains: in creativity, in relationships, and in a broader sense of existence surpassing the individual's experience of being. Considering that these issues are most important at the end of life, psychotherapies inspired by Frankl's work can be considered as beneficial in palliative care (Breitbart et al. 2004). (See Appendix 1–B, "Existential Psychotherapies," in Chapter 1.)

Nonspecific or Common Elements and Concerns in All Psychotherapies

Although each narrowly focused intervention requires that a clinician have specific technical skills and familiarity with the method, nonspecific or common elements across all the different psychotherapies have been identified that influence psychotherapeutic outcome regardless of the technique. Among these common elements are, for example, "learning factors," referring to the fact that human beings can learn from experience.

TABLE 11–2. Key assumptions of humanistic psychology
Human beings cannot be divided into components.
They belong to a unique human context.
Consciousness includes awareness of oneself in the context of other people.
Persons are intentional and have choices and responsibilities.
Human beings search for meaning, value, and creativity.

An important question with regard to psychotherapy is whether technique or relational aspects are more important for outcome. In clinical practice, both technical skills (e.g., analysis and feedback concerning material provided by the patient, adequate identification of the patient's capacity and limits for growth) and relational aspects (e.g., empathy, authenticity, flexibility, tolerance) are important. Moreover, technique and relational competencies are interrelated (Stiefel and Bernard 2008).

Psychotherapy research indicates that an important part (50%) of outcome variance remains unexplained (Lambert and Ogles 2004). However, various factors contributing to outcome variance have been identified: psychopathology or severity of the symptoms of the patient (about 25%), relational aspects (about 10%), variables related to the therapist (about 10%), and technical skills (about 5%) (Beutler et al. 2004). These findings do not imply that technique and specific skills can be replaced by "sympathy"; technical skills and theoretical knowledge are important tools allowing a therapist to understand and thus be able to fully develop the relational aspects, such as empathy, which greatly depends on the comprehension of a given situation. However, these studies on outcome challenge the ideology of psychotherapeutic "schools" and question the constant reinvention of "new" psychotherapeutic approaches, which are especially prevalent in palliative care (Stiefel and Bernard 2008).

Clinicians should keep in mind that dying patients often suffer from cognitive impairment, which may interfere with psychotherapeutic approaches that require a certain level of concentration. For such patients, other interventions that might be more appropriate than verbal psychotherapeutic ones include providing a holding environment that respects their limitations; taking care to avoid over- or understimulating them; containing, mentalization, and other nonspecific elements that are present in any patient encounter (as discussed earlier in this section of the chapter); facilitating the presence of family members (especially during the night); and using body-centered approaches (massage, relaxation, etc.).

Support of the Supporters

Up to 30% of oncologists suffer from psychiatric morbidity and report high levels of emotional exhaustion and professional demotivation and low levels of personal achievement, indicating burnout (Ramirez et al. 1996). Work-related stress in cancer care is related to heavy clinical and administrative duties, unpredictable work schedules, and exposure to suffering and death (Shanafelt et al. 2006). Although patient volume, as well as administration and organization of work, can only be influenced on an institutional level, the oncology clinician can reflect on his or her way of facing suffering and death and try to cope with it more adequately, thus reducing stress in the patient encounter.

To face the dying patient represents a kind of archetypal situation that provokes stress in any clinician, challenges one's professional and personal identity, and calls for support. In this section, we discuss key issues for the support of the supporter (Stiefel 2008).

Coping With Limits

For some clinicians, guiding the patient at the end of life is extremely stressful; this is especially the case for those who have great difficulty respecting their own limits. Facing the limits of cure may then trigger strong emotions, such as guilt or rage, and provoke reactions, such as massive denial of the patient's suffering or acting out by pursuing treatments that do more harm than good.

Being able to recognize and respect limits, which are part of life and of the medical profession, requires that oncology clinicians 1) reflect on their attitudes toward limits, 2) identify their personal and professional experiences with limits, and 3) question their own professional identity (Stiefel and Guex 1996). Clinicians need to consider how they have experienced and reacted to limits in childhood and adulthood, how they understand their professional duties, and how they deal with the fact that not all cancer patients can be cured. If a clinician, for example, facing situations of therapeutic impotence, finds himself confronted with intense feelings of anger or despair due to ancient but still active memories of having been obliged as a kid to helplessly witness the long and painful agony of his dying mother, he will have to work on his past if he intends to continue to work with patients for whom curative treatment is not longer possible. Based on our experience with communication skills training (CST)—which includes in Switzerland several individual sessions of supervisions, during which exactly such issues are often reported by clinicians—focusing on the interrelations between personal and professional experiences can be very helpful. If a clinician's personal experiences are interfering considerably with his or her professional duties, a personal psychotherapy may be indicated; otherwise, professional burnout may sooner or later paralyze a clinician who struggles with unresolved issues from the past.

Winnicott (1993) argues that people cannot ask for, and do not themselves have to be, "perfect mothers": it is sufficient to be a "good-enough mother" who provides adequate care and is sensitive to the infant's needs. For our discussion, "mother" can be replaced by "clinician." In health care, the clinician's duty is to cure patients and to care for those who cannot be cured. If the clinician denies or ignores the limits of curative power, he or she might expose patients to a danger, for example by continuing aggressive treatments in palliative situations.

Continual reflection on one's personal way of facing limits and on how the institutional and cultural context deals with limits is therefore an important task of the oncology clinician in order to adequately care for the patients for whom curative treatment is not possible (anymore). Such reflection is important not only for the patient, but also for the clinician's psychological well-being. Feeling constantly pressured by situations of patient transition to palliative care may induce feelings of helplessness, impotence, guilt, or rage, which are difficult to endure and may lead to high levels of stress and distress, professional burnout, and/or psychiatric disorders such as depression or substance abuse. In contrast, by being able to accept the limits of medicine, the clinician will diminish work-related stress, increase job satisfaction, and feel more adequate in the care of the palliative patient. In many cancer centers, however, this topic is ignored despite the fact that attention to it could play an important role in reducing professional stress. Creating a professional environment that allows open discussions of these issues and provides the clinicians with access to collective and/or individual supervision of their experiences can be most beneficial.

Deconstruction of Ego Ideals

Progression of disease also represents a source of considerable psychological distress for the clinician, such as when facing patients who are desperately searching for new treatments and innovative drugs, patients who are in denial or feeling hopelessness, or family members who put considerable pressure on the patient and/or health care providers. Caring for patients at the end of life not only challenges the capacities of the clinician's "ego," which should harbor medical, psychological, and human experience and competence, but also stimulates his or her "ego ideal." The ego ideal—a source for professional achievements—creates the desire for how a clinician would like to be. If there is a considerable gap between how one is and how one wishes to be and if one does not reflect on ego ideals, then psychological distress arises in the clinician (Stiefel 2008). During a professional career, the process of deconstructing ego ideals without resigning or becoming cynical is important, although it is rarely discussed and in some settings is even avoided by creating an institutional illusion of "winning the war on cancer." In contrast, clinicians who are able to mourn their ego ideals and who are satisfied with their actual capacities feel less pressure and can establish trustful and supporting relationships with their patients. As a senior oncologist stated,

> It was quite sad for me to slowly adjust my ambitions to the reality of what we can do in oncology. Of course we are constantly shifting between feelings of power and impotence, and of course we should never give up; but pushing the limits should be restricted to research and not an attitude in the clinical treatment of far advanced cancer. After adjusting my ambitions to reality, I finally felt liberated by the idea that I no longer have to do more than I can; I feel more comfortable to talk with patients whose diseases progress and I am now able to listen. And that's what counts in these situations.

Empathy, Identification, Countertransference, and Collusion

Communication with dying patients is often limited to short conversations, because patients are exhausted or tend to withdraw from relationships when facing the end of life. Therefore, the nonverbal communication and attitudes of the clinician, largely influenced by his or her own emotional state, become crucial. Death and dying evoke empathy in the clinician. *Empathy*, which can be defined as understanding, being aware of, being sensitive to, and experiencing the feelings and thoughts of another, implies not only closeness to the patient, but also the capacity to distance oneself again and concentrate on oneself.

Not only empathy, however, is triggered by the patient's suffering (Table 11–3). If adequate distance is lacking, *identification* may occur, with the consequence that there is no distinction between the physician and the patient: the physician experiences "being the patient," and the patient has the impression of not being able to count any longer on a competent and professional health care provider. Empathy has to be distinguished not only from identification, but also from *countertransference* (Gabbard 1994), defined as an interpersonal experience with roots in the clinician's own biography. Countertransference colored by positive or negative emotions is especially frequent in distressful situations, such as end of life, and influences the clinician's attitude, perhaps by leading him or her to avoid a patient (negative countertransference) or to favor a patient excessively while

---

TABLE 11–3. **Empathy and other frequent phenomena occurring in the clinician-patient relationship**

Empathy: the capacity to be sensitive to the experiences of another

Identification: the lack of adequate distance to the patient

Countertransference: an interpersonal experience of the clinician with roots in his or her own biography

Collusion: the patient and the physician struggle with the same, largely unconscious and unresolved issues

---

neglecting other patients in need (positive countertransference). Finally, *collusion* (Gabbard 1994) must be distinguished from empathy. Collusion— often perceived as extremely strong emotional experiences—occurs when patient and physician are both struggling with the same, largely unconscious, problems. Collusion may occur with regard to unresolved losses in the past leading to highly emotional reactions; for example, a request for assisted suicide anticipating the loss of life may provoke the physician to immediately comply or to react aggressively, refusing to even discuss what might have caused the request.

The way the oncology clinician encounters the dying patient is also influenced by the clinician's own representation of death. Without reflecting on his or her own death and on the meaning of death, the oncologist will not be able to adequately accompany the patient, because the clinician will be guided more by his or her own representations than by what the patient experiences. The following dialogue among members of an oncology team illustrates various ways of perceiving death:

> MEDICAL ONCOLOGIST: For me, death represents a crevasse. There is nothing more after death—just a dark and lonely hole.
> ONCOLOGY NURSE: I think that after the patient has died, he will be gone for an eternal journey in the galaxy.
> PSYCHIATRIST: How do you separate from dying patients?
> MEDICAL ONCOLOGIST: I never say good-bye to them. I try to avoid this topic and I sometimes even avoid the patient.
> ONCOLOGY NURSE: When I feel that my patient might pass away while I'm off duty, I tell her before I leave that I hope she will have a peaceful journey.

These different representations of death influence the care provided and demonstrate how confusing and distressing it might be for a patient to be subjected to a variety of attitudes by carers. Clinicians who are aware of and able to question their own representations of death and attitudes toward the dying patient do not confuse their own ideas with the patient's experience of death and can join in the way the patient feels and not in the way they imagine the patient is feeling or the way they want the patient to feel.

Clarification of their own representations therefore enables clinicians to realize that patients have a variety of feelings and thoughts about death and dying and many of them face death without fear but with a feeling of inner peace; and they will also perceive that the wish for a "good death for everyone" is an illusion based on the carers' need to avoid their own suffering. Some patients want to clarify some issues, others do not; some want to solve conflicts and others do not; and some want to say goodbye to loved ones and others do not. It might be adequate to question the patient's attitudes, especially at the end of life, but no patient should be burdened with the clinician's own expectations and needs, and everyone should have the right to die in his or her own way. The fact that clinicians allow themselves to encounter the patient's experience of terminal illness will ultimately help them to reduce their own fears about death and reduce the stress evoked by the encounter with the dying.

Communication Challenges and Training

Patient interviews are stressful, especially when communicating about end-of-life issues. This was illustrated in a study by Bernard et al. (2010), showing that a 15-minute (simulated) patient interview in CST was associated with a high number and variety of defense mechanisms emerging in oncology clinicians. A subgroup of clinicians who participated in CST showed an increase in mature defenses after training, resulting in lower levels of anxiety. Defense mechanisms—operating without consciousness and triggered by anxiety-provoking situations in order to contribute to the individual's adaptation—therefore are indicators for stress.

Defenses, especially immature defenses such as projection and denial, may temporarily reduce threatening emotions, but they also 1) diminish the clinician's capacity to integrate all aspects of a given situation, 2) weaken the working alliance with the patient, and 3) hamper the clinician's ability to respond to the patient's needs, thus complicating the relationship, which in turn leads to increased stress. In addition, even if a defensive attitude is protective, it might contribute in the long run to psychological distress and disturbances (Gabbard 1994).

Physicians with a defensive attitude who show difficulties in containing their own emotions use so-called blocking behaviors (Maguire and Pitceathly 2002), which are unconscious communication strategies aimed at suppressing the patient's emotional expression. Blocking behaviors occur, for example, in unbalanced interviews with an overwhelming length of speaking time by the physician, a focus on biomedical aspects, abrupt transitions from emotions to medical information, cynical remarks or nonverbal behaviors indicating time pressure, or a detached attitude.

Given the fact that CST is effective with regard to skills improvement, development of such training programs can only be welcomed. This training should include self-reflection, most efficiently developed in individual supervision, which is an integrated part of the Swiss CST, mandatory for specialization in oncology (Stiefel et al. 2010b). Self-reflection elements in CST enable the clinician to identify, describe, and question his or her own defenses, which will lead to patient encounters that are less contaminated by the clinician's own preoccupations.

Besides the fact that training should include self-reflection elements, there are also minimal requirements, as defined in a consensus statement on CST (Stiefel et al. 2010a) based on a systematic review (Barth and Lannen 2011) and adapted by the European Society for Medical Oncology (2010). In this paper, among other recommendations, it is stated that CST should 1) last at least 3 days to ensure transfer of skills into practice; 2) be provided in small groups (4–6 persons per facilitator), allowing active participation and interactivity; 3) be run by trained and competent facilitators; and 4) integrate role play, group discussions, and didactic material, including prepared videos with patients and actors. If these criteria are respected, CST can be of great help toward improving clinicians' skills. In contrast, courses that try to do it "the quick way" are at best useless, and might even be counterproductive.

Conclusion

Supporting the dying patient is one of the most challenging tasks for the oncology clinician. It demands not only human and psychological competencies, but also constant reflection on the clinician's own representations about death and dying, the capacity to contain painful emotions, acceptance of limits and support, and the motivation for continuous postgraduate education with regard to psycho-oncological and communicational aspects of cancer care.

Key Clinical Points

- Adjustment to existential threat is influenced by different variables, such as biography, emotions, representations, defenses, coping, context, and support; all of these should be evaluated, because they might be sources of distress and targets of support.

- Psychological challenges of the dying patient include loss of control, facing uncertainty and separation, and dealing with unresolved issues of the past. Different psychotherapeutic interventions, if indicated, can be of great help to the dying patient.

- To encounter dying patients is stressful for oncology clinicians. Support of the supporters consists of helping clinicians to accept limits, to reflect on their ego ideals, and to consider empathy, identification, countertransference, and collusion arising in their relationships with these patients.

- Communication skills training (CST) not only can improve clinicians' skills but, by means of self-reflection elements, can also contribute to clinicians' psychological well-being; however, CST needs to fulfill minimal requirements in order to be effective.

References

Barth J, Lannen P: Efficacy of communication skills training in oncology: a systematic review and meta-analysis. Ann Oncol 22:1030–1040, 2011

Beck AT: Cognitive therapy: a 30-year retrospective. Am Psychol 46:368–376, 1991

Beck AT, Rush AJ, Shaw B, et al: Cognitive Therapy of Depression. New York, Guilford, 1979

Bernard M, de Roten Y, Despland JN, et al: Communication skills training and clinicians' defenses in oncology: an exploratory, controlled study. Psychooncology 19:209–215, 2010

Beutler LE, Malik M, Alimohamed S, et al: Therapist variables, in Bergin and Garfield's Handbook of Psychotherapy and Behavior Change, 5th Edition. Edited by Lambert MJ. New York, Wiley, 2004, pp 227–306

Bowlby J: A Secure Base: Parent-Child Attachment and Healthy Human Development. New York, Basic Books, 1988

Breitbart W, Gibson C, Poppito SR, et al: Psychotherapeutic interventions at the end of life: a focus on meaning and spirituality. Can J Psychiatry 49:366–372, 2004

Bugental JFT: The third force in psychology. Journal of Humanistic Psychology 4:19–25, 1964

Erikson E: Eight Stages of Men: Childhood and Society. New York, WW Norton, 1950, pp 219–233

European Society for Medical Oncology: Recommendations for a global curriculum in medical oncology. 2010. Available at: http://www.esmo.org/education-research/recommendations-for-a-global-core-curriculum-in-mo.html. Accessed July 31, 2012.

Gabbard GO: Psychodynamic Psychiatry in Clinical Practice. Washington, DC, American Psychiatric Publishing, 1994

Guex P, Stiefel F, Rousselle I: Psychotherapy with patients with cancer. Psychother Rev 2:269–273, 2000

Hollon SD, Beck AT: Cognitive and cognitive behavioral therapies, in Bergin and Garfield's Handbook of Psychotherapy and Behavior Change. Edited by Lambert MJ. New York, Wiley, 2004, pp 447–542

Kaplan HI, Sadock BJ: Kaplan and Sadock's Synopsis of Psychiatry: Behavioral Sciences/Clinical Psychiatry, 8th Edition. Baltimore, MD, Williams & Wilkins, 1998

Kissane DW, Bloch S, Dowe DL, et al: The Melbourne Family Grief Study, I: perceptions of family functioning in bereavement. Am J Psychiatry 153:650–658, 1996a

Kissane DW, Bloch S, Dowe DL, et al: The Melbourne Family Grief Study, II: psychosocial morbidity and grief in bereaved families. Am J Psychiatry 153:659–666, 1996b

Kübler-Ross E: On Death and Dying. New York, Macmillan, 1969

Lambert MJ, Ogles BM: The efficacy and effectiveness of psychotherapy, in Bergin and Garfield's Handbook of Psychotherapy and Behavior Change, 5th Edition. Edited by Lambert MJ. New York, Wiley, 2004, pp 139–193

Lewin K: The theoretical basis of dynamic psychiatry, in Psychodynamic Psychiatry in Clinical Practice: the DSM-IV Edition. Edited by Gabbard GO. Washington, DC, American Psychiatric Publishing, 2005, pp 29–63

Maguire P, Pitceathly C: Key communication skills and how to acquire them. BMJ 325:687–700, 2002

Minuchin P: Relationships within the family: a systems perspective on development, in Relationships Within Families: Mutual Influences. Edited by Hinde RA, Stevenson-Hinde J. New York, Wiley, 1988, pp 7–26

Pavlov IP, Gantt WH: Lectures on Conditioned Reflexes: Twenty-Five Years of Objective Study of the Higher Nervous Activity (Behaviour) of Animals. New York, Liverwright Publishing, 1928

Penedo FJ, Dahn JR, Molton I, et al: Cognitive-behavioral stress management improves stress management skills and quality of life in men recovering from treatment of prostate carcinoma. Cancer 100:192–200, 2004

Penedo FJ, Molton I, Dahn JR, et al: A randomized clinical trial of group-based cognitive-behavioral stress management in localized prostate cancer: development of stress management skills improves quality of life and benefit finding. Ann Behav Med 31:261–270, 2006

Ramirez AJ, Graham J, Richards MA, et al: Mental health of hospital consultants: the effects of stress and satisfaction at work. Lancet 347:724–728, 1996

Razavi D, Stiefel F: Common psychiatric disorders in cancer patients, I: adjustment disorders and depressive disorders. Support Care Cancer 2:223–232, 1994

Richman J: From despair to integrity: an Eriksonian approach to psychotherapy for the terminally ill. Psychotherapy 32:317–322, 1995

Sameroff AJ: Developmental systems: context and evolution, in Handbook of Child Psychology: History, Theory, and Methods. Edited by Mussen PH, Kessen W. New York, Wiley, 1983, pp 237–294

Seligman MEP, Csikszentmihalyi M: Positive psychology: an introduction. Am Psychol 55:5–14, 2000

Shanafelt T, Chung H, White H, et al: Shaping your career to maximize personal satisfaction in the practice of oncology. J Clin Oncol 24:4020–4026, 2006

Stiefel F: Support of the supporters. Supportive Care Cancer 16:123–126, 2008

Stiefel F, Bernard M: Psychotherapeutic interventions in palliative care, in Psychosocial Issues in Palliative Care, 2nd Edition. Edited by Lloyd-Williams M. New York, Oxford University Press, 2008, pp 161–178

Stiefel F, Guex P: Palliative and supportive care: at the frontier of medical omnipotence. Ann Oncol 7:135–138, 1996

Stiefel F, Razavi D: Common psychiatric disorders in cancer patients, II: anxiety and acute confusional states. Support Care Cancer 2:233–237, 1994

Stiefel F, Razavi D: Informing about diagnosis, relapse, and progression of disease: communication with the terminally ill cancer patient, in Communication in Cancer Care: Recent Results in Cancer Research. Edited by Stiefel F. Berlin, Germany, Springer Verlag, 2006, pp 37–46

Stiefel F, Guex P, Real O: An introduction to psycho-oncology with special emphasis to its historical and cultural context, in Topics in Palliative Care, Vol. 3. Edited by Bruera E, Portenoy R. New York, Oxford University Press, 1998, pp 175–189

Stiefel F, Krenz S, Zdrojewski C, et al: Meaning in life assessed with the "Schedule for Meaning in Live Evaluation" (SMILE): a comparison between a cancer patient and student sample. Supportive Care Cancer 16:1151–1155, 2008

Stiefel F, Barth J, Bensing J, et al: Communication skills training in oncology: a position paper based on a consensus meeting among European experts in 2009. Ann Oncol 21:204–207, 2010a

Stiefel F, Bernhard J, Bianchi G, et al: The Swiss model, in Handbook of Communication in Oncology and Palliative Care. Edited by Kissane D, Bultz B, Butow P, et al. New York, Oxford University Press, 2010b, pp 642–648

Turk DC, Feldman CS: A cognitive-behavioral approach to symptom management in palliative care: augmenting somatic interventions, in Handbook of Psychiatry in Palliative Medicine. Edited by Chochinov HM, Breitbart W. New York, Oxford University Press, 2000, pp 223–240

Viederman M: The supportive relationship, the psychodynamic life narrative, and the dying patient, in Handbook of Psychiatry in Palliative Medicine. Edited by Chochinov HM, Breitbart W. New York, Oxford University Press, 2000, pp 215–222

Weisman A: Coping With Cancer. New York, McGraw-Hill, 1979

Winnicott DW: Babies and Their Mothers. Reading, MA, Addison-Wesley, 1993

CHAPTER 12

Psycho-Oncology and Optimal Standards of Cancer Care

Developments, Multidisciplinary Team Approach, and International Guidelines

Luigi Grassi, M.D.
Rosangela Caruso, M.D.
Maria Giulia Nanni, M.D.

The authors are deeply indebted to Elisabeth Andtritsch (Austria), Pia Dellson (Sweden), Haryana Dhillon (Australia), Maria Die-Trill (Spain), Joachim Weis and Andrea Schumacher (Germany), Deborah McLeod (Canada), Lucia M. Silva Monteiro (Portugal), Kazuhiro Yoshiuchi (Japan), Mecheline van der Linden (The Netherlands), Brigitta Wössmer (Switzerland), Lea Baider (Israel), and Sedat Ozkan (Turkey) as representatives of the national societies of psycho-oncology within the International Federation of Psycho-Oncology Societies (www.ipos-society.org) whose contribution in delineating the role of psychosocial oncology in their own countries has been invaluable. Updated information involving more countries is available in Grassi and Watson (2012) and on the Federation website.

> Anyone who has had an extensive experience in the treatment of cancer is aware that there are great differences among patients.... There is solid evidence that the course of the disease in general is affected by emotional distress.... Could this not be an area for another discipline in medicine[?]...Thus, we as doctors may begin to emphasize treatment of the patient as a whole as well as the disease from which the patient is suffering.
>
> Eugene Pendergrass (Presidential Address, American Cancer Society, 1959)

Cancer is a group of very different multidetermined diseases with treatments that have become extremely complex. Cancer is also a devastating illness with physical, emotional, interpersonal, and social implications that should be constantly monitored across the disease trajectory (Grassi et al. 2010). For these reasons, the only possible way to achieve optimal cancer care and outcome is having, as Pendergrass stated many years ago in his presidential address to the American Cancer Society, a holistic approach that involves considering and treating the patient as a whole (Pendergrass 1961).

Nowadays, this holistic approach is attained through an integration of different professionals working together in multidisciplinary teams (MDTs), instead of having a single professional working alone with a patient. According to Fleissig et al. (2006), not using MDTs in oncology services can result in problems such as nonuniform access to specialist care, frequent reports of inadequacies in cancer services, a disjointed referral system, large variations in frequency of individual treatments used, and variations in caseloads for particular doctors treating cancer. In contrast, the objective of MDTs is essentially to improve the consistency and continuity of care, the coordination and cost effectiveness of care, the communication between health professionals, and, consequently, the clinical outcomes. This would favor recruitment into clinical trials, satisfaction and psychological well-being of patients, job satisfaction and psychological well-being of team members, and educational opportunities for health professionals (Fleissig et al. 2006). In fact, reviews about the effects of teamwork confirmed that working in MDTs reduces hospitalization time, costs, and unanticipated admissions; favors better accessibility for patients; and improves coordination of care. Moreover, findings indicate enhanced satisfaction, acceptance of treatment, and improved health outcomes for patients, as well as enhanced job satisfaction, greater role clarity, and enhanced well-being among team members (Mickan 2005; Mickan and Rodger 2005).

However, MDTs are entities whose complexities derive from the fact that they do not consist of professionals who work independently and occasionally meet and discuss issues with one another but rather are organized as a group of professionals who work side by side sharing all the processes of care (J. F. Holland et al. 2010). Therefore, MDTs need to be well organized in order to work coherently and consistently, and some aspects, including team philosophy, leadership, dynamics, communication, and workload, are essential areas and dimensions that should be taken into account for effective and successful MDT care.

Some principles have been described (Turner 2010) as helping strategies to facilitate the integration and functioning of the professionals in MDTs. In particular, the aims and purposes of the work team should be clear and relevant for the patients and the organization; the intrinsic goals should be shared and agreed upon by the members of the team; the leaders of the team should be able to create and maintain the structure, manage possible conflicts, and coordinate the several tasks by giving feedback; communication should be clear and based on regular patterns; and a sense of cohesion should develop through the work team, with mutual respect sustained for the various professions represented and for the characteristics of individual members.

Following all these principles is not an easy task, and problems in reciprocal interaction are often reported. Team malfunctioning is possible when MDT members do not know the specific roles and activities expected of each component of the team (Catt et al. 2005; Jenkins et al. 2001). Other vulnerabilities and challenges that occur when working in teams, and that should be carefully evaluated, include personality conflicts, power struggles, distortion in communication, competitiveness, role confusion, splitting mechanisms, and unrealistic expectations (Loscalzo and von Gunten 2010; Loscalzo et al. 2010). If not properly addressed, these issues may contribute to the development of burnout, such as emotional exhaustion and depersonalization, which affects about one-third of cancer care professionals, and poor personal accomplishment in work activity, which affects at least one-quarter (Sherman et al. 2006; Trufelli et al. 2008).

Psycho-Oncology as Part of the Multidisciplinary Approach to Cancer

Although MDTs may differ from each other based on types and sites of cancer, stages of cancer, and kind of treatment, MDTs in cancer settings usually comprise multiple health care professionals who, by working together, provide the expertise derived from various specialties. Most cancer care MDTs include geneticists, radiologists, surgeons, medical oncologists, nurses, and palliative care physicians. However, the development of psycho-oncology, as a specialty discipline that focuses on the psychological, social, and spiritual factors that affect the quality of life of cancer patients and their loved ones, has substantiated the need for MDTs to also have psycho-oncologists, as specialist clinical professionals involved in the care of cancer patients and their families.

Psycho-oncology is *de facto* an area of multidisciplinary interest, because it shares its boundaries with the major specialties of oncology (e.g., medical oncology, hematology, radiation oncology, surgery, palliative care), psychiatry and psychology, and biological sciences (e.g., epidemiology, immunology, biology, pathology, genetics) (J.C. Holland 2003, 2004). Although the emotional impact of cancer and cancer treatment on patients and their families, the complex psychological implications of terminal illness, and the psychophysiological factors implicated in cancer first gained the attention of a small group of psychiatrists in the 1950s and 1960s (Bhanson 1969; Bhanson and Kissen 1966; Blumberg et al. 1954; Kübler-Ross 1969; Sutherland 1956), it was the oncologists' need for more precise indications about the psychosocial, behavioral, and rehabilitative issues in cancer care that led to growth of the field of psycho-oncology in the United States in the early 1970s (Cullen et al. 1977). This growth was definitely sanctioned by the American Cancer Society, which funded research projects and conferences on psychosocial research in the late 1970s and early 1980s (American Cancer Society 1982, 1984; Cohen et al. 1982). The increasing emergence of cancer-center advocacy groups was a concomitant factor in the growth of psycho-oncology, fueled by several studies which reported psychological and emotional implications and consequences of cancer that were felt by patients as important needs but were not being properly addressed by health care professionals (J.C. Holland, 2002).

In fact, a bulk of data have indicated that 30%–40% of cancer patients fail to adapt emotionally to their illness or treatments and therefore develop psychological disorders—mainly depressive, anxiety, and adjustment disorders as defined in ICD-10 (World Health Organization 1992) and DSM-IV (American Psychiatric Association 1994) taxonomic systems (Caruso et al. 2012; Mitchell et al. 2011). A further 15%–25% present with other significant clinical conditions such as health anxiety, irritable mood, demoralization, or general emotional distress, which are usually identified not through the categorical systems such as DSM-IV and ICD-10, but instead with other systems (e.g., Diagnostic Criteria for Psychosomatic Research) (Fava et al. 1995, 2001; Grassi et al. 2007).

The implications and the impact of psychosocial disorders (both the classical psychiatric diagnoses and the psychosocial conditions deserving

clinical attention) for the patients and the families are of paramount importance in oncology. Several studies have demonstrated that clinically significant distress is associated with maladaptive coping, reduction of quality of
life, impairment in social relationships, risk of suicide, longer rehabilitation
time, poor adherence to treatment, abnormal illness behavior, family dysfunction and psychosocial morbidity, and possibly shorter survival (Grassi
et al. 2005; Robson et al. 2010).

Significant levels of emotional distress have also been reported to affect
family members equally with or even more than cancer patients, and evidence shows that unrecognized and unmet psychosocial needs are an important predictor of psychological morbidity in caregivers (Baider et al.
2000; Glajchen 2004; Pitceathly and Maguire 2003). In fact, emotional disorders can be shown among cancer patients' caregivers in every phase of the
illness, even though most literature has concentrated on grief and bereavement (Grassi 2007).

In spite of these findings, data have accumulated showing that far less
than 30% of distressed cancer patients and families needing intervention are
recognized in clinical settings by oncology health professionals and thus
referred to mental health or, more specifically, psycho-oncology services
(Grassi and Riba 2009). This means that the majority of patients and family
members are left in a condition having extremely negative consequences for
their quality of life.

Thus, the inclusion of psycho-oncologists in MDTs results in favoring
the assessment of psychological, social, and spiritual consequences of cancer and in providing more global and complete care to the patients and
caregivers (Grassi and Giraldi 2012; J.C. Holland and Weiss 2008, 2010).
Psycho-oncologists also help in managing the problems that emerge from
working in cancer MDTs, including the problem of burnout (Price et al.
2006; Vachon 2010).

Developing Psycho-Oncology Services and Programs in Cancer Settings

For the reasons cited above, the organization of psycho-oncology services or
programs has become reality in many institutions and departments. Several
examples are available according to the specific country's health system and
the type of setting (e.g., cancer or mental health; academic or nonacademic).

Creating a psycho-oncology service or program is not an easy process
because doing so requires competence and enthusiasm, as well as the capac-

ity to understand the dynamics of the context in which the program will be set up. A major problem is that funding for mental health and behavioral research in cancer has been extremely poor in comparison with funding for biomedical research. However, some changes have occurred in the last decade as multiple experiences have accumulated with regard to the integration of psychosocial programs in oncology.

According to J.C. Holland (1998), in developing a psycho-oncology service or program, several steps are necessary:

- **Step 1**—Making a proposal for the development of the service. A proposal for the creation of a specific service should be clearly written and should contain a precise and enthusiastic *mission statement* (e.g., humanistic approach to cancer and quality of life), a defined *rationale* (e.g., evidence-based literature on psychosocial issues in cancer care; information about the service and its centrality in terms of consultation, research, multiprofessional collaboration), a specification of the *functions* (e.g., types of clinical services, training, and teaching programs available; clinical research projects), and a *table of organization* (e.g., the disciplines involved in the unit and the contact persons).
- **Step 2**—Recruitment of staff in the psycho-oncology service. The optimal staff consists of mental health professionals (e.g., psychiatrists, psychologists) with training in psycho-oncology, and social workers, nurses, and volunteers with experience in working in MDTs.
- **Step 3**—Recruitment of community resources and organizations. The psycho-oncology service should liaise with cancer organizations and psychological support/mental health services in the community.
- **Step 4**—Planning to sustain morale. The risk is that psycho-oncology can be devalued by the oncology staff and institution because of stigma and/or unfamiliarity with the area. Therefore, proper strategies (e.g., attendance of psycho-oncologists at oncology conferences, discussing cases together, availability to learn the oncology way of work and vice versa, invitation of oncologists to psycho-oncology activities) can improve the collaboration.
- **Step 5**—Education and research. It is necessary that psycho-oncologists become part of local training courses in medicine, nursing, social work, psychology, and all the areas involved in cancer care, in order to have the opportunity to effectively interact with and become integrated into the educational programs of the institution.
- **Step 6**—Interfacing with oncology specialties and advocacy movements. The psycho-oncology program can represent an important opportunity to liaise with both cancer specialties (e.g., surgery, radiation, medical oncology, hematology) and advocacy movements.

The activities provided by psycho-oncology programs are based on three pillars: clinical care, education, and research. *Clinical care* of cancer patients and their families is the main aim of psycho-oncology services. Psychosocial assessment and psychological/psychiatric consultation are the most common clinical activities both in inpatient and outpatient psycho-oncology units. Many different forms of psychosocial interventions, from psychopharmacological to counseling and psychotherapy, are also usually part of psycho-oncology services and programs.

Education is intertwined with clinical care and is a second specific aim of psycho-oncology services and programs. From a general point of view, it can be structured at three levels. The first is the basic training of health care professionals on the most important and clinically useful areas of psychosocial oncology, including communication, screening for emotional distress, and decision making. For this purpose, the online multilingual core curriculum in psycho-oncology developed by the International Psycho-Oncology Society (IPOS) (2010) (www.ipos-society.org/education/core_curriculum/core_curriculum.aspx) represents an interesting and helpful basic tool to be recommended to all cancer care professionals. A second level is related to providing certain health care professionals (e.g., social workers, nurses) with more specific training on communication and counseling, psychoeducational models, and psychological support. A third level involves training programs in psychosocial oncology addressed to clinical psychologists and psychiatrists to teach them the specific interventions (e.g., mental health assessment, psychotherapy, psychopharmacology) for cancer patients and their families.

Lastly, *research* is an extremely important activity within psycho-oncology programs or services. The meaning and the role of psycho-oncology as a discipline are substantially related to what evidence-based research has indicated over the last 30 years. Research has grown exponentially in almost all areas of oncology. Given that mental health intersects with and has a relationship with every other discipline, psychosocial dimensions can be studied from all the perspectives and can involve, for their intrinsic nature, the majority of cancer fields and activities (e.g., screening campaigns, genetic oncology, survivorship, palliative care).

Some models of psycho-oncology services or programs have been described in the literature (Grassi and Travado 2012; Hutchinson et al. 2006; Levin et al. 2004; McQuellon et al. 1996). Others are mainly deducible through the details presented at Web sites of many different institutions, both academic and non-academic.

From Research and Clinical Experience to Guidelines and Recommendations on Psychosocial Care of Cancer Patients

The immense psycho-oncology literature and research gathered over the last quarter century has become the platform in many countries for the development of guidelines, recommendations, and/or proposals to their governments about the need for and the ethical value of offering psychosocial care to cancer patients (Grassi and Riba 2012). These efforts have been endorsed by the national scientific societies of psycho-oncology as well as by advocacy movements, whose roles have been and remain extremely important in the optimization of health care services (Johansen and Grassi 2010). Although the status of these developments, so far, is quite variable across countries, the general view is that psycho-oncology should be part of the organization of cancer care systems to adequately respond to the needs of cancer patients and their families (Grassi and Watson 2012). In the following subsections, we discuss the situation in some countries around the world.[1]

The Experience in the United States and Canada

In the United States, the National Comprehensive Cancer Network (NCCN; www.nccn.org) was established in 1997 with the aims of creating guidelines for treatment of cancer, including the integration of psychosocial care into routine cancer care. In particular, the NCCN Distress Management Panel, consisting of multidisciplinary health care professions (i.e., psychiatry, oncology, psychology, social work, nursing), clergy, and patient associations, developed the guidelines on distress. The destigmatizing term *distress* was chosen to describe the "multifactorial unpleasant emotional experience of a psychological (cognitive, behavioral, emotional), social, and/or spiritual nature that may interfere with the ability to cope effectively with cancer, its physical symptoms and its treatment" (p. 6). Since the first edition of the Dis-

---

[1]The information presented in this section was current as of July 2011. The data serve as examples of experiences in some countries and are not representative of all the possible perspectives on psycho-oncology around the world. More information and updates of the documents are available from the IPOS Federation website, at www.ipos-society.org/about/federation/federation_documents.aspx.

tress Management guidelines (J.C. Holland 1997), several more have been published until the most recent version 2.2013 (www.nccn.org). An ultrashort 0–10 visual analogue scale, the Distress Thermometer (DT), was developed as a rapid screening instrument to assess the emotional dimensions of cancer, and a list of possible physical, emotional, spiritual, family, and practical problems can be used as a further tool. The NCCN Distress Management guidelines cover recognition and monitoring of cancer patients' level of distress using the DT during their visits at cancer centers, identification of the nature of distress and its clinical meaning (e.g., through a DSM or ICD diagnosis when possible), and the management of the specific clinical conditions according to practice algorithms. The work of the panel has been recognized throughout the world, where the DT has rapidly become one of the "gold standard" instruments for the rapid screening of distress in cancer care contexts. Distress is identified nowadays as the "sixth vital sign," having the same importance as blood pressure, temperature, heart frequency, breath, and pain (Bultz and Carlson 2006; Bultz and Johansen 2011; Bultz et al. 2012).

Also in the United States (www.apos-society.org), under the request of the National Institutes of Health (NIH), the Institute of Medicine (IOM) of the National Academy of Sciences established a working group with the main aim of studying how and how much the psychosocial needs of cancer patients were addressed, reviewing the available training programs and identifying the barriers to accessing cancer-related mental health services. The main conclusion of the group's report (Adler and Page 2008) is that there is enough evidence supporting the inclusion of psychosocial health services in cancer care and that "attending to psychosocial needs should be an integral part of quality cancer care. All components of the health care system that are involved in cancer care should explicitly incorporate attention to psychosocial needs into their policies, practices, and standards addressing clinical health care" (pp. 8–9). The document indicates that communication is a *sine qua non* for all activities in cancer care and highlights the need for the training of health care providers in all aspects of communication. Furthermore, it confirms the need for psychosocial screening to rapidly identify cancer patients needing specific intervention from psycho-oncology services and to provide psychosocial treatment integrated with the medical treatment when needed. The IOM's 10 proposed basic strategic recommendations to reach optimal standard of cancer care are summarized in Table 12–1.

The general recommendation of the NCCN and the IOM reports is that addressing psychosocial needs should be an integral part of quality cancer care, with all components of the health care system explicitly incorporating attention to psychosocial needs into their policies, practices, and standards addressing clinical care (Holland and Weiss 2008).

TABLE 12–1.   Summary of recommendations for psycho-oncology standard of care

---

Recommendation 1—*The standard of care:* All cancer care should ensure the provision of appropriate psychosocial health services by facilitating basic communication between doctors (medical team) and patients and families; identifying the patients' psychosocial health needs; implementing psychosocial treatment plans; and following up on, reevaluating, and adjusting the plans.

Recommendation 2—*Health care providers:* All cancer care providers should ensure that every patient receives care meeting the standard for psychosocial health care.

Recommendation 3—*Patient and family education:* Patient education and advocacy organizations should educate patients with cancer and their family caregivers to expect, and to request when necessary, that their cancer care meets the standard for psychosocial care.

Recommendation 4—*Support for dissemination and uptake:* Organizations, institutions, and agencies should conduct large-scale demonstrations and evaluations of approaches to psychosocial health care in accordance with the standard of care.

Recommendation 5—*Support from payers:* Group purchasers of insurance should include provisions in their contracts that ensure coverage and reimbursement for identifying the psychosocial needs of cancer patients.

Recommendation 6—*Quality oversight:* Organizations, institutions, and agencies should fund research on performance measures for psychosocial cancer care and create oversight mechanisms that can be used to measure and report the quality of ambulatory oncology care.

Recommendation 7—*Workforce competencies:* Educational organizations, licensing bodies, and professional societies should examine their standards and certification criteria that identify competencies in delivering psychosocial health care in accordance with the model that integrates medical and psychosocial care.

Recommendation 8—*Standardized nomenclature:* To facilitate research on quality measurement of psychosocial interventions, organizations and agencies should create and lead an initiative to develop a standardized, transdisciplinary taxonomy and nomenclature for psychosocial health services.

TABLE 12–1. Summary of recommendations for psycho-oncology standard of care *(continued)*

Recommendation 9—*Research priorities:* Organizations sponsoring research in oncology care should include, among their funding priorities, a number of psychosocial areas (e.g., development of reliable, valid, and efficient tools and strategies to ensure that all cancer patients receive care that meets the standard of psychosocial care; identification of effective evidence-based psychosocial services to treat mental health problems and to assist patients in adopting and maintaining healthy behaviors).

Recommendation 10—*Promoting uptake and monitoring progress:* National cancer organizations should monitor progress toward improved delivery of psychosocial services in cancer care and report findings at least biannually to oncology providers, consumer organizations, group purchasers and health plans, and quality oversight organizations.

Source. Adapted from Adler and Page 2008; Holland and Weiss 2008.

In Canada, the Canadian Association of Psychosocial Oncology (CAPO; www.capo.ca) published the "National Standards for Psychosocial Oncology" in 1999, the first document of its kind worldwide. The document has been revised (Canadian Association of Psychosocial Oncology 2010) with the inclusion of standards of care, organizational standards, educational standards, and integration of all phases of the cancer control trajectory, including prevention and survivorship. The recommendations and conclusions of CAPO on the standards regarding the principles of practice, professional issues, and organization and structure of psychosocial oncology programs have been endorsed by the Canadian Association of Provincial Cancer Agencies, the Canadian Cancer Society, the Canadian Strategy for Cancer Control, and the Canadian Council on Health Services Accreditation. Furthermore, clinical guidelines, "A Pan-Canadian Practice Guideline: Screening, Assessment and Care of Psychosocial Distress (Depression, Anxiety) in Adults With Cancer," have been developed with the specific aim of informing "Canadian health authorities, program leaders, administrators and professional health care providers about the optimum screening, assessment and psychosocial-supportive care of adult patients with cancer who are identified as experiencing depression and/or anxiety" (Howell et al. 2010, p. 3). In 2005, the Canadian Strategy for Cancer Control added emotional distress as the sixth vital sign, implying that monitoring of emotional distress is a vital indicator of a patient's state of being, needs, and progress through the disease, and published the "National Psychosocial Oncology Education Framework" (Canadian Strategy for Cancer Control 2007). The

"Pan-Canadian Clinical Practice Guideline: Assessment of Psychosocial Health Care Needs of the Adult Cancer Patient" currently represents the platform for the development of psychosocial oncology services throughout Canada (Howell et al. 2009). Recently, a renewal of federal funding for 5 more years to the Canadian Partnership Against Cancer (2012–2017) was approved, and psychosocial oncology has been addressed within the partnership under the Cancer Journey Action Portfolio. Within this portfolio, two central strategic initiatives developed under the first mandate, and to be extended and sustained under this second 5-year mandate, are 1) integrated person-centered care, including navigation, palliative and end-of-life care, and screening for distress, and 2) survivorship.

The Experience in Europe

In Europe, the experience in psychosocial oncology dates back to the 1980s when scientific societies were established in many countries, such as France, Germany, Italy, Spain, and the United Kingdom, with the consequent implementation and dissemination of psycho-oncology clinical, research, and educational activities (Dolbeault et al. 1999; Keller et al. 2003). Only recently, however, have some important indications been presented by the European Council (European Union 2008) that clearly acknowledge the significance of psychosocial aspects in cancer care. More specifically, the council indicates that "to attain optimal results, a patient-centered comprehensive interdisciplinary approach and optimal psycho-social care should be implemented in routine cancer care, rehabilitation and post-treatment follow-up for all cancer" (para. 5), stressing in particular the "healthcare and psycho-social needs of children and their families" (para. 8). The document emphasizes that "cancer treatment and care is multidisciplinary, involving the cooperation of oncological surgery, medical oncology, radiotherapy, chemotherapy as well as psycho-social support and rehabilitation and, when cancer is not treatable, palliative care," and that "services providing care to the individual patient and support to the patient's family must be effectively coordinated" (para. 11). It also recognizes that implementation of comprehensive strategies is important for lung cancer survivors because many "suffer severe medical, psychological or social consequences" (para. 17). All member states of the European Union are invited by the European Council "to take into account the psycho-social needs of patients and improve the quality of life for cancer patients through support, rehabilitation and palliative care" (para. 19).

However, differences in programs across European countries demonstrate that the National Cancer Plans are still not homogeneous in incorporating psychosocial guidelines or in promoting the routine application of psychosocial care in oncology settings (Grassi and Watson 2012). The

European Partnership for Action Against Cancer maintains a Web site (www.epaac.eu/national-cancer-plans) with links to the National Cancer Plans for many of the European Union member states.

In Austria, the Austrian Platform of Psycho-Oncology (www.oeppo.com) is working on developing a National Cancer Plan. Currently, the organization is evaluating the status of psycho-oncological services offered all over the country, the national data regarding the prevalence and incidence of psychological disorders in patients with cancer, and the recommendations in education in psycho-oncology.

In Germany, psycho-oncology is established in the National Cancer Plan. Working groups defined the main goals for complete cancer care (e.g., Working Group 4, Patient Orientation, on patient communication, patient competence, and shared decision making; Working Group 2, Patient Care, on psychosocial care of cancer patients). Guidelines for psycho-oncology are also in progress, with extensive literature research in the fields of intervention and comorbidity through the involvement of national societies (www.dapo-ev.de).

In Italy, psycho-oncology services have long been established in cancer institutes and some hospitals and health agencies. The Italian Society of Psycho-Oncology (www.siponazionale.it) has had an influence in enlightening the national institutions about the need for a psychosocial approach in cancer care. In the report on cancer rehabilitation promoted by the Federation of Cancer Patients Associations and supported by the Ministry of Health and Social Policy, the recommendation regarding the right of all cancer patients to receive proper psychosocial support was particularly stressed (www.favo.it). The National Cancer Plan 2010–2012 and the ministry's document "Reducing the Burden of Cancer 2011–2013" have followed this recommendation (www.salute.gov.it). Psycho-oncology and the need for comprehensive psychosocial care of cancer patients is formally recognized and acknowledged in several paragraphs of these documents. The way in which psycho-oncology services within the national and regional/local health services should be routinely implemented, however, has yet to be determined.

In the Netherlands, psycho-oncology has been part of the responsibility of a specific working group on the integration of psychosocial care since 2005 and is one of the seven prioritized themes that the Dutch National Cancer Control Programme (NCCP) Steering Committee elected from among 150 themes. Psychosocial oncologists are part of the organization and structure of cancer control in the country and have helped in increasing the attention on cancer care, including follow-up screening that includes an assessment of the patient's psychosocial situation and the later effects of treatments, relapses, and metastases (www.nvpo.nl). Furthermore, an objective of the NCCP 2005–2010 working group on patient education and psychosocial care was that the psychosocial problems affecting patients and their relatives should be prevented and appropriately treated.

In Portugal, the 2007 Portuguese Cancer Program has acknowledged the importance of cancer psychosocial issues, including the need to implement psycho-oncology units in the main cancer centers or to integrate psychosocial professionals in other oncology services throughout the country (www.appo.pt). Multidisciplinary psycho-oncology units are available in main cancer institutes as well as in most palliative care units. More effort is needed to implement psycho-oncology services in all hospitals and community systems.

In Spain, a major improvement in psycho-oncology has been the inclusion of the Spanish Society of Psycho-Oncology (www.sepo.es) as a part of the National Cancer Strategy, as well as the inclusion, in the chapter on quality of life, of a specific action of promoting the access to psycho-oncology care to patients and families who may benefit from it. Psycho-oncology has also been included in the chapters on care of children and adolescents and on palliative care.

In Sweden, the National Cancer Strategy was published by the government in 2009, as the starting point of a process of development of the national organization for cancer care in which the development of a competence center for psychosocial support and cancer rehabilitation, as well as programs to include these aspects in routine cancer care, is demanded (www.swedpos.se).

In Switzerland, psychosocial support and psycho-oncology are among the 10 main topics of the National Cancer Programme for Switzerland 2011–2015 (2011; www.psychoonkologie.ch). For the psycho-oncology topic, several goals should be pursued, including 1) the development of national standards and guidelines for the psychosocial support of patients and relatives (including children with cancer and children with family members suffering from cancer), with a standardized distress screening to be implemented into the primary oncological treatment, and the qualification of psycho-oncology professionals clearly worked out, including the standards for their education; 2) the development of national guidelines for the financing of psycho-oncological options within primary care; and 3) the integration of psycho-oncology care within oncology primary care by increasing awareness, education, and networking.

In the United Kingdom (www.bpos.org), the National Institute for Health and Clinical Excellence (NICE; www.nice.org.uk), an independent organization responsible for providing national guidance on promoting good health and preventing and treating ill health, prepared a series of guidelines for various areas of public health and clinical practice, including oncology. In 2004, within the cancer service guidance, NICE published guidelines on "improving supportive and palliative care for adults with cancer," with the objective of ensuring that cancer patients, as well as their families and caregivers, are well informed, cared for, and supported. Specifically, the guidelines recommend that people with cancer be involved in cancer services; that there be good communication, and that people with cancer be involved in decision making; that information be available free of charge; that people with cancer be offered a range of physical, emotional, spiritual, and social support; that services be available to help people living with the aftereffects of cancer to manage the effects themselves; that people with advanced cancer have access to a range of services to improve their quality of life; that there be support for people dying from cancer; that the needs of families and other caregivers of people with cancer be met; and that there be a trained workforce to provide these services.

The Experience in Australia

In Australia, the national guidelines on the implementation of psycho-oncology models of care were established at the beginning of 2000 (www.pocog.org.au; www.cosa.org.au/groups/psycho-oncology.html). More specifically, in Western Australia (WA), the WA Health Cancer Services Framework by the WA Cancer Services Taskforce (Turner et al. 2005) published recommendations. The most relevant are that the number of and access to clinical psychologists and counseling psychologists for public patients should increase, as should the public, specialist, and general practitioner awareness of these systems (Initiative 12); that each tumor collaborative should have links to a specialist clinical psychology service (Initiative 13); that supportive care should be an integral component of cancer care (Initiative 6); that referral to psychosocial support services should be actively managed (Initiatives 11, 43); and that consumer awareness of options for accessing psychosocial support should increase (Initiative 16). Comprehensive clinical guidelines have also been prepared in Australia (www.nhmrc.gov.au), and a manual titled "Psychosocial Clinical Practice Guidelines: Providing Information Support and Counselling for Women With Breast Cancer" was published by the National Breast Cancer Centre (2000). Subsequently, a multidisciplinary steering group prepared the "Clinical Practice Guidelines for the Psychosocial Care of Adults with Cancer," which were published by the National Breast Cancer Centre and National Cancer Control Initiative (2003) and were approved by the National Health and Medical Research Council (Turner et al. 2005). Some principles and the relative patients' rights for psycho-oncology care, adapted from the Department of Health, Western Australia (2008), are summarized in Table 12–2.

TABLE 12–2.   Patients' rights for psycho-oncology care in cancer settings

---

1. Right to have social, psychological, emotional, spiritual, and functional needs treated as an integral part of overall cancer care for all cancer patients

2. Right to have equitable access to psychosocial care for all cancer patients and their families and caregivers

3. Right to a patient-centered approach addressing individual needs and priorities of all patients and their families and caregivers

4. Right that psychosocial well-being remains a priority across the cancer journey

5. Right to privacy and confidentiality and to receive cancer care in settings that are family friendly and that recognize the special needs of families with young children or specific cultural background

6. Right that psychosocial care is a shared responsibility of all clinicians

7. Right to have access to multidisciplinary input to optimize patient care

8. Right that all cancer clinicians develop and practice effective communication skills and assessment for psychosocial issues

9. Right that clinicians providing specialized psychosocial support have experience in the cancer field

10. Right that assessment and intervention strategies used in the provision of psychosocial care are evidence based

11. Right that clinical supervision, quality improvement processes assessing the effectiveness of interventions and service performance/ achievement of core aims and objectives, and benchmarking service performance are part of regular care

12. Right that consumers of cancer services may participate in service development and quality improvement activities

---

Source.   Adapted from the Department of Health, Western Australia: *Psycho-Oncology Model of Care.* Perth, Australia, WA Cancer and Palliative Care Network, Department of Health, Western Australia, 2008.

The Experience in Other Countries

Some groups in other parts of the world are also working on developing guidelines for psychosocial oncology.

In Israel, for example, the Standards for the Field of Psycho-Oncology were formulated and developed by the Israel Psycho-Oncology Society, and approved by the Israel National Oncology Council and Israel Ministry of Health in 2003 (Table 12–3).

In Japan, the Cancer Control Act was enacted in June 2006 and implemented in April 2007. The Ministry of Health, Labour and Welfare and every prefecture are responsible for planning to provide quality palliative care to cancer patients from an early stage and for expanding the use of morphine and other drugs to help ease patients' suffering. All comprehensive cancer centers and affiliated hospitals in Japan are expected to have a palliative care team in which a psycho-oncologist is included as an essential member (www .jpos-society.org). The Ministry of Health, Labour and Welfare is funding training for psycho-oncologists and communication skills training for oncologists.

Significant changes are also occurring in many other countries, such as China, Korea, Taiwan (www.tpos-society.org), and Turkey, where psychosocial oncology is or is becoming a structured part of multidisciplinary care in cancer (Watson and Grassi 2012).

TABLE 12–3. **Standards for psycho-social-oncological services to patients and their families in Israel**

General position

1. Referral for psycho-oncological services is made upon the request of the patient and family, or by the medical team and community services.

2. The psycho-oncological team is responsible for identifying patients at high risk for psychosocial distress.

3. Intervention plans [are] based on knowledge and understanding of the relevant medical profile (stage, genetics, course of the disease, nature of the therapy), patient needs and the familial/social and cultural context.

4. The caregiving team strives to develop tailored intervention skills capable of providing patients and their families with tools to cope with emotional distress and process information, and skills for making decisions throughout the course of the disease.

TABLE 12–3.   Standards for psycho-social-oncological services to patients and their families in Israel *(continued)*

5.   The psycho-oncological unit provides patients and their families with information regarding all community resources of potential use to help in coping with the disease and its treatment.

6.   Psycho-oncological interventions are based on up-to-date knowledge and outcome research. It is recommended that emphasis be placed on short-term interventions focused on coping with the disease, as well as on couples, family and group interventions.

Integration of the multidisciplinary team

1.   The psycho-oncology team is an integral part of discussions and meetings of the institute/department/clinic staff.

2.   The psycho-oncological team contributes to the knowledge base of other relevant professions with regard to the psycho-oncological aspects of cancer.

3.   The psycho-oncological team is responsible for managing joint interventions in cooperation with the institute's physicians, nurses and other professionals.

4.   The psycho-oncological team is part of the palliative care unit and contributes to the arsenal of therapeutic skills and knowledge available to other professions involved in treating the terminal cancer patients and their caregivers.

5.   The psycho-oncological team works to advance treatment and care for the terminal patients and their families.

6.   The psycho-oncology unit serves as a framework in which every professional and every relevant profession can function effectively in an integrative manner. Interdisciplinary overlap should not obscure the unique contribution of each discipline.

7.   The psycho-oncology unit develops consistent procedures for interaction with other hospital departments, units and institutes that care for cancer patients, as part of a comprehensive approach (e.g., departments of genetics, neurosurgery, surgery and geriatrics, breast clinics).

Source.   Adapted from the Standards for the Field of Psycho-Oncology, formulated and developed by the Israel Psycho-Oncology Society and approved by the Israel National Oncology Council and Israel Ministry of Health in 2003. From: http://www.ipos-society.org/about/federation/federation_documents.aspx.

Conclusion

The development of psycho-oncology over the last 30 to 40 years has had a major role in enlightening the general population, oncology health professionals, and health care administrators about the need for psychosocial care in cancer. With the increased awareness about the importance of psychosocial issues in medical illness, the development of psychosomatic medicine as a subspecialty of psychiatry (Gitlin et al. 2004), and the frequently reported statements about the importance of mental health to the quality of life of any individual ("No Health Without Mental Health"; Prince et al. 2007), it is not possible today to organize cancer care without a specific investment in psycho-oncology ("No Cancer Health Without Mental Health"; Clarke 2010).

The literature, however, also includes complaints about the fact that very few programs are truly integrated in terms not only of multidisciplinary professions but also of synergisms between all constituents of a patient, family, and community–oriented approach (i.e., including all health professionals and advocacy groups) (Loscalzo et al. 2010). Another problem is that psychosocial oncology departments or programs continue to be understaffed and underfunded, with consequences in the delivery of psycho-oncology activities. This is a complex phenomenon that, on the one hand, reinforces the problem of stigma and scarce interest in mental health in general and, on the other, suggests that the literature regarding the cost-effectiveness of mental health intervention in terms of large cost savings (e.g., reduced medical utilization, faster return to work, fewer visits to general practitioners and specialists) should be made more visible to administrators. This is also the case for psychosocial oncology, because data exist showing that psychosocial interventions are not only effective, but also economical, allowing the health system to save money if emotional distress and the other psychological complications determined by cancer are properly treated (Carlson and Bultz 2004).

Therefore, more effort is necessary before psychosocial care for patients and their families is the standard in all cancer treatment centers as well as in the community, particularly, but not exclusively, in developing countries, where psycho-oncology has not yet or not completely been established or not become an integral part of care (J.C. Holland et al. 2011). In places where psychosocial oncology has been funded and developed, the introduction of psycho-oncologists in MDTs and the establishment of psycho-oncology departments, divisions, or units have favored the use of psychosocial screening procedures and the application of the clinical principles relative to psychosocial assessment and intervention for cancer patients and their families, with an increase in the quality of care, the outcome of the disease, and the satisfaction of the patients, their families, and the staff itself (Walker et al. 2003). Furthermore, as expected, various types of psychosocial interventions delivered by trained psycho-oncology professionals are effective in reducing psychological suffering and symptoms, and in improving quality of life, especially in patients with anxiety and depression (Andrykowski and Manne 2006; Manne and Andrykowski 2006; Osborn et al. 2006).

For these reasons, the main message launched by the International Psycho-Oncology Society (IPOS; 2010) in its "Statement on Standards and Clinical Practice Guidelines in Cancer" is that "quality cancer care must integrate the psychosocial domain into routine care" and that "distress should be measured as the 6th Vital Sign after temperature, blood pressure, pulse, respiratory rate and pain" (www.ipos-society.org). This statement has been endorsed by a number of organizations and associations throughout the world, including the IPOS Federation of Psycho-Oncology Societies, the International Union Against Cancer, the World Psychiatric Association, and many other scientific societies and advocacy movements throughout the world. Only with the implementation of psycho-oncology standards of care in all oncology health care settings can people with cancer or long-term survivors of cancer and their families receive a holistic approach in which all the dimensions of suffering—physical, emotional, spiritual, and social—are at the center of assessment and treatment.

Key Clinical Points

- A multidisciplinary approach to cancer, including the psychosocial approach, favors better accessibility for patients; reduces hospitalization time, costs, and unanticipated admissions; and improves coordination of care. As a result, patients perceive enhanced satisfaction, acceptance of treatment, and improved physical and psychological health outcomes.

- About 30%–40% of cancer patients fail to adapt to their illness or treatments and present with emotional distress and psychological disorders—mainly depressive and adjustment disorders—as a consequence of cancer and treatments.

- Psycho-oncology is a part of the multidisciplinary approach to cancer. It is not possible today to organize cancer care without a specific investment in psycho-oncology.

- More effort is necessary to have psychosocial care for patients and their families as a standard of care in all cancer treatment centers and in the community, especially in developing countries.

- As stated by the International Psycho-Oncology Society (2010), "Quality cancer care must integrate the psychosocial domain into routine care and distress should be measured as the 6th Vital Sign after body temperature, blood pressure, pulse, respiratory rate and pain" (www.ipos-society.org).

* Various standards for psychosocial service to patients and their families are proposed in different countries.

References

Adler NE, Page AEK: Cancer Care for the Whole Patient: Meeting Psychosocial Health Needs, National Institute of Medicine Committee on Psychosocial Services to Cancer Patients/Families in a Community Setting. Washington, DC, National Academies Press, 2008

American Cancer Society: American Cancer Society Working Conference: The psychological, social and behavioral medicine aspects of cancer: research and professional education needs and directions for the 1980s. Minneapolis, Minnesota, July 29–31, 1981. Cancer 50(suppl): 1919–1978, 1982

American Cancer Society: American Cancer Society Workshop Conference on Methodology in Behavioral and Psychosocial Cancer Research. St. Petersburg, Florida, April 21, 22, and 23, 1983. Cancer 53(suppl): 2217–2384, 1984

American Psychiatric Association: Diagnostic and Statistical Manual of Mental Disorders, 4th Edition. Washington, DC, American Psychiatric Association, 1994

Andrykowski MA, Manne SL: Are psychological interventions effective and accepted by cancer patients? I. Standards and levels of evidence. Ann Behav Med 32:93–97, 2006

Baider L, Cooper CL, De-Nour K (eds): Cancer and the Family, 2nd Edition. Sussex, UK, Wiley, 2000

Bhanson CB (ed): Second conference on psychophysiological aspects of cancer. Ann NY Acad Sci 164:313–634, 1969

Bhanson CB, Kissen DM (eds): Psychophysiological aspects of cancer. Ann NY Acad Sci 125:775–1055, 1966

Blumberg EM, West PM, Ellis FW: A possible relationship between psychological factors and human cancer. Psychosom Med 16:277–286, 1954

Bultz BD, Carlson LE: Emotional distress: the sixth vital sign—future directions in cancer care. Psychooncology 15:93–95, 2006

Bultz BD, Johansen C: Screening for distress, the 6th vital sign: where are we, and where are we going? Psychooncology 20: 569–571, 2011

Bultz B, Loscalzo MJ, Clark KL: Screening for distress, the 6th vital sign, as the connective tissue of health care systems: a roadmap to integrated interdisciplinary person-centred care, in Clinical Psycho-Oncology: An International Perspective. Edited by Grassi L, Riba M. Chichester, UK, Wiley, 2012, pp 83–96

Canadian Association of Psychosocial Oncology: Standards of psychosocial health services for persons with cancer and their families. May 2010. Available at: www.capo.ca/pdf/CAPOstandards.pdf. Accessed August 1, 2012.

Canadian Strategy for Cancer Control: National Psychosocial Oncology Education Framework. Toronto, ON, Canada, 2007

Carlson LE, Bultz BD: Efficacy and medical cost offset of psychosocial interventions in cancer care: making the case for economic analyses. Psychooncology 13:837–849, 2004

Caruso R, Morelli AC, Nanni MG, et al: Psychiatric disorders related to cancer: prevalence, etiology and recognition. Neuropathological Diseases 1:7–39, 2012

Catt S, Fallowfield L, Jenkins V, et al: The informational roles and psychological health of members of 10 oncology multidisciplinary teams in the UK. Br J Cancer 93:1092–1097, 2005

Clarke DM: No cancer health without mental health. Med J Aust 193(suppl):S43, 2010

Cohen J, Cullen JW, Martin LR: Psychosocial Aspects of Cancer. New York, Raven, 1982

Cullen J, Fox B, Isom R: Cancer: The Behavioral Dimensions. New York, Raven, 1977

Dolbeault S, Szporn A, Holland JC: Psycho-oncology: where have we been? Where are we going? Eur J Cancer 35:1554–1558, 1999

Department of Health, Western Australia: Psycho-Oncology Model of Care. Perth, Australia, WA Cancer and Palliative Care Network, Department of Health, Western Australia, 2008

European Union: Council Conclusions on reducing the burden of cancer. Luxembourg, 10 June 2008. Available at: http://www.consilium.europa.eu/ueDocs/cms_Data/docs/pressData/en/lsa/101031.pdf. Accessed August 1, 2012.

Fava GA, Freyberger HJ, Bech P, et al: Diagnostic criteria for use in psychosomatic research. Psychother Psychosom 63:1–8, 1995

Fava GA, Mangelli L, Ruini C: Assessment of psychological distress in the setting of medical disease. Psychother Psychosom 70:171–175, 2001

Fleissig A, Jenkins V, Catt S, et al: Multidisciplinary teams in cancer care: are they effective in the UK? Lancet Oncol 7:935–943, 2006

Gitlin DF, Levenson JL, Lyketsos CG: Psychosomatic medicine: a new psychiatric subspecialty. Acad Psychiatry 28:4–11, 2004

Glajchen M: The emerging role and needs of family caregivers in cancer care. J Support Oncol 2:145–155, 2004

Grassi L: Bereavement in families with relatives dying of cancer. Curr Opin Support Pall Care 1:43–49, 2007

Grassi L, Giraldi T: Psycho-oncology: integrating science into clinical care. Neuropathological Diseases 1:1–5, 2012

Grassi L, Riba M: New frontiers and challenges of psychiatry in oncology and palliative care, in Advances in Psychiatry, Vol. 3. Edited by Christodoulou GN, Jorge M, Mezzich J. Geneva, Switzerland, World Psychiatric Association, 2009, pp 105–114

Grassi L, Riba M: Introducing multicultural psycho-oncology, in Clinical Psycho-Oncology: An International Percspective. Edited by Grassi L, Riba M., Chichester, UK, Wiley, 2012, pp 3–9

Grassi L, Travado L: Developing a psycho-oncology program in cancer settings—experiences from Southern Europe: the models of Ferrara and Lisbon. Neuropathological Diseases 1:161–178, 2012

Grassi L, Holland JC, Johansen C, et al: Psychiatric concomitants of cancer, screening procedures and training of health care professionals in oncology: the paradigms of psycho-oncology in the psychiatry field, in Advances in Psychiatry, Vol 2. Edited by Christodoulou GN, Jorge M, Mezzich J. Geneva, Switzerland, World Psychiatric Association, 2005, pp 59–66

Grassi L, Biancosino B, Marmai L, et al: Psychological factors affecting oncology conditions, in Psychological Factors Affecting Medical Conditions: A New Classification for DSM-V. Edited by Porcelli P, Sonino N. Basel, Germany, Karger, 2007, pp 57–71

Grassi L, Nanni MG, Caruso R: Emotional distress in cancer: screening policy, clinical limitations and educational needs. J Med Pers 8:51–59, 2010

Grassi L, Watson M, and IPOS Federation of Psycho-Oncology Societies' co-authors: Psychosocial care in cancer: an overview of psychosocial programmes and national cancer plans of countries within the International Federation of Psycho-Oncology Societies. Psychooncology 21:1027–1033, 2012

Holland JC: Preliminary guidelines for the treatment of distress. Oncology 11:109–114, 1997

Holland JC: Establishing a psycho-oncology unit in a cancer center, in Psycho-Oncology. Edited by Holland JC, Breitbart W, Jacobson PB, et al. New York, Oxford University Press, 1998, pp 1049–1054

Holland JC: History of psycho-oncology: overcoming attitudinal and conceptual barriers. Psychosom Med 64:206–221, 2002

Holland JC: American Cancer Society Award lecture. Psychological care of patients: psycho-oncology's contribution. J Clin Oncol 21(23 Suppl):253s–265s, 2003

Holland JC: IPOS Sutherland Memorial Lecture: an international perspective on the development of psychosocial oncology. Psychooncology 13:445–459, 2004

Holland J, Weiss T: The new standard of quality cancer care: integrating the psychosocial aspects in routine cancer from diagnosis through survivorship. Cancer J 14:425–428, 2008

Holland JC, Weiss TR: Principles of psycho-oncology, in Holland-Frei Cancer Medicine, 8th edition. Edited by Hong WK, Bast RC Jr, Hait WN, et al. Hamilton, ON, Canada, BC Decker, 2010, pp 793–809

Holland JC, Andersen B, Breitbart WS, et al: Distress management. J Natl Compr Canc Netw 8:448–485, 2010

Holland J, Watson M, Dunn J: The IPOS new International Standard of Quality Cancer Care: integrating the psychosocial domain into routine care. Psychooncology 20:677–680, 2011

Holland JF, Frei III E, Hong WK, et al: Multidisciplinary management, in Holland-Frei Cancer Medicine, 8th Edition. Edited by Hong WK, Bast RC Jr, Hait WN, et al. Hamilton, ON, Canada, BC Decker, 2010, pp 823–829

Howell D, Currie S, Mayo S, et al: A Pan-Canadian Clinical Practice Guideline: Assessment of Psychosocial Health Care Needs of the Adult Cancer Patient. Toronto, ON, Canada, Canadian Partnership Against Cancer (Cancer Journey Action Group) and the Canadian Association of Psychosocial Oncology, 2009

Howell D, Keller-Olaman S, Oliver T, et al: A Pan-Canadian Practice Guideline: Screening, Assessment and Care of Psychosocial Distress (Depression, Anxiety) in Adults With Cancer. Toronto, ON, Canada, Canadian Partnership Against Cancer (Cancer Journey Action Group) and the Canadian Association of Psychosocial Oncology, 2010. Available at: http://www.capo.ca. Accessed August 30, 2012.

Hutchison SD, Steginga SK, Dunn J: The tiered model of psychosocial intervention in cancer: a community based approach. Psychooncology 15:541–546, 2006

International Psycho-Oncology Society (IPOS): Statement on standards and clinical practice guidelines in cancer care. July 2010. Available at: http://www.ipos-society.org/about/news/standards_news.aspx. Accessed August 1, 2012.

Jenkins VA, Fallowfield LJ, Poole K: Are members of multidisciplinary teams in breast cancer aware of each other's informational roles? Qual Health Care 10:70–75, 2001

Johansen C, Grassi L: International psycho-oncology: present and future, in Psycho-Oncology, 2nd Edition. Edited by Holland JC, Breitbart WS, Jacobsen PB, et al. New York, Oxford University Press, 2010, pp 655–659

Keller M, Weis J, Schumacher A, Griessmeier B.: Psycho-oncology in a united Europe: changes and challenges. Crit Rev Oncol Hematol 45:109–117, 2003

Kübler-Ross E: On Death and Dying. New York, Macmillan, 1969

Levin T, Weiner JS, Saravay SM, et al: Two-year evaluation of the logic model for developing a psycho-oncology service. Psychiatr Serv 55:427–433, 2004

Loscalzo MJ, von Gunten CF: Interdisciplinary team work in palliative care: compassionate expertise for serious complex illness, in Handbook of Psychiatry in Palliative Medicine, 2nd edition. Edited by Chochinov HM, Breitbart W. New York, Oxford University Press, 2009, pp 172–185

Loscalzo MJ, Bultz BD, Jacobsen PB: Building psychosocial programs: a roadmap to excellence, in Psycho-Oncology, 2nd Edition. Edited by Holland JC, Breitbart WS, Jacobsen PB, et al. New York, Oxford University Press, 2010, pp 569–574

Manne SL, Andrykowski MA: Are psychological interventions effective and accepted by cancer patients? II. Using empirically supported therapy guidelines to decide. Ann Behav Med 32:98–103, 2006

McQuellon RP, Hurt GJ, DeChatelet P: Psychosocial care of the patient with cancer. A model for organizing services. Cancer Pract 4:304–311, 1996

Mickan SM: Evaluating the effectiveness of health care teams. Aust Health Rev 29:211–217, 2005

Mickan SM, Rodger SA: Effective health care teams: a model of six characteristics developed from shared perceptions. J Interprof Care 19:358–370, 2005

Mitchell AJ, Chan M, Bhatti H, et al: Prevalence of depression, anxiety, and adjustment disorder in oncological, haematological, and palliative-care settings: a meta-analysis of 94 interview-based studies. Lancet Oncol 12:160–174, 2011

National Breast Cancer Centre: Psychosocial clinical practice guidelines: information, support and counselling for women with breast cancer. National Health and Medical Research Council National Breast Cancer Center Psychosocial Working Group, Commonwealth of Australia, 2000. Available at: http://www.nhmrc.gov.au/guidelines/publications/cp61. Accessed January 22, 2013.

National Breast Cancer Centre and National Cancer Control Initiative: Clinical Practice Guidelines for the Psychosocial Care of Adults With Cancer. Camperdown, Australia, National Breast Cancer Centre, 2003

National Cancer Programme for Switzerland 2011–2015, Abridged Version. January 2011. Available at: http://www.oncosuisse.ch/file/oncosuisse/nkp/2011-2015/kurzversion/NKP_Kurzversion_e.pdf. Accessed August 30, 2012.

Osborn RL, Demoncada AC, Feuerstein M: Psychosocial interventions for depression, anxiety, and quality of life in cancer survivors: meta-analyses. Int J Psychiatry Med 36:13–34, 2006

Pendergrass EP: Host resistance and other intangibles in the treatment of cancer. Am J Roentgenol 85: 891–896, 1961

Pitceathly C, Maguire P: The psychological impact of cancer on patients' partners and other key relatives: a review. Eur J Cancer 39:1517–1524, 2003

Price M, Butow P, Kirsten L: Support and training needs of cancer support group leaders: a review. Psychooncology 15:651–663, 2006

Prince M, Patel V, Saxena S, et al: No health without mental health. Lancet 370:859–877, 2007

Robson A, Scrutton F, Wilkinson L, et al: The risk of suicide in cancer patients: a review of the literature. Psychooncology 19:1250–1258, 2010

Sherman AC, Edwards D, Simonton S, et al: Caregiver stress and burnout in an oncology unit. Palliat Support Care 4:65–68, 2006

Sutherland AM: Psychological impact of cancer and its therapy. Med Clin North Am 40:705–720, 1956

Trufelli DC, Bensi CG, Garcia JB, et al: Burnout in cancer professionals: a systematic review and meta-analysis. Eur J Cancer Care (Engl) 17:524–531, 2008

Turner J: Working as a multidisciplinary team, in Handbook of Communication in Oncology and Palliative Care. Edited by Kissane DW, Bultz BD, Butow PM, et al. New York, Oxford University Press, 2010, pp 245–257

Turner J, Zapart S, Pedersen K, et al: Clinical practice guidelines for the psychosocial care of adults with cancer. Psychooncology 14:159–173, 2005

Vachon MLS: Oncology staff stress and related interventions, in Handbook of Psycho-Oncology, 2nd Edition. Edited by Holland JC, Breitbart WS, Jacobsen PB, et al. New York, Oxford University Press, 2010, pp 575–581

Walker MS, Ristvedt SL, Haughey BH: Patient care in multidisciplinary cancer clinics: does attention to psychosocial needs predict patient satisfaction? Psychooncology 12:291–300, 2003

World Health Organization: International Statistical Classification of Diseases and Related Health Problems, 10th Revision. Geneva, World Health Organization, 1992

Index

Page numbers printed in *boldface* type refer to table or figures.

Antidepressants. *See also* Selective
  serotonin reuptake inhibitors;
  Tricyclic antidepressants
  as "antistress pill," 178–179
  benefits of for cancer patients, 180–
    181
  demoralization in cancer patients
    and, 108
  depression in cancer patients and,
    102, 105
  research on in cancer patients, **182–
    183**
  somatic symptoms and, 190
Antipsychotics, 187. *See also* Atypical
  antipsychotics
Anxiety. *See also* Death anxiety
  angst and, 219
  correlation of demoralization and
    depression with, 101
  existential issues and, 218–219
  genetic testing and, 154, 156–157
  hypnotherapy and, 135, 137
  prevalence of in cancer patients, 2
  psychopharmacology for, 181
  reactions to cancer diagnosis and,
    13, **14**
  relaxation techniques and, 127
Apathy, and psychopharmacology,
  185–186, **189**
Appetite, as somatic symptom,
  191
Appraisal, and evaluation phase of
  coping process, 9–10, 51
Apprehension, and
  psychopharmacology, 181, 184,
  189
Approach strategies, of coping, 10
Aromatase inhibitors, 191
Aripiprazole, 187
Ars Moriendi (the art of dying), 4, 20
Assessment. *See also* Diagnosis;
  Psychometric assessment; Quality
  of life; Screening
  for identification of psychological
    distress, 124

for risk of hereditary cancers, 149,
  150
Atypical antipsychotics, 185. *See also*
  Antipsychotics
Australia
  gynecological cancer risk
    management in, 161
  hereditary breast and ovarian
    cancer syndrome rates in, 152,
    160
  psycho-oncology services in, 329,
    330
Austria
  gynecological cancer risk
    management in, 161
  psycho-oncology services in, 327
Austrian Platform of Psycho-Oncology,
  327
Authentic guilt, 221–222
Avoidant strategies, of coping, 10

BALANCE, and cultural history, **84**
Bargaining phase, and reactions to
  diagnosis of advanced cancer, 17
Basal cell nevus syndrome, **147**
Bech-Rafaelsen Melancholia Scale,
  242
Beck, Aaron T., 100
Beck Depression Inventory (BDI), 98,
  242, 244, 246
Becker, Ernest, 218
Behavioral activation strategies, for
  depression, 105–106
Being-in-the-world, and existential
  issues, 214, 223
Being-towards-death, and hospice care,
  212, 218–219
Benzodiazepines, 181, 184, 185, 191
Bevacizumab, 69
Binswanger, Ludwig, 214–215
Biography, and dying patient, 290, 292.
  See also Life review
Biological factors, and reactions to
  cancer diagnosis, 8
Bladder cancer, 25–26